NETTER'S
ESSENTIAL SYSTEMS-BASED ANATOMY

NETTER'S
ESSENTIAL SYSTEMS-BASED ANATOMY

VIRGINIA T. LYONS, PhD

Associate Professor of Medical Education

Associate Dean for Preclinical Education

Geisel School of Medicine at Dartmouth

Hanover, New Hampshire

Illustrations by

FRANK H. NETTER, MD

Contributing Illustrators

CARLOS A. G. MACHADO, MD

DRAGONFLY MEDIA GROUP

KRISTEN WIENANDT MARZEJON, MS, MFA

JAMES A. PERKINS, MS, MFA

JOHN A. CRAIG, MD

ELSEVIER

Elsevier
1600 John F. Kennedy Blvd.
Ste 1600
Philadelphia, PA 19103-2899

NETTER'S ESSENTIAL SYSTEMS-BASED ANATOMY ISBN: 978-0-323-69497-1
Copyright © 2022 by Elsevier, Inc. All rights reserved.

ISBN: 978-0-323-69497-1

Publisher: Elyse O'Grady
Content Strategist: Marybeth Thiel
Publishing Services Manager: Catherine Jackson
Senior Project Manager: Kate Mannix
Design Direction: Patrick Ferguson

Printed in India

Last digit is the print number: 9 8 7 6 5 4 3 2

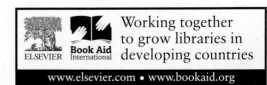

Working together
to grow libraries in
developing countries

www.elsevier.com • www.bookaid.org

In memory of my father, Richard Calvin Taylor, 1942–2020
A man of integrity who frequently told me at the dinner table that I was smart and could achieve whatever I set my mind to. These were exactly the words a young girl needed to hear from her Dad.

ABOUT THE AUTHOR

Virginia T. Lyons, PhD, is an Associate Professor of Medical Education and the Associate Dean for Preclinical Education at the Geisel School of Medicine at Dartmouth. She received her BS in Biology from Rochester Institute of Technology and her PhD in Cell Biology and Anatomy from the University of North Carolina at Chapel Hill. Dr. Lyons has devoted her career to education in the anatomical sciences, teaching gross anatomy, histology, embryology, and neuroanatomy to medical students and other health professions students. She has led courses and curricula in human gross anatomy and embryology for more than 20 years and is a strong advocate for incorporating engaged pedagogies into preclinical medical education. Dr. Lyons has been recognized with numerous awards for teaching and mentoring students, including an Arnold Gold Humanism in Medicine Award. She was chosen as an inaugural member of academies of educators at two different institutions and was elected to the Dartmouth chapter of the Alpha Omega Alpha Honor Medical Society. Dr. Lyons is the co-author of the Geisel Human Anatomy Learning Modules website, which is accessed by students worldwide to aid their understanding of anatomical structures and their appearance on various imaging modalities utilized in the clinical environment. She also serves as the Discipline Editor for Anatomy on the Aquifer Sciences Curriculum Editorial Board, working to integrate anatomical concepts into virtual patient cases that are used in multiple settings including clerkships and residency training.

ABOUT THE ARTISTS

Frank H. Netter, MD

Frank H. Netter was born in 1906 in New York City. He studied art at the Art Student's League and the National Academy of Design before entering medical school at New York University, where he received his MD degree in 1931. During his student years, Dr. Netter's notebook sketches attracted the attention of the medical faculty and other physicians, allowing him to augment his income by illustrating articles and textbooks. He continued illustrating as a sideline after establishing a surgical practice in 1933, but he ultimately opted to give up his practice in favor of a full-time commitment to art. After service in the United States Army during World War II, Dr. Netter began his long collaboration with the CIBA Pharmaceutical Company (now Novartis Pharmaceuticals). This 45-year partnership resulted in the production of the extraordinary collection of medical art so familiar to physicians and other medical professionals worldwide.

In 2005, Elsevier, Inc. purchased the Netter Collection and all publications from Icon Learning Systems. There are now more than 50 publications featuring the art of Dr. Netter available through Elsevier, Inc.

Dr. Netter's works are among the finest examples of the use of illustration in the teaching of medical concepts. The 13-book *Netter Collection of Medical Illustrations*, which includes most of the more than 4,000 paintings created by Dr. Netter, became and remains one of the most famous medical works ever published. *Netter's Atlas of Human Anatomy*, first published in 1989, presents the anatomical paintings from the Netter Collection. Now translated into 16 languages, it is the anatomy atlas of choice among medical and health professions students the world over.

The Netter illustrations are appreciated not only for their aesthetic qualities, but, more importantly, for their intellectual content. As Dr. Netter wrote in 1949, "...clarification of a subject is the aim and goal of illustration. No matter how beautifully painted, how delicately and subtly rendered a subject may be, it is of little value as a medical illustration if it does not serve to make clear some medical point." Dr. Netter's planning, conception, point of view, and approach are what inform his paintings and what makes them so intellectually valuable.

Frank H. Netter, MD, physician and artist, died in 1991.

Learn more about the physician-artist whose work has inspired the Netter Reference Collection: https://netterimages.com/artist-frank-h-netter.html.

Carlos A.G. Machado, MD

Carlos Machado was chosen by Novartis to be Dr. Netter's successor. He continues to be the main artist who contributes to the Netter Collection of medical illustrations.

Self-taught in medical illustration, cardiologist Carlos Machado has contributed meticulous updates to some of Dr. Netter's original plates and has created many paintings of his own in the style of Netter as an extension of the Netter Collection. Dr. Machado's photorealistic expertise and his keen insight into the physician/patient relationship inform his vivid and unforgettable visual style. His dedication to researching each topic and subject he paints places him among the premier medical illustrators at work today.

Learn more about his background and see more of his art at: https://netterimages.com/artist-carlos-a-g-machado.html.

PREFACE

According to the Association of American Medical College's report on preclinical curriculum structure (accessed Dec 2020), more than 88% of reporting medical schools utilize an organ systems-based approach for some or all of their preclinical curriculum. In this approach, content in the anatomical sciences is often integrated into systems-based courses rather than being presented in a stand-alone fashion. Unlike the anatomical disciplines of histology and embryology, gross anatomy has been traditionally taught in a regional fashion, where students concurrently examine structures from numerous body systems within a particular area of the body. Most anatomical textbooks and other educational resources are organized in this manner and thus are not ideal for students learning in a systems-based curriculum.

Netter's Essential Systems-Based Anatomy is designed to provide a foundational resource for students learning gross anatomy in a curriculum organized by organ systems. Each chapter begins with an introduction to a particular system of the body that provides a broad overview of the function of the system and the structures that comprise it. Subsequent pages are organized into concise topics that feature informative illustrations from the Netter collection. Text is meant to be succinct and high-yield, avoiding extraneous detail and focusing on key points. Optimal learning occurs when information is presented in the context that it will be used, thus clinical relevance is emphasized. The end of each chapter includes questions that allow learners to evaluate their knowledge and apply it to clinical scenarios.

My goal was to create a textbook that uses plain language, is accessible to all levels of learners, and emphasizes the visual nature of learning anatomy. I am a proponent of learning anatomy in an incremental fashion, beginning with foundational information relevant to all health providers; learning more detailed information in the clinical environment; and finally focusing on particular areas of anatomy if it is relevant to a student's chosen career. I hope learners will find this a useful introduction to the wonder that is human anatomy.

ACKNOWLEDGMENTS

I never imagined that I would write a book, and I couldn't have done it without the encouragement I received from Elyse O'Grady, who championed my idea, and the patience and understanding of Marybeth Thiel when my optimism about meeting deadlines didn't correlate with reality. I am extremely fortunate to have had the opportunity to work with Dr. Carlos Machado, who is a talented and meticulous artist but also one of the kindest individuals that I have met. Throughout my career I have worked with many supportive and dedicated educators, and I would like to acknowledge my first mentor, Dr. Richard Doolittle, who provided opportunities for me to explore anatomy education as a career and was a wonderful role model. I would like to thank Drs. Noelle Granger and Bill Henson, who encouraged me to pursue my goals in education and provided opportunities for me to become involved in scholarly projects as a graduate student and newly minted faculty member. I am grateful for extensive advice and support from Dr. Brian Catlin, who embraces my passion for innovation and has contributed his time and expertise to numerous educational projects in the anatomical courses at Dartmouth. I have benefited from his knowledge of surgical anatomy and clinical relevance, and I cherish our friendship. I would like to thank my family for their patience and understanding, especially my husband Patrick, who provides unconditional love and support for all my pursuits and accepts my tendency to overextend myself. Finally, I am eternally grateful to my parents who supported my education, instilled in me a strong work ethic, and provided plenty of love and encouragement along the way.

CONTENTS

CHAPTER 1

INTRODUCTION

1.1 ANATOMICAL POSITION AND BODY PLANES

The study of anatomy has been compared with learning a new language. In addition to learning terms for various structures and functions, health care professionals need to communicate about the position of structures in the body and how they relate to one another. Anatomic relationships are described with reference to the **anatomical position,** a universally accepted body position where:

- The individual is standing erect with the head, eyes, and chest facing forward
- The upper limbs are extended at the side of the body with the palms facing forward
- The lower limbs are extended with the toes facing forward

Thus, to describe the relationship of an individual's head to their feet, the term superior would be used regardless of whether he or she is standing or lying on a table.

In mathematics, the relationships between the sides of a three-dimensional shape such as a cube are described as being aligned on *x, y,* and *z* axes. Similar to this, anatomical relationships can be described using **anatomic planes** that are "imaginary slices" through the body aligned on orthogonal axes. The three major planes are:

- **Sagittal Plane:** any anterior to posterior vertical plane that divides the body into right and left parts. Some specific sagittal planes are the **median (midsagittal) plane** that divides the body into equal right and left halves; the **midclavicular plane** that passes through the midpoint of the clavicle; and the **scapular line** that intersects the inferior angle of the scapula.
- **Axial (Transverse) Plane:** any horizontal plane that separates the body into superior and inferior parts. One specific axial plane is the **transumbilical plane** that passes through the umbilicus (navel). Slices in the axial plane are often called "cross-sections."
- **Coronal Plane:** any right-to-left vertical plane that separates the body into anterior and posterior parts. The **midaxillary line** is a specific plane that passes through the axilla (armpit) and divides the body into equal anterior and posterior parts.

Clinical Focus

Computed tomography (CT) and magnetic resonance imaging (MRI) are two imaging techniques that obtain data in one or more anatomic planes and use a computer to produce a radiologic image. These techniques are especially useful in clinical practice because they can detect small differences in density between soft tissue structures.

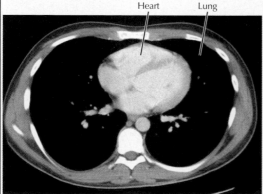

Heart   Lung

A CT scan in the axial plane at the level of the heart (*Image courtesy Nancy McNulty, M.D.*)

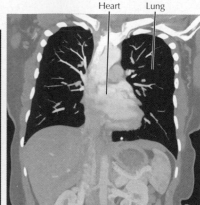

Heart   Lung

Data from sequential axial CT scans can be reformatted by a computer to produce an image in a different plane, such as this one in the coronal plane.

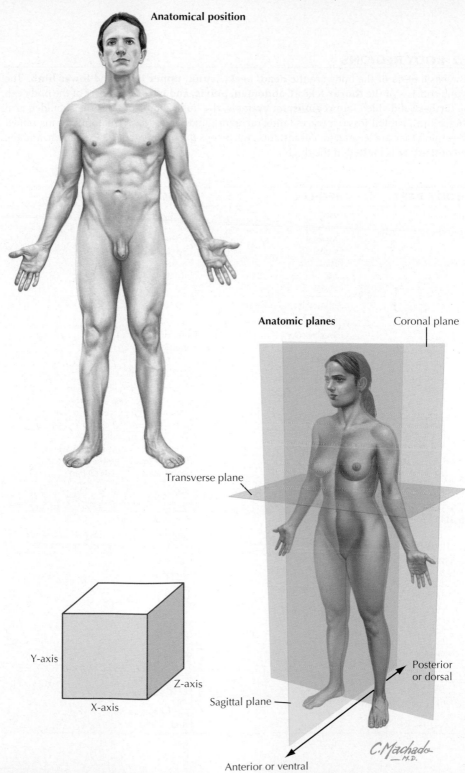

Anatomical position

Anatomic planes

Coronal plane

Transverse plane

Y-axis

Z-axis

X-axis

Sagittal plane

Posterior or dorsal

Anterior or ventral

C. Machado
M.D.

Figure 1.1 ANATOMICAL POSITION AND BODY PLANES

1.2 BODY REGIONS

The basic parts of the body are the **head, neck, trunk, upper limb,** and **lower limb.** The trunk consists of the **thorax** (chest), **abdomen, pelvis,** and **back.** Each part of the body can be further subdivided into **regions;** for example, the upper limb contains the shoulder, arm (brachium), cubital fossa, forearm (antebrachium), and hand. Many anatomic terms reflect the region they are located in. For instance, the biceps *brachii* is a muscle in the arm, and the *femoral* artery is located in the thigh.

BODY PART	REGION	ASSOCIATED WITH
Head	Frontal	Forehead
	Temporal	Temple; side of head anterior to ear
	Occipital	Posterior head
	Orbital	Eye
	Nasal	Nose
	Oral	Mouth
	Mental	Chin
Neck	Anterior/lateral/posterior cervical	Parts of the neck
Thorax	Infraclavicular	Inferior border of clavicle
	Presternal	Anterior sternum
	Pectoral	Chest
	Mammary	Breast
Abdomen	Epigastric	Upper abdomen, medial part (epi = above; gastric = stomach)
	Hypochondriac	Upper abdomen, below ribcage (hypo = below; chondro = cartilage)
	Umbilical	Navel or "belly button"
	Hypogastric	Lower abdomen, medial part (hypo = below; gastric = stomach)
	Lumbar	Lower abdomen, lateral part
Pelvis	Inguinal	Groin
	Perineal	Genitalia, anus
Back	Vertebral	Vertebral column
	Scapular	Scapula
	Lumbar	Lumbar vertebral column (lower back)
Upper limb	Deltoid	Shoulder
	Axillary	Armpit
	Brachium	Arm
	Cubital	Anterior elbow
	Antebrachium	Forearm
	Carpal	Wrist
	Palmar	Palm of hand
Lower limb	Gluteal	Buttocks
	Femoral	Thigh
	Patellar	Anterior knee
	Popliteal	Posterior knee
	Crural	Leg
	Plantar	Bottom of foot
	Calcaneal	Heel

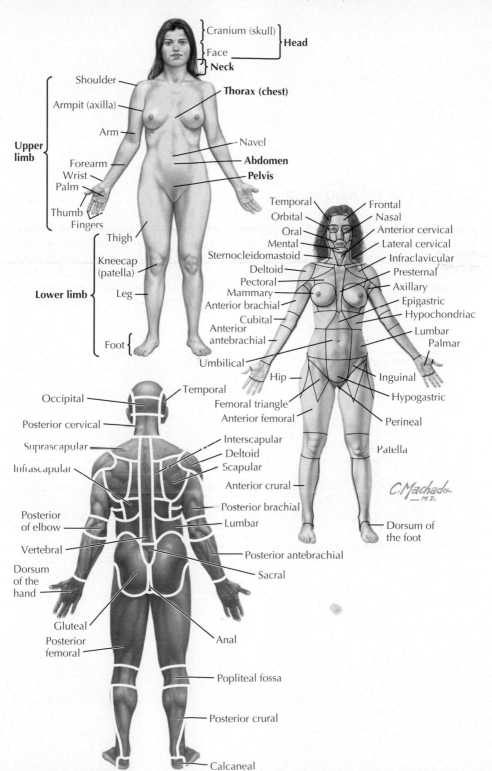

Figure 1.2 BODY REGIONS

1.3 TERMS OF RELATIONSHIP

The three-dimensional organization of the body is an important component of the study of anatomy; thus structures are frequently described by their relationships to other structures. The following table includes some of the most common terms of relationship. **Cranial** (toward the head) and **caudal** (toward the tail) are similar terms to **superior** and **inferior,** although by convention they are generally used for the embryo rather than the adult. Likewise, **ventral** and **dorsal** are equivalent terms to **anterior** and **posterior,** respectively. The terms **proximal** and **distal** are especially useful in the limbs where the point of origin is where the limb is attached to the trunk.

TERMS OF RELATIONSHIP	DEFINITION
Superior	Toward the head
Inferior	Toward the feet
Anterior	Toward the front of the body
Posterior	Toward the back of the body
Medial	Closer to the midline of the body
Lateral	Farther from the midline of the body
Superficial/external	Closer to the surface of the body or toward the outside
Deep/internal	Farther from the surface of the body or toward the inside
Proximal	Toward the point of origin
Distal	Away from the point of origin
Ipsilateral	On the same side of the body
Contralateral	On the opposite side of the body

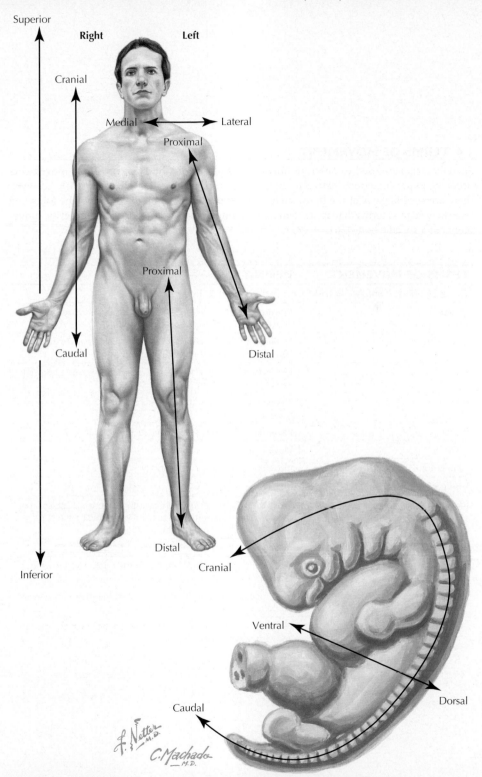

Figure 1.3 TERMS OF RELATIONSHIP

1.4 TERMS OF MOVEMENT

Specific terms are used to describe **movements of various body parts.** Most movements occur at joints (junctions between components of the musculoskeletal system); however, there are several parts of the body, such as the eye, that move independently. The following table lists general terms that apply to more than one body part and terms that describe movements of a specific body part.

TERMS OF MOVEMENT	DEFINITION
General Terms That Apply to More Than One Body Part	
Flexion	Movement typically in the sagittal plane that decreases the angle between two body parts (bending)
Extension	Movement typically in the sagittal plane that increases the angle between two body parts (straightening)
Abduction	Movement typically in the coronal plane that moves a body part away from the midline
Adduction	Movement typically in the coronal plane that moves a body part toward the midline
Rotation	Movement of a body part around its longitudinal axis
Elevation	Movement of a body part superiorly
Depression	Movement of a body part inferiorly
Movements of a Specific Body Part	
Pronation/supination	Rotation of the radius medially over the ulna, which causes the palm to face posteriorly, and rotation of the radius laterally, which returns the limb to anatomical position
Protrusion/retrusion	Movement of the mandible anteriorly and posteriorly
Protraction/retraction	Movement of the scapula away from the midline and toward the midline
Inversion/eversion	Movement of the sole of the foot toward the midline and away from the midline
Dorsiflexion/plantarflexion	Movement of the toes of the foot toward the anterior leg and away from the anterior leg

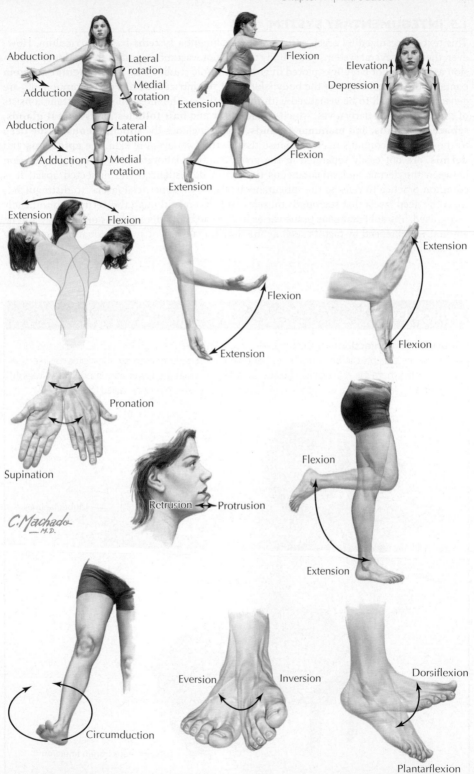

Figure 1.4 TERMS OF MOVEMENT

1.5 INTEGUMENTARY SYSTEM

This text is organized by organ systems to compliment a systems-based curriculum. However, there are several systems of the body that do not warrant a significant amount of discussion as they cannot be fully explored in gross anatomic studies. The **integumentary system** contains the largest organ of the body (skin), but the intricate details of its components are generally too small to be visualized with the naked eye. The integumentary system consists of the **skin** and its derivatives, which include **hair** and **hair follicles, nails, sweat glands, sebaceous glands,** and **mammary glands.** It also includes the **subcutaneous tissue** deep to the skin that contains mainly adipose tissue. The two layers of skin, the **epidermis** and **dermis,** are not easily separated in the gross anatomy laboratory. However, the junction between the dermis and subcutaneous tissue can be visualized and dissected apart. It is common practice to refer to the subcutaneous tissue as "superficial fascia" to distinguish it from the deep fascia that surrounds muscles and viscera, although this term is not officially recognized. The subcutaneous tissue varies in thickness in different areas of the body and its amount is influenced by factors such as the nutritional state of an individual or the climate they live in.

Clinical Focus

Subcutaneous injections are a common way to administer medications such as insulin and fertility drugs, and patients can be educated to perform the procedure at home. Ideal sites for injection are locations where the subcutaneous tissue is thickest, such as the lower abdomen, gluteal region, thigh, or arm. In the clinical environment the subcutaneous tissue is often called "Sub-Q."

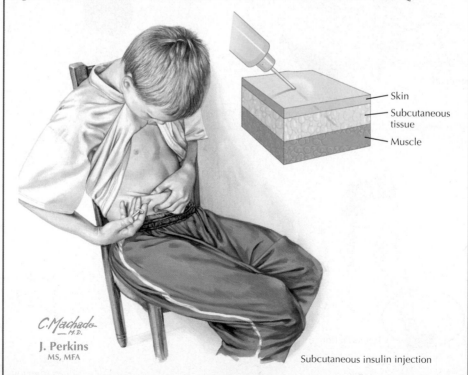

C. Machado
—M.D.

J. Perkins
MS, MFA

Skin

Subcutaneous tissue

Muscle

Subcutaneous insulin injection

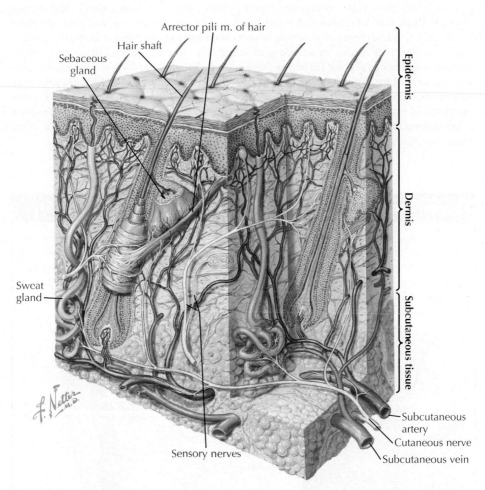

Sebaceous gland

Hair shaft

Arrector pili m. of hair

Epidermis

Dermis

Subcutaneous tissue

Sweat gland

Subcutaneous artery

Cutaneous nerve

Subcutaneous vein

Sensory nerves

Figure 1.5 INTEGUMENTARY SYSTEM

1.6 FASCIA, SYNOVIUM, AND SEROUS MEMBRANES

Fascia is essentially a "packing material" that supports and insulates structures in the body. The subcutaneous tissue discussed previously is a type of fascia mainly composed of loose connective tissue and adipose. In contrast, **deep fascia** consists of dense connective tissue that is lacking fat. Deep fascia has many roles, including forming intermuscular septa that create functional compartments in the limbs; ensheathing muscles, organs, and neurovascular structures; and forming thick retinacula to hold tendons in place at the wrist and ankle. Similar to fascia, **synovial membranes** are composed of connective tissue and have a supportive function. These membranes line the inner surfaces of joint capsules and secrete **synovial fluid** that lubricates and nourishes the articular surfaces of the joint. Synovial membranes also line the internal surface of sacs called **bursae** (see clinical focus) that reduce friction between structures associated with joints. For example, some bursae lie between tendons and bones to prevent friction as the tendon slides back and forth during muscle contraction. Other bursae are subcutaneous to allow skin to slide freely over bony prominences such as the elbow. **Serous membranes** also form or line compartments, although they are composed of squamous epithelial cells ("mesothelium") that secrete a lubricating substance called **serous fluid.** Serous membranes line body cavities and the outer surfaces of many organs so these structures can move freely against one another.

Clinical Focus

Fascia can limit the spread of infection between anatomic compartments and can form adhesions around inflamed tissue to contain it. Bursae may become inflamed (**bursitis**) from compression (e.g., of a subcutaneous bursa) or excessive repetitive motion of the joint they are associated with. Swelling is typical of an inflamed bursa, and it may be necessary to drain the excess fluid from the sac.

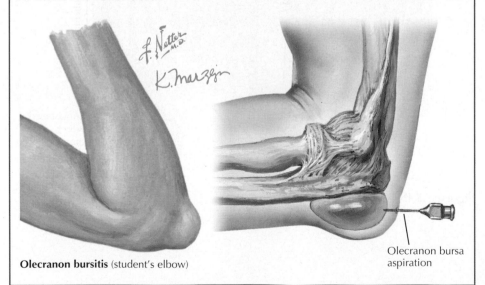

Olecranon bursa aspiration

Olecranon bursitis (student's elbow)

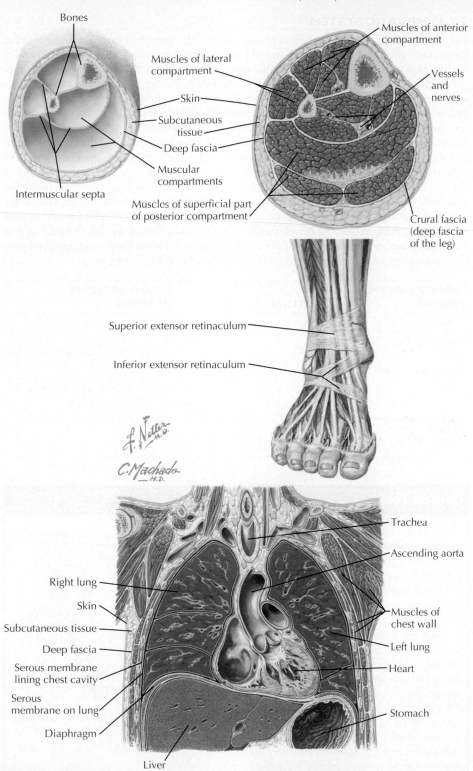

Bones

Muscles of lateral compartment

Muscles of anterior compartment

Skin

Vessels and nerves

Subcutaneous tissue

Deep fascia

Muscular compartments

Intermuscular septa

Muscles of superficial part of posterior compartment

Crural fascia (deep fascia of the leg)

Superior extensor retinaculum

Inferior extensor retinaculum

Trachea

Ascending aorta

Right lung

Skin

Muscles of chest wall

Subcutaneous tissue

Left lung

Deep fascia

Heart

Serous membrane lining chest cavity

Serous membrane on lung

Diaphragm

Stomach

Liver

Figure 1.6 FASCIA, SYNOVIUM, AND SEROUS MEMBRANES

1.7 LYMPHATIC SYSTEM

During circulation, fluid moves between capillaries and the interstitial space due to hydrostatic and osmotic pressures. Typically the amount of fluid that leaves capillaries is greater than the amount that is reabsorbed; thus one of the primary functions of the **lymphatic system** is to collect this excess fluid and return it to the circulation. During this process, the lymphatic system plays an important role in bodily defense because it filters the fluid and traps foreign particles before they enter the circulation. **Lymphatic capillaries** in the interstitial space collect the fluid (**lymph**), and it flows into larger collecting vessels and finally into lymphatic ducts. There are two lymphatic ducts in the body, the **right lymphatic duct** and the **thoracic duct,** and these are the only lymphatic vessels large enough to be seen well at the gross level. The right lymphatic duct receives lymphatic drainage from the upper right side of the body, while the thoracic duct drains the remaining parts. The two lymphatic ducts return lymph to the circulation by merging with the junction between the subclavian and internal jugular veins at the base of the neck. **Lymph nodes** are encapsulated clusters of immune cells that are interspersed between lymphatic vessels. As lymph passes through a lymph node, foreign material such as bacteria, viruses, cellular debris, and cancer cells is filtered out of the lymph and acted on by the immune system. Major groups of lymph nodes are listed in the following table.

GROUP OF LYMPH NODES	LOCATION	MAJOR REGIONS DRAINED
Cervical	Adjacent to internal jugular vein	Head and neck
Axillary	Axilla	Breast, upper limb, thoracic and abdominal walls superior to umbilicus
Mediastinal	Mediastinum	Thoracic viscera
Inguinal	Groin	Lower limb, perineum, abdominal wall inferior to umbilicus
Aortic (preaortic and lumbar)	Adjacent to abdominal aorta	Abdominal viscera, retroperitoneum, gonads
Iliac	Adjacent to iliac vessels	Pelvic viscera

Clinical Focus

Lymph nodes often become enlarged (**lymphadenopathy**) when the body is fighting an infection, because the immune cells within the nodes proliferate in response to trapped bacteria or viruses. Lymphatic vessels can become inflamed (**lymphangitis**) and may produce red streaks under the skin. A lymph node that traps a large number of cancer cells can become a secondary cancer site. Thus the path of lymphatic drainage is relevant when evaluating metastatic disease because evaluation of lymph nodes can provide information regarding the extent of metastasis. At times it is necessary to remove lymph nodes and lymphatic vessels that are infiltrated by cancer cells. This may result in edema (swelling) due to insufficient lymphatic drainage.

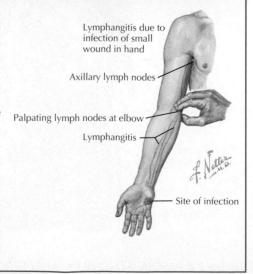

Lymphangitis due to infection of small wound in hand

Axillary lymph nodes

Palpating lymph nodes at elbow

Lymphangitis

Site of infection

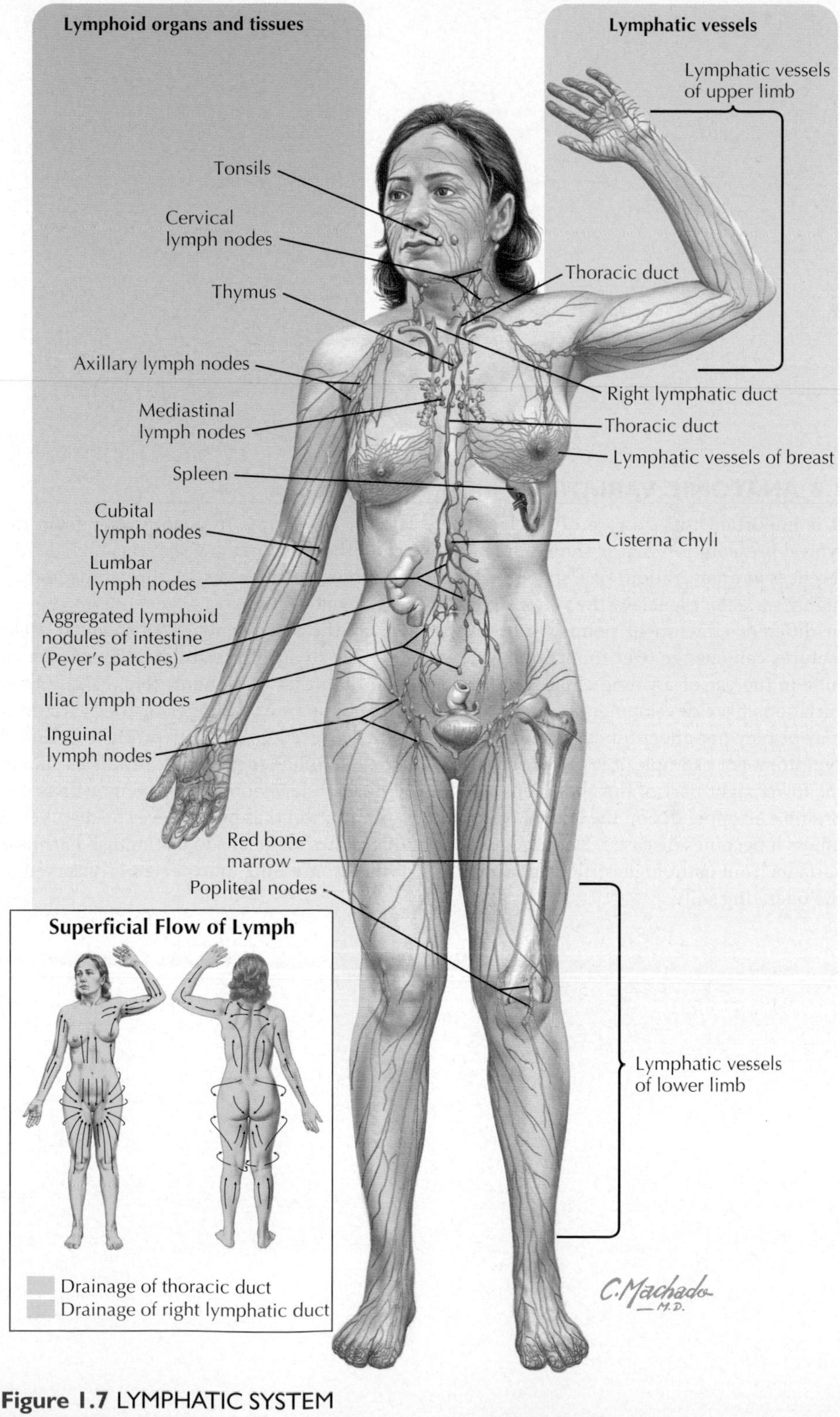

Lymphoid organs and tissues

Tonsils

Cervical lymph nodes

Thymus

Axillary lymph nodes

Mediastinal lymph nodes

Spleen

Cubital lymph nodes

Lumbar lymph nodes

Aggregated lymphoid nodules of intestine (Peyer's patches)

Iliac lymph nodes

Inguinal lymph nodes

Red bone marrow

Popliteal nodes

Lymphatic vessels

Lymphatic vessels of upper limb

Thoracic duct

Right lymphatic duct

Thoracic duct

Lymphatic vessels of breast

Cisterna chyli

Lymphatic vessels of lower limb

Superficial Flow of Lymph

Drainage of thoracic duct
Drainage of right lymphatic duct

C. Machado M.D.

Figure 1.7 LYMPHATIC SYSTEM

1.8 ANATOMIC VARIATION

It is important to be aware of the fact that anatomic structures frequently vary from the typical presentation that is shown in textbooks and other resources. Variations include differences in organization, size, shape, or location of structures. The vasculature of the body is highly variable, especially the venous system. Muscles may have extra heads, missing heads, or different attachment points. Bones are shaped by the forces applied to them, so their features can change over time. Some variations are due to age; for example, the eustachian tube in the ear of a young child is more horizontal than that of an adult (Fig. 2.32). Other variations have developmental causes, such as possessing an extra finger or toe. Variations may or may not affect function, and many are not discovered unless they produce a clinical symptom. For example, it is common knowledge that an inflamed appendix produces pain in the lower right part of the abdomen. However, abnormal development of the intestines can produce an appendix on the left side of the body—a variation that might never be discovered unless it becomes diseased. Knowledge of variations allows clinicians to distinguish harmless variants from pathologic structures, for instance when something unexpected is observed in the operating suite.

Variations in vasculature pattern

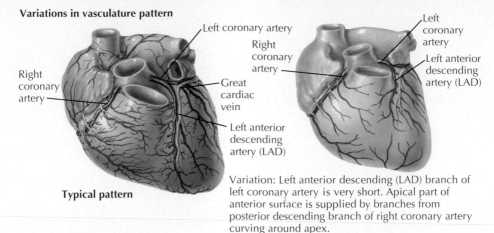

Typical pattern

Variation: Left anterior descending (LAD) branch of left coronary artery is very short. Apical part of anterior surface is supplied by branches from posterior descending branch of right coronary artery curving around apex.

Variations in organ shape

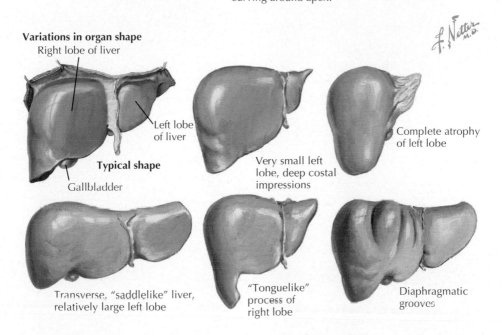

Right lobe of liver

Left lobe of liver

Typical shape

Gallbladder

Very small left lobe, deep costal impressions

Complete atrophy of left lobe

Transverse, "saddlelike" liver, relatively large left lobe

"Tonguelike" process of right lobe

Diaphragmatic grooves

Variations in organ position

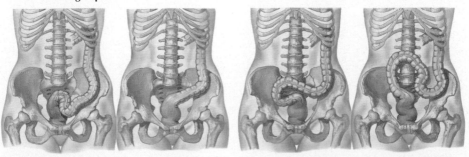

Typical

Short, straight, obliquely into pelvis

Looping to right side

Ascending high into abdomen

Figure 1.8 ANATOMIC VARIATION

NERVOUS SYSTEM

2.1 THE NERVOUS SYSTEM

The nervous system has two structural divisions—the **central nervous system** (CNS) and the **peripheral nervous system** (PNS). The CNS consists of the brain and spinal cord. The PNS consists of all of the nervous tissue located outside of the CNS—nerves that function as communication links between the body and CNS, and ganglia containing neuronal cell bodies. The two types of peripheral nerves are **cranial nerves** and **spinal nerves.** The nervous system can also be classified functionally by the types of structures it innervates. The **somatic nervous system** innervates structures involved with moving and supporting the body, namely skin, skeletal muscle, tendons, bones, and ligaments. In contrast, the **autonomic nervous system (ANS)** innervates visceral structures involved with maintaining homeostasis via processes such as digestion and circulation. Visceral structures include smooth muscle that lines organs and blood vessels, cardiac muscle of the heart, arrector pili muscles in the skin, and glands. The ANS has three components: a **parasympathetic division** that promotes internal functions when the body is at rest ("resting and digesting" division); a **sympathetic division** that prepares the body for intense situations such as stress and exercise ("fight or flight" division); and the **enteric nervous system,** which is a collection of neurons in the wall of the digestive tract that regulate processes such as gastrointestinal motility and blood flow.

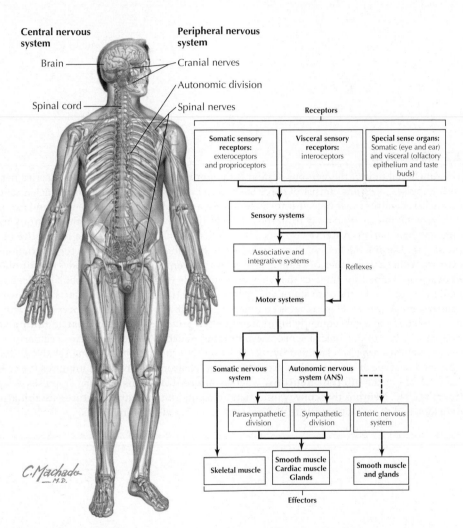

Figure 2.1 THE NERVOUS SYSTEM

2.2 NEURONS

The functional unit of the nervous system is the **neuron,** which is the cell that carries nervous impulses. Neurons consist of three basic parts: a cell body that contains a nucleus and organelles; dendrites that receive information from a stimulus or another neuron; and axons that transmit information away from the cell body. It is important to realize that neurons are different from nerves. A **nerve** consists of multiple neurons surrounded by a connective tissue sheath. Despite the fact that neurons all have the same basic parts, structural variations exist regarding the number of cellular processes that connect to the cell body. **Multipolar neurons** are named for the fact that they have multiple (more than two) cellular processes joining the cell body; they are abundant in both the central and peripheral parts of the nervous system. A type of neuron that is common in the PNS has one cellular process connected to the cell body that subsequently bifurcates into two processes—these are **pseudounipolar neurons.** A few of the special senses have **bipolar neurons,** which have two cellular processes. Neurons are also classified by the direction their impulse is traveling relative to the CNS, and the type of structure they are innervating. Neurons that conduct impulses towards the CNS are called **afferent neurons,** whereas **efferent neurons** conduct impulses away from the CNS. Neurons that convey information to and from somatic structures are **somatic neurons,** and those that innervate visceral structures are **visceral neurons.**

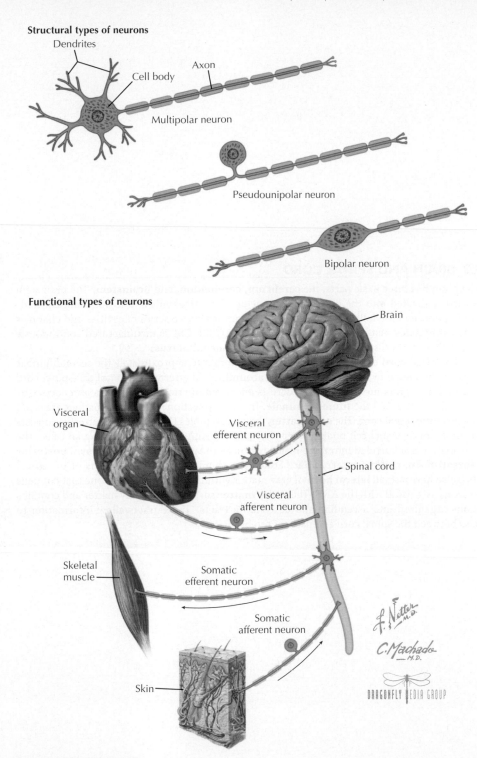

Structural types of neurons

Dendrites

Cell body

Axon

Multipolar neuron

Pseudounipolar neuron

Bipolar neuron

Functional types of neurons

Brain

Visceral organ

Visceral efferent neuron

Visceral afferent neuron

Spinal cord

Skeletal muscle

Somatic efferent neuron

Somatic afferent neuron

Skin

Figure 2.2 NEURONS

2.3 BRAIN AND SPINAL CORD

The brain has three basic parts, the **cerebrum, cerebellum,** and **brainstem.** The brainstem is further divided into the diencephalon (includes the thalamus and hypothalamus), mid-brain, pons, and medulla. The interior of the brain features a series of cavities and channels called **ventricles** that contain cerebrospinal fluid (CSF). CSF is manufactured continuously by collections of cells in the ventricles called the **choroid plexus.**

The **spinal cord** extends from the base of the brain to approximately the second lumbar vertebra in adults; in infants it terminates around L3. The terminal part of the spinal cord is called the **conus medullaris.** The cord is anchored inferiorly to the dura and coccyx by a thin filament called the **filum terminale.** In a cross-sectional view, two distinct areas are visible in the spinal cord. The **gray matter,** which resembles the shape of a butterfly, consists primarily of neuronal cell bodies, interneurons, and supporting cells called glial cells. The gray matter is subdivided into three major regions—the **anterior (ventral) horn, posterior (dorsal) horn,** and the **intermediate zone.** The thoracic and sacral regions of the spinal cord also have a small **lateral horn** of gray matter within the intermediate zone that contains neurons associated with the ANS. The **white matter** surrounds the gray matter and contains axons organized into ascending and descending tracts. These tracts allow information to pass between the spinal cord and parts of the brain.

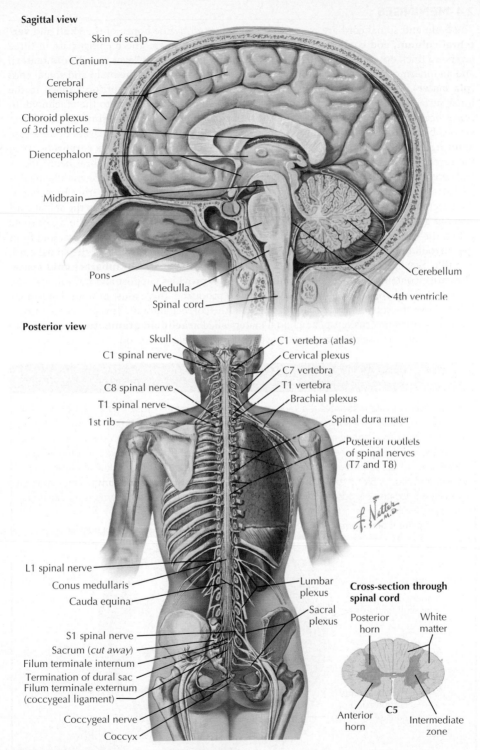

Sagittal view

Skin of scalp

Cranium

Cerebral hemisphere

Choroid plexus of 3rd ventricle

Diencephalon

Midbrain

Pons

Medulla

Spinal cord

Cerebellum

4th ventricle

Posterior view

Skull

C1 spinal nerve

C8 spinal nerve

T1 spinal nerve

1st rib

C1 vertebra (atlas)

Cervical plexus

C7 vertebra

T1 vertebra

Brachial plexus

Spinal dura mater

Posterior rootlets of spinal nerves (T7 and T8)

L1 spinal nerve

Conus medullaris

Cauda equina

S1 spinal nerve

Sacrum (*cut away*)

Filum terminale internum

Termination of dural sac
Filum terminale externum (coccygeal ligament)

Coccygeal nerve

Coccyx

Lumbar plexus

Sacral plexus

Cross-section through spinal cord

Posterior horn

White matter

Anterior horn

C5

Intermediate zone

Figure 2.3 BRAIN AND SPINAL CORD.

2.4 MENINGES

The brain and spinal cord are protected and supported by the bones of the **skull** and **vertebral column,** and connective tissue layers called **meninges.** The meninges are in three layers—a thick outermost layer (**dura mater**), a thin intermediate layer (**arachnoid mater**), and an innermost layer that is intimately applied to the surface of the brain and spinal cord (**pia mater**). The cranial dura has two layers—an outer periosteal portion applied to the inner surface of the cranium, and an inner meningeal portion adjacent to the arachnoid. In some locations these two layers separate, forming channels called **dural sinuses** that collect venous blood from the cerebral veins. In other locations two meningeal layers of dura fuse to form supportive partitions between parts of the brain, including the **falx cerebri** between the cerebral hemispheres and the **tentorium cerebelli** between the cerebral hemispheres and cerebellum. The dura mater of the brain receives arterial supply from the middle meningeal artery (a branch of the maxillary artery, see Fig. 2.5) and innervation from branches of the trigeminal nerve and cervical spinal nerves. The dura mater surrounding the spinal cord exists as a single layer that has extensions called **dural sleeves** that encircle the nerve roots within the vertebral canal. In contrast to the cranial dura, the spinal dura is separated from the surrounding bone by an **epidural space** that contains fat and veins of the spinal cord. The thin, weblike arachnoid is separated from the pia mater by the **subarachnoid space.** This space contains **cerebrospinal fluid (CSF)** that provides support and buoyancy to the brain and spinal cord. Because CSF is continually produced, there must be a mechanism for CSF to leave the subarachnoid space to maintain the correct amount. This process is accomplished by small protrusions of arachnoid mater called **arachnoid granulations** that project into the venous sinuses and facilitate movement of CSF into the blood.

Clinical Focus

Meningitis is inflammation of the meninges that is most often caused by a viral or bacterial infection. The inflammation and swelling associated with meningitis may obstruct the flow of CSF, leading to a condition called **hydrocephalus** (excess CSF within the brain that may compress brain tissue). The middle meningeal artery travels between the cranium and periosteal layer of dura mater. Rupture of this vessel, for example due to a skull fracture, causes an accumulation of blood external to the dura called an **epidural hematoma**. This condition is fatal if not treated because the blood compresses the brain and compromises its function.

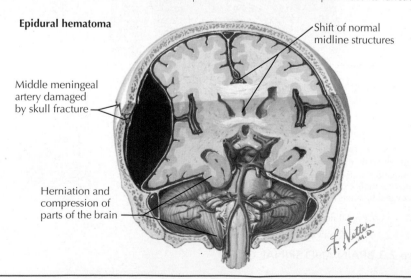

Epidural hematoma

Shift of normal midline structures

Middle meningeal artery damaged by skull fracture

Herniation and compression of parts of the brain

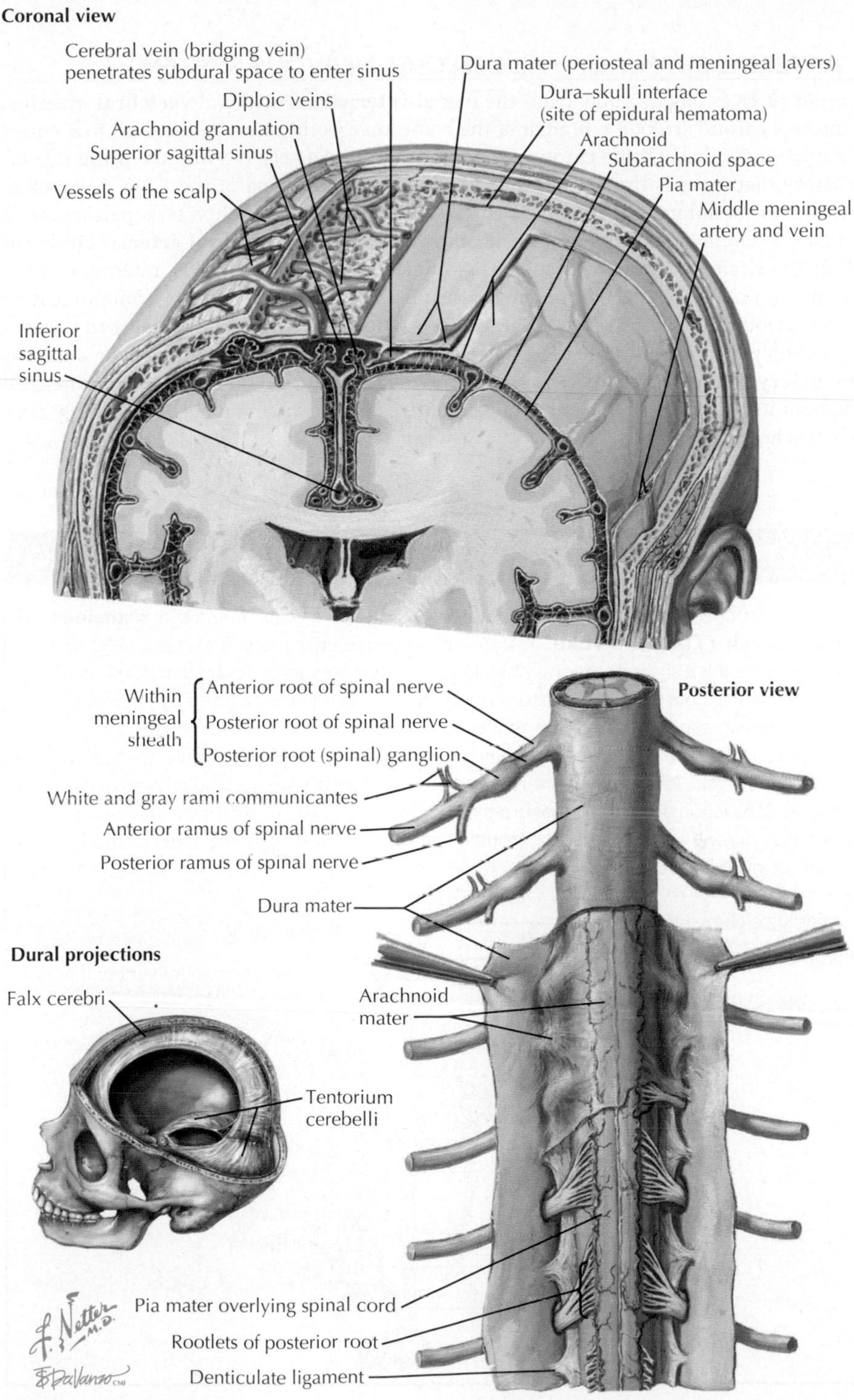

Coronal view

Cerebral vein (bridging vein) penetrates subdural space to enter sinus

Diploic veins

Arachnoid granulation
Superior sagittal sinus

Vessels of the scalp

Dura mater (periosteal and meningeal layers)

Dura–skull interface (site of epidural hematoma)

Arachnoid
Subarachnoid space
Pia mater

Middle meningeal artery and vein

Inferior sagittal sinus

Within meningeal sheath
{ Anterior root of spinal nerve
Posterior root of spinal nerve
Posterior root (spinal) ganglion

Posterior view

White and gray rami communicantes
Anterior ramus of spinal nerve
Posterior ramus of spinal nerve

Dura mater

Dural projections

Falx cerebri

Arachnoid mater

Tentorium cerebelli

Pia mater overlying spinal cord

Rootlets of posterior root

Denticulate ligament

Figure 2.4 MENINGES

2.5 ARTERIAL SUPPLY OF THE CENTRAL NERVOUS SYSTEM

The brain receives blood supply from the paired **internal carotid** and **vertebral arteries.** The internal carotid artery is a branch of the common carotid artery in the neck that enters the cranial cavity through the carotid canal. The vertebral artery is a branch of the subclavian artery that ascends the neck within the transverse foramina of the C1–C6 vertebrae and traverses the foramen magnum to enter the cranial cavity. Both vessels participate in the collateral circulation of the brain via connections with the **cerebral arterial circle (of Willis).** The circle is composed of four pairs of arteries (anterior cerebral, internal carotid, posterior communicating, posterior cerebral) and a small unpaired anterior communicating branch that joins the two anterior cerebral vessels. Due to its length, the spinal cord receives arterial supply from a multitude of vessels. The vertebral arteries give off a single **anterior spinal artery** and paired **posterior spinal arteries** that descend on the surface of the cord throughout its length. The vessels are supplemented by segmental branches that mainly arise from branches of the aorta.

Clinical Focus

If the blood supply to the brain is interrupted, a patient may experience a **transient ischemic attack (TIA)** or **stroke**. A transient ischemic attack is sometimes called a "mini stroke" because it is a short, temporary blockage of blood flow to the brain that does not cause permanent damage but exhibits symptoms of stroke. A TIA is usually caused by atherosclerosis in a blood vessel supplying the brain that induces clot formation and produces an embolus that lodges in a vessel. The condition can be temporary if the body is able to dissolve the clot; however, if the clot causes permanent obstruction, then a stroke results. A stroke usually causes loss of function due to death of brain cells. Common signs of a stroke include numbness or weakness on one side of the body, trouble speaking or understanding speech, sudden loss of vision, or difficulty walking.

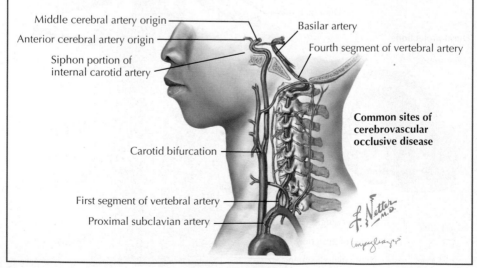

Middle cerebral artery origin

Anterior cerebral artery origin

Siphon portion of
internal carotid artery

Basilar artery

Fourth segment of vertebral artery

**Common sites of
cerebrovascular
occlusive disease**

Carotid bifurcation

First segment of vertebral artery

Proximal subclavian artery

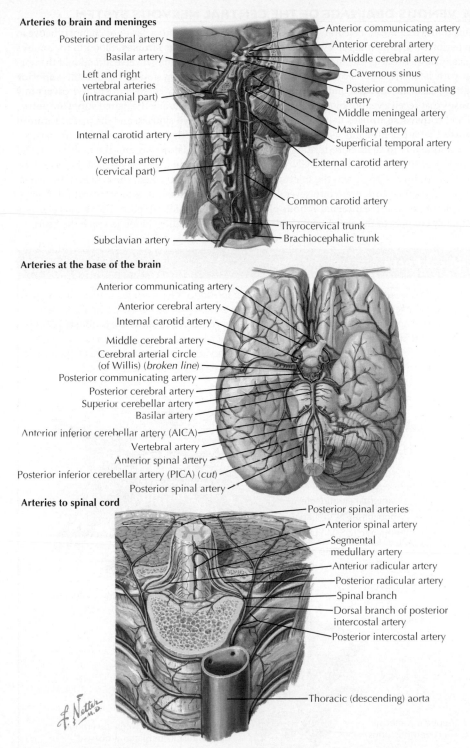

Arteries to brain and meninges

Posterior cerebral artery
Basilar artery
Left and right vertebral arteries (intracranial part)
Internal carotid artery
Vertebral artery (cervical part)
Subclavian artery

Anterior communicating artery
Anterior cerebral artery
Middle cerebral artery
Cavernous sinus
Posterior communicating artery
Middle meningeal artery
Maxillary artery
Superficial temporal artery
External carotid artery
Common carotid artery
Thyrocervical trunk
Brachiocephalic trunk

Arteries at the base of the brain

Anterior communicating artery
Anterior cerebral artery
Internal carotid artery
Middle cerebral artery
Cerebral arterial circle (of Willis) (*broken line*)
Posterior communicating artery
Posterior cerebral artery
Superior cerebellar artery
Basilar artery
Anterior inferior cerebellar artery (AICA)
Vertebral artery
Anterior spinal artery
Posterior inferior cerebellar artery (PICA) (*cut*)
Posterior spinal artery

Arteries to spinal cord

Posterior spinal arteries
Anterior spinal artery
Segmental medullary artery
Anterior radicular artery
Posterior radicular artery
Spinal branch
Dorsal branch of posterior intercostal artery
Posterior intercostal artery
Thoracic (descending) aorta

Figure 2.5 ARTERIAL SUPPLY OF THE CENTRAL NERVOUS SYSTEM

2.6 VENOUS DRAINAGE OF THE CENTRAL NERVOUS SYSTEM

Veins of the brain (e.g., cerebral veins, cerebellar veins) drain into a series of channels between the periosteal and meningeal layers of dura called **dural venous sinuses.** Blood in the sinuses typically flows towards the internal jugular vein; however, flow may reverse direction if the normal path is obstructed, because the sinuses lack valves. Major sinuses include the **superior sagittal, inferior sagittal,** and **straight sinuses** within the falx cerebri; the paired **cavernous sinuses** that receive venous blood from the orbit as well as the brain; the paired **superior petrosal** and **transverse sinuses** that funnel blood into the sigmoid sinuses; and the paired **sigmoid sinuses** that are continuous with the internal jugular veins. The cavernous sinuses are particularly unique due to their close relationship to multiple cranial nerves and the internal carotid arteries. CN III, CN IV, CN V_1 and CN V_2 are all located within the lateral wall of the cavernous sinus. In contrast, CN VI and the internal carotid artery pass through the center of the sinus. Veins of the spinal cord drain into several vertebral venous plexuses associated with the vertebral column, such as the **internal venous plexus** within the epidural space. The venous plexuses ultimately connect to the azygos and caval venous systems to allow blood to reach the heart.

Clinical Focus

Infections in the nasal cavity or paranasal sinuses can spread to the cavernous sinuses via the ophthalmic veins. Microorganisms, most commonly *Staphylococcus aureus*, get trapped in the trabeculae of the sinuses and inflammation leads to clot formation (**cavernous sinus thrombosis [CST]**). Swelling in the sinus can compress the adjacent cranial nerves leading to symptoms such as sensory loss or visual problems. In addition, because venous blood cannot flow freely through the sinus, it backs up in the ophthalmic veins causing swelling in the orbit and proptosis.

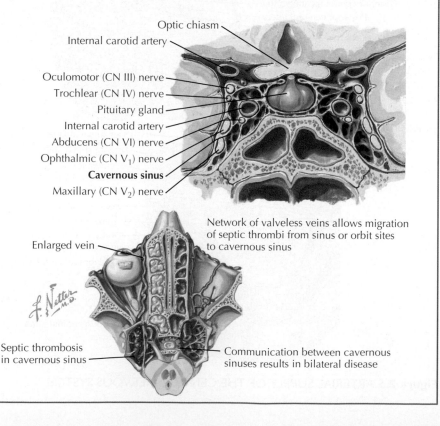

Optic chiasm

Internal carotid artery

Oculomotor (CN III) nerve

Trochlear (CN IV) nerve

Pituitary gland

Internal carotid artery

Abducens (CN VI) nerve

Ophthalmic (CN V_1) nerve

Cavernous sinus

Maxillary (CN V_2) nerve

Network of valveless veins allows migration of septic thrombi from sinus or orbit sites to cavernous sinus

Enlarged vein

Septic thrombosis in cavernous sinus

Communication between cavernous sinuses results in bilateral disease

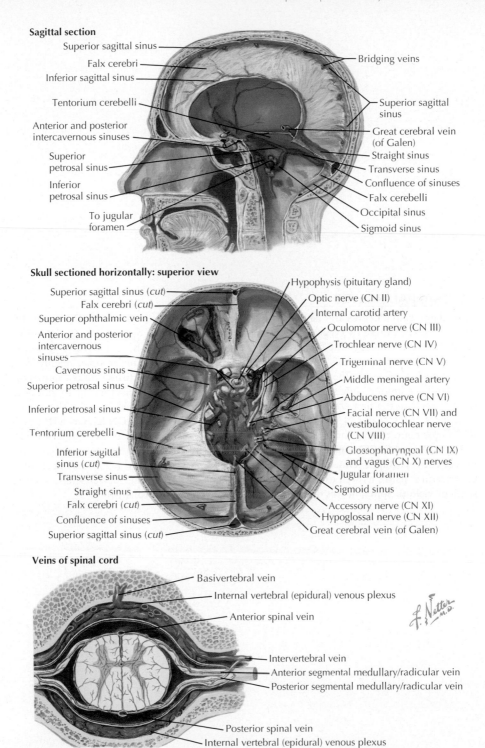

Sagittal section

Superior sagittal sinus

Falx cerebri

Inferior sagittal sinus

Tentorium cerebelli

Anterior and posterior intercavernous sinuses

Superior petrosal sinus

Inferior petrosal sinus

To jugular foramen

Bridging veins

Superior sagittal sinus

Great cerebral vein (of Galen)

Straight sinus

Transverse sinus

Confluence of sinuses

Falx cerebelli

Occipital sinus

Sigmoid sinus

Skull sectioned horizontally: superior view

Superior sagittal sinus (*cut*)

Falx cerebri (*cut*)

Superior ophthalmic vein

Anterior and posterior intercavernous sinuses

Cavernous sinus

Superior petrosal sinus

Inferior petrosal sinus

Tentorium cerebelli

Inferior sagittal sinus (*cut*)

Transverse sinus

Straight sinus

Falx cerebri (*cut*)

Confluence of sinuses

Superior sagittal sinus (*cut*)

Hypophysis (pituitary gland)

Optic nerve (CN II)

Internal carotid artery

Oculomotor nerve (CN III)

Trochlear nerve (CN IV)

Trigeminal nerve (CN V)

Middle meningeal artery

Abducens nerve (CN VI)

Facial nerve (CN VII) and vestibulocochlear nerve (CN VIII)

Glossopharyngeal (CN IX) and vagus (CN X) nerves

Jugular foramen

Sigmoid sinus

Accessory nerve (CN XI)

Hypoglossal nerve (CN XII)

Great cerebral vein (of Galen)

Veins of spinal cord

Basivertebral vein

Internal vertebral (epidural) venous plexus

Anterior spinal vein

Intervertebral vein

Anterior segmental medullary/radicular vein

Posterior segmental medullary/radicular vein

Posterior spinal vein

Internal vertebral (epidural) venous plexus

Figure 2.6 VENOUS DRAINAGE OF THE CENTRAL NERVOUS SYSTEM

2.7 CRANIAL NERVES

Cranial and spinal nerves are the two types of peripheral nerves in the body. The major difference between these two types of nerves is where they connect to the CNS. By definition, cranial nerves connect to the brain, and spinal nerves connect to the spinal cord. However, there is one exception to this general rule because the 11th cranial nerve arises mainly from the cervical spinal cord. The **cranial nerves** are numbered 1 to 12 (using roman numerals) and also have unique names. For example, the terms "CN I" and "olfactory nerve" are both used to refer to the first cranial nerve. Of the 12 cranial nerves, three convey only sensory neurons (**CN I, CN II, CN VIII**). Five nerves (**CN III, CN IV, CN VI, CN XI, CN XII**) transmit motor neurons that innervate skeletal muscles. The remaining four nerves (**CN V, CN VII, CN IX,** and **CN X**) contain both sensory and motor neurons. Sensory neurons in cranial nerves convey what is sometimes referred to as "ordinary sensation" (e.g., touch, pressure, temperature, pain), as well as "special sensation" (sensations of the special senses such as smell or vision). Spinal nerves do not convey special sensory neurons.

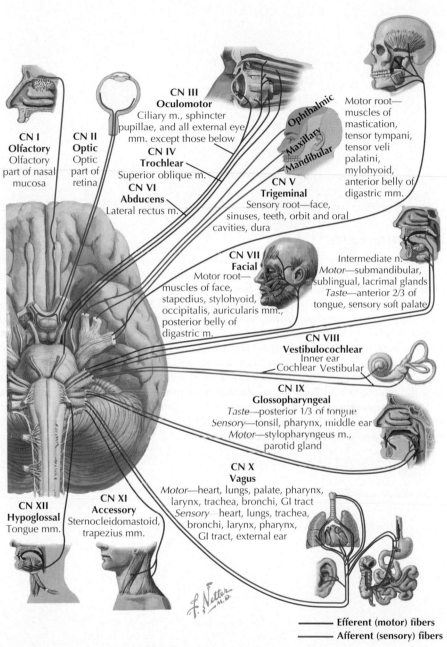

CN I
Olfactory
Olfactory
part of nasal
mucosa

CN II
Optic
Optic
part of
retina

CN III
Oculomotor
Ciliary m., sphincter
pupillae, and all external eye
mm. except those below

CN IV
Trochlear
Superior oblique m.

CN VI
Abducens
Lateral rectus m.

Ophthalmic

Maxillary

Mandibular

CN V
Trigeminal
Sensory root—face,
sinuses, teeth, orbit and oral
cavities, dura

Motor root—
muscles of
mastication,
tensor tympani,
tensor veli
palatini,
mylohyoid,
anterior belly of
digastric mm.

CN VII
Facial
Motor root—
muscles of face,
stapedius, stylohyoid,
occipitalis, auricularis mm.,
posterior belly of
digastric m.

Intermediate n.
Motor—submandibular,
sublingual, lacrimal glands
Taste—anterior 2/3 of
tongue, sensory soft palate

CN VIII
Vestibulocochlear
Inner ear
Cochlear Vestibular

CN IX
Glossopharyngeal
Taste—posterior 1/3 of tongue
Sensory—tonsil, pharynx, middle ear
Motor—stylopharyngeus m.,
parotid gland

CN X
Vagus
Motor—heart, lungs, palate, pharynx,
larynx, trachea, bronchi, GI tract
Sensory—heart, lungs, trachea,
bronchi, larynx, pharynx,
GI tract, external ear

CN XII
Hypoglossal
Tongue mm.

CN XI
Accessory
Sternocleidomastoid,
trapezius mm.

—— Efferent (motor) fibers
—— Afferent (sensory) fibers

Figure 2.7 CRANIAL NERVES

2.8 CRANIAL BASE

Cranial nerves arise from the brain inside the cranial cavity, thus must travel through openings in the skull to reach their targets. The inferior part of the skull that is in contact with the ventral surface of the brain is called the **cranial base.** The base contains three cranial fossae (anterior, middle, and posterior) that are separated by the lesser wing of the sphenoid and petrous ridge of the temporal bone. Cranial nerves I and II travel through openings in the **anterior cranial fossa,** specifically the small foramina in the **cribriform plate** and **optic canal,** respectively. The **middle cranial fossa** contains the **superior orbital fissure,** which is a large crack that conveys CN III, CN IV, CN VI, and branches of the first division of CN V_1 the ophthalmic nerve. The other two divisions of the trigeminal nerve also exit the skull within the middle cranial fossa via the **foramen rotundum** (CN V_2) and **foramen ovale** (CN V_3). The remaining six cranial nerves travel through openings in the **posterior cranial fossa,** namely the **internal acoustic meatus** (CN VII, CN VIII), **jugular foramen** (CN IX, CN X, CN XI), and the **hypoglossal canal** (CN XII).

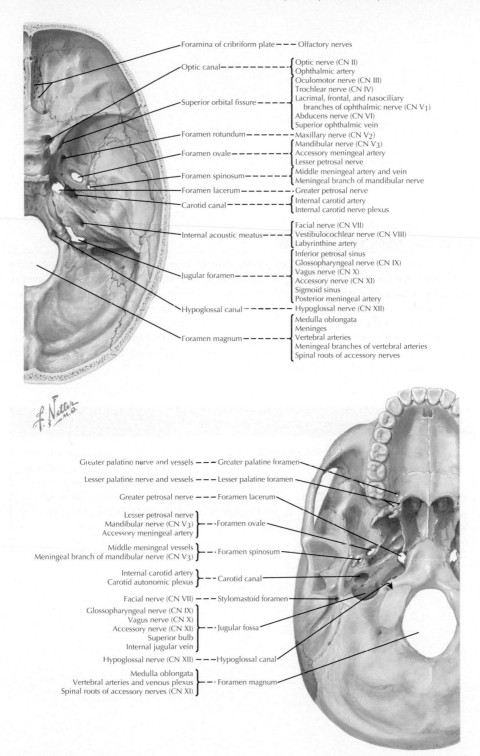

Foramina of cribriform plate – – – Olfactory nerves

Optic canal – – – – – – { Optic nerve (CN II)
Ophthalmic artery

Oculomotor nerve (CN III)
Trochlear nerve (CN IV)
Superior orbital fissure – – – – – { Lacrimal, frontal, and nasociliary
branches of ophthalmic nerve (CN V₁)
Abducens nerve (CN VI)
Superior ophthalmic vein

Foramen rotundum – – – – – – Maxillary nerve (CN V₂)

Foramen ovale – – – – – – – { Mandibular nerve (CN V₃)
Accessory meningeal artery
Lesser petrosal nerve

Foramen spinosum – – – – – { Middle meningeal artery and vein
Meningeal branch of mandibular nerve

Foramen lacerum – – – – – – · Greater petrosal nerve

Carotid canal – – – – – – { Internal carotid artery
Internal carotid nerve plexus

Internal acoustic meatus – – – { Facial nerve (CN VII)
Vestibulocochlear nerve (CN VIII)
Labyrinthine artery

Jugular foramen – – – – – – { Inferior petrosal sinus
Glossopharyngeal nerve (CN IX)
Vagus nerve (CN X)
Accessory nerve (CN XI)
Sigmoid sinus
Posterior meningeal artery

Hypoglossal canal – – – – – Hypoglossal nerve (CN XII)

Foramen magnum – – – – – – { Medulla oblongata
Meninges
Vertebral arteries
Meningeal branches of vertebral arteries
Spinal roots of accessory nerves

Greater palatine nerve and vessels – – – Greater palatine foramen

Lesser palatine nerve and vessels – – – Lesser palatine foramen

Greater petrosal nerve – – – Foramen lacerum

Lesser petrosal nerve
Mandibular nerve (CN V₃)   } – – Foramen ovale
Accessory meningeal artery

Middle meningeal vessels
Meningeal branch of mandibular nerve (CN V₃) } – – Foramen spinosum

Internal carotid artery
Carotid autonomic plexus   } – – Carotid canal

Facial nerve (CN VII) – – – Stylomastoid foramen

Glossopharyngeal nerve (CN IX)
Vagus nerve (CN X)
Accessory nerve (CN XI)   } – – Jugular fossa
Superior bulb
Internal jugular vein

Hypoglossal nerve (CN XII) – – – Hypoglossal canal

Medulla oblongata
Vertebral arteries and venous plexus   } – – Foramen magnum
Spinal roots of accessory nerves (CN XI)

Figure 2.8 CRANIAL BASE

2.9 OLFACTORY NERVE (CN I)

The first cranial nerve is composed of a collection of afferent neurons in the roof of the nasal cavity that convey olfactory information (sensation of smell). These neurons, known as **olfactory cells,** are located in a specialized portion of the nasal epithelium called the **olfactory mucosa.** Cilia on the olfactory cells have receptors for odorant molecules, and binding of molecules generates action potentials in the olfactory axons that pass through small holes in the **cribriform plate** of the ethmoid bone to enter the cranial cavity. These axons terminate by synapsing with neurons in the olfactory bulbs, which then convey information to olfactory areas in the brain via the olfactory tract.

Clinical Focus

Loss of the sense of smell is called **anosmia.** Temporary anosmia can be caused by conditions that obstruct the nasal passages and prevent odors from reaching the olfactory epithelium (e.g., nasal congestion, nasal polyps) or by agents that damage olfactory cells (e.g., viruses, medications, noxious chemicals). Olfactory cells are continually replaced over an individual's lifetime; thus the loss of smell due to cell damage is usually temporary. Head trauma (e.g., fractures of the cribriform plate) or damage to brain tissue (e.g., tumors) may cause permanent anosmia.

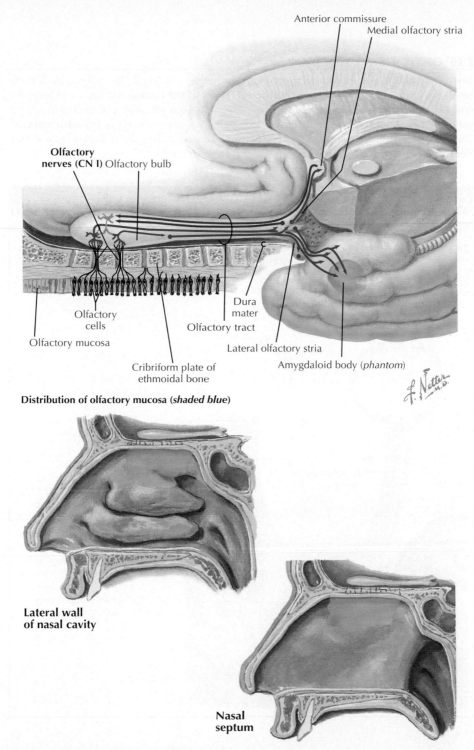

Distribution of olfactory mucosa (*shaded blue*)

Lateral wall
of nasal cavity

Nasal
septum

Figure 2.9 OLFACTORY NERVE (CN I)

2.10 OPTIC NERVE (CN II)

The second cranial nerve contains special afferent neurons for sight. The cell bodies of these bipolar neurons are located in the **ganglion cell layer of the retina,** and the axons leave the eyeball as the **optic nerve.** The optic nerve passes between the orbit and cranial cavity via the **optic canal.** Once in the cranial cavity, the two optic nerves merge at the **optic chiasm.** This connection allows sharing of neurons between the two nerves that aids binocular vision. Neurons continue to targets in the brain via the optic tracts.

Clinical Focus

The optic nerve can become inflamed **(optic neuritis)** in association with infections such as measles, tuberculosis, and Lyme disease. This often causes pain and temporary loss of vision until the infection resolves. Inflammation of the optic nerve and vision loss is also common with demyelinating diseases such as multiple sclerosis (MS). The pituitary gland is very closely associated with the optic chiasm; thus pituitary tumors can exert pressure on the chiasm resulting in visual impairment.

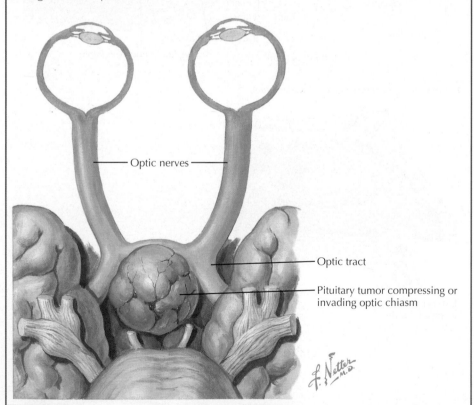

Optic nerves

Optic tract

Pituitary tumor compressing or invading optic chiasm

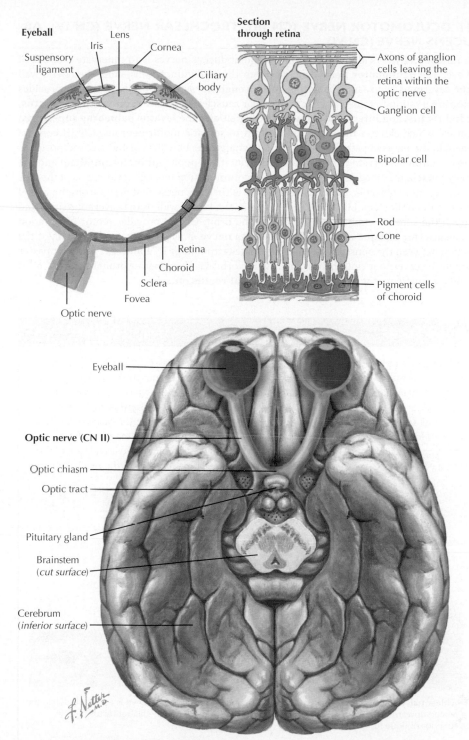

Eyeball

Suspensory ligament
Iris
Lens
Cornea
Ciliary body
Retina
Choroid
Sclera
Fovea
Optic nerve

Section through retina

Axons of ganglion cells leaving the retina within the optic nerve
Ganglion cell
Bipolar cell
Rod
Cone
Pigment cells of choroid

Eyeball

Optic nerve (CN II)

Optic chiasm
Optic tract
Pituitary gland
Brainstem (*cut surface*)
Cerebrum (*inferior surface*)

Figure 2.10 OPTIC NERVE (CN II)

2.11 OCULOMOTOR NERVE (CN III), TROCHLEAR NERVE (CN IV), ABDUCENS NERVE (CN VI)

The function of the oculomotor, trochlear, and abducens nerves is to innervate muscles of the eye. The **oculomotor nerve** emerges from the midbrain, travels along the lateral wall of the cavernous sinus, and enters the orbit through the superior orbital fissure. It provides motor innervation to four of the six extraocular muscles: **superior rectus, inferior rectus, medial rectus,** and **inferior oblique.** It also innervates the **levator palpebrae superioris,** a muscle which elevates the eyelid. In addition to somatic motor neurons, CN III conveys preganglionic parasympathetic neurons that synapse in the ciliary ganglion. The postganglionic neurons innervate the constrictor muscle of the pupil (**sphincter pupillae**) and the **ciliary muscle** that mediates the process of accommodation (changing the shape of the lens to focus on near objects). The **trochlear nerve** is the only nerve that arises from the dorsal aspect of the brainstem. Like CN III, it travels in the lateral wall of the cavernous sinus and through the superior orbital fissure to reach the orbit. CN IV provides motor innervation to the **superior oblique muscle.** The **abducens nerve** emerges from the brainstem at the junction between the pons and medulla (alternate terminology is "abducent" nerve). It passes through the cavernous sinus before entering the orbit via the superior orbital fissure. CN VI provides somatic motor innervation to the **lateral rectus muscle.**

Clinical Focus

The cranial nerves that innervate the extraocular muscles are all associated with the cavernous sinus and thus may be affected by pathologies such as cavernous sinus thrombosis (see Clinical Focus 2.6). Damage to CN III produces ptosis due to the loss of levator palpebrae function; a fixed and dilated pupil that will not accommodate due to the loss of parasympathetic innervation; and an eye that is directed down and out since only the superior oblique and lateral rectus are functioning. Loss of superior oblique function with CN IV damage results in an adducted and slightly elevated eye since depression and abduction of the eye is weakened. Damage to CN VI impacts the function of the lateral rectus; thus abduction of the eye is impaired.

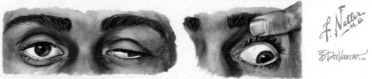

Oculomotor palsy: affected eye exhibits ptosis and a dilated pupil. The eye is abducted and depressed, due to the pull of the two extraocular muscles that are functioning.

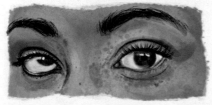

Trochlear palsy: affected eye is hypertropic (deviated upwards) and extorted due to the loss of superior oblique function.

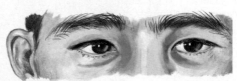

Abducens palsy: affected eye is adducted due to the loss of abduction by the lateral rectus muscle.

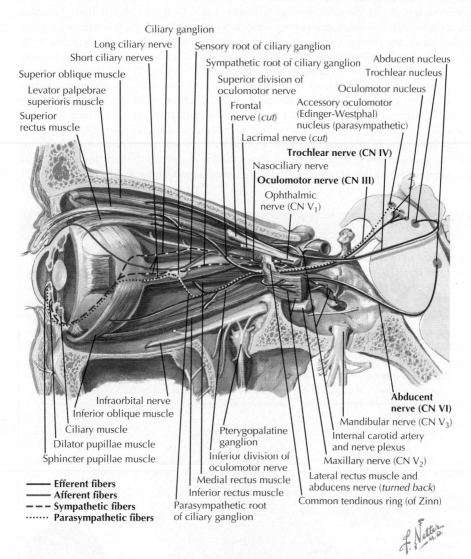

Ciliary ganglion
Long ciliary nerve
Short ciliary nerves
Superior oblique muscle
Levator palpebrae
superioris muscle
Superior
rectus muscle

Sensory root of ciliary ganglion
Sympathetic root of ciliary ganglion
Superior division of
oculomotor nerve
Frontal
nerve (cut)
Lacrimal nerve (cut)

Abducent nucleus
Trochlear nucleus
Oculomotor nucleus
Accessory oculomotor
(Edinger-Westphal)
nucleus (parasympathetic)

Trochlear nerve (CN IV)
Nasociliary nerve
Oculomotor nerve (CN III)
Ophthalmic
nerve (CN V₁)

Infraorbital nerve
Inferior oblique muscle
Ciliary muscle
Dilator pupillae muscle
Sphincter pupillae muscle

——— Efferent fibers
——— Afferent fibers
– – – Sympathetic fibers
······· Parasympathetic fibers

Pterygopalatine
ganglion
Inferior division of
oculomotor nerve
Medial rectus muscle
Inferior rectus muscle
Parasympathetic root
of ciliary ganglion

**Abducent
nerve (CN VI)**
Mandibular nerve (CN V₃)
Internal carotid artery
and nerve plexus
Maxillary nerve (CN V₂)
Lateral rectus muscle and
abducens nerve (turned back)
Common tendinous ring (of Zinn)

Figure 2.11 OCULOMOTOR NERVE (CN III), TROCHLEAR NERVE (CN IV),
ABDUCENS NERVE (CN VI)

2.12 TRIGEMINAL NERVE (CN V)

After emerging from the pons, the trigeminal nerve divides into three divisions designated CN V_1, CN V_2, and CN V_3. The **trigeminal ganglion,** which contains sensory cell bodies of afferent neurons in CN V, is located at the junction of the trigeminal nerve and its three divisions. CN V_1, the **ophthalmic nerve,** enters the superior orbital fissure and divides into three branches that pass into the orbit (frontal, nasociliary, and lacrimal nerves). These branches contain only sensory neurons that convey information mainly from the cornea, conjunctiva, lacrimal gland, anterior part of the nasal cavity, and the skin of the upper face and forehead. CN V_2, the **maxillary nerve,** travels through the foramen rotundum and enters a deep region of the face called the pterygopalatine fossa. Here it gives off branches that convey sensory neurons primarily from the midportion of the face, posterior part of the nasal cavity, upper teeth and gums, nasopharynx, and palate. CN V_3, the **mandibular nerve,** leaves the cranial cavity through the foramen ovale and enters the infratemporal fossa. The mandibular nerve is the only division of the trigeminal nerve that contains motor neurons; these innervate the muscles of mastication (chewing) as well as a few additional small muscles in the head. CN V_3 also conveys sensory neurons from the lower third of the face, lower teeth and gums, anterior two-thirds of the tongue and the lateral aspect of the scalp.

Clinical Focus

Trigeminal neuralgia is a chronic pain condition caused by injury to the trigeminal nerve. Facial pain varies in nature from constant aching or burning sensations, to sudden intense stabbing feelings. Pain can be triggered by touching sensitive regions of the face, such as when shaving or applying lotion. The exact cause is unknown; however, compression of the trigeminal nerve by blood vessels in the brain may be involved. Demyelinating diseases such as multiple sclerosis can also cause trigeminal neuralgia. Another source of facial pain is **herpes zoster (shingles)**, which is caused by reactivation of the varicella zoster virus (VZV) in the trigeminal ganglion. Initial infection with VZV usually causes chicken pox, and then the virus remains dormant for many years within the sensory ganglia of the body. If the virus in the trigeminal ganglion becomes reactivated, it can produce painful blisters within the sensory distribution of one or more divisions of the trigeminal nerve.

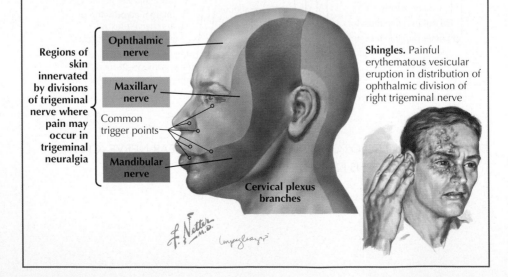

Regions of skin innervated by divisions of trigeminal nerve where pain may occur in trigeminal neuralgia

Ophthalmic nerve

Maxillary nerve

Common trigger points

Mandibular nerve

Cervical plexus branches

Shingles. Painful erythematous vesicular eruption in distribution of ophthalmic division of right trigeminal nerve

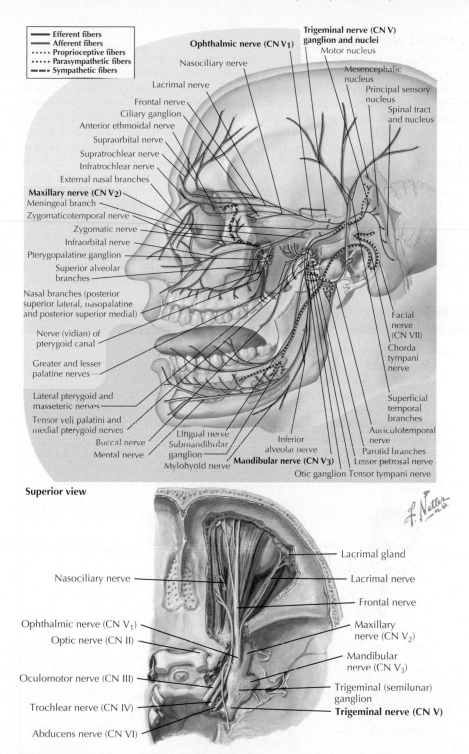

Efferent fibers
Afferent fibers
Proprioceptive fibers
Parasympathetic fibers
Sympathetic fibers

Trigeminal nerve (CN V)
ganglion and nuclei

Ophthalmic nerve (CN V₁)
Motor nucleus

Nasociliary nerve
Mesencephalic nucleus

Lacrimal nerve
Principal sensory nucleus

Frontal nerve
Spinal tract and nucleus

Ciliary ganglion

Anterior ethmoidal nerve

Supraorbital nerve

Supratrochlear nerve

Infratrochlear nerve

External nasal branches

Maxillary nerve (CN V₂)
Meningeal branch

Zygomaticotemporal nerve

Zygomatic nerve

Infraorbital nerve

Pterygopalatine ganglion

Superior alveolar branches

Nasal branches (posterior superior lateral, nasopalatine and posterior superior medial)

Facial nerve (CN VII)

Nerve (vidian) of pterygoid canal

Chorda tympani nerve

Greater and lesser palatine nerves

Lateral pterygoid and masseteric nerves

Superficial temporal branches

Tensor veli palatini and medial pterygoid nerves

Auriculotemporal nerve

Buccal nerve

Lingual nerve
Submandibular ganglion

Inferior alveolar nerve

Parotid branches

Mental nerve

Mandibular nerve (CN V₃)

Lesser petrosal nerve

Mylohyoid nerve

Otic ganglion Tensor tympani nerve

Superior view

Lacrimal gland

Nasociliary nerve

Lacrimal nerve

Frontal nerve

Ophthalmic nerve (CN V₁)

Maxillary nerve (CN V₂)

Optic nerve (CN II)

Mandibular nerve (CN V₃)

Oculomotor nerve (CN III)

Trigeminal (semilunar) ganglion

Trochlear nerve (CN IV)

Trigeminal nerve (CN V)

Abducens nerve (CN VI)

Figure 2.12 TRIGEMINAL NERVE (CN V)

2.13 FACIAL NERVE (CN VII)

The seventh cranial nerve emerges from the brainstem at the medullary-pontine junction, leaves the cranial cavity through the internal acoustic meatus, travels through the temporal bone, and exits the skull via the stylomastoid foramen. While in the temporal bone, the facial nerve gives off three branches. The first is the **greater petrosal nerve,** which conveys parasympathetic neurons that supply the lacrimal gland. These neurons join sympathetic fibers to form the nerve of the pterygoid canal, synapse in the pterygopalatine ganglion, and ultimately travel to the orbit to reach their target. The sensory ganglion of the facial nerve, the **geniculate ganglion,** is located in the region where the greater petrosal nerve arises. The next branch that arises from the facial nerve is the **nerve to stapedius** that innervates the stapedius muscle. The third branch, the **chorda tympani nerve**, conveys taste sensations from the anterior two-thirds of the tongue and parasympathetic neurons that innervate the submandibular and sublingual salivary glands. The distal part of the facial nerve emerges from the skull through the **stylomastoid foramen.** The bulk of the nerve then traverses the parotid gland before dividing into five terminal branches that supply the muscles of facial expression: **temporal, zygomatic, buccal, marginal mandibular,** and **cervical.** This group of muscles includes muscles that close the eyes and mouth, wrinkle the forehead, and produce a smile.

Clinical Focus

Idiopathic facial paralysis (IFP), more commonly known as Bell palsy, is caused by inflammation of the facial nerve within the facial canal. The inflammation is likely caused by a viral infection; research suggests that viruses such as herpes simplex, varicella zoster, cytomegalovirus, and Epstein-Barr are all potential causes. Typically only one facial nerve is affected, so symptoms of facial muscle weakness or paralysis typically present on one side of the face. Common signs include loss of wrinkles on one side of the forehead, loss of the ability to completely close one eye, inability to elevate one corner of the mouth during smiling, and drooling due to the inability to close one side of the mouth. If inflammation extends into the proximal part of the facial canal, the patient may experience loss of taste or increased sensitivity to sound due to compression of the chorda tympani nerve and nerve to stapedius.

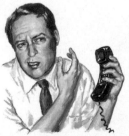

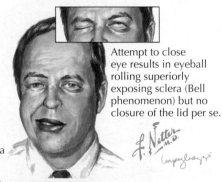

Attempt to close eye results in eyeball rolling superiorly exposing sclera (Bell phenomenon) but no closure of the lid per se.

Hyperacusis. This may be early or initial symptom of a peripheral VII nerve palsy: patient holds phone away from ear because of painful sensitivity to sound. Loss of taste also may occur on affected side.

Left Peripheral VII Facial Weakness. Patient unable to wrinkle forehead; eyelid droops very slightly; cannot show teeth at all on affected side in attempt to smile; and lower lip droops slightly.

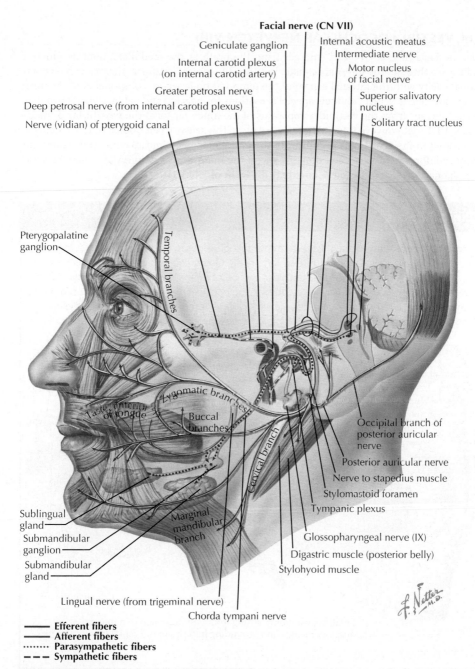

Facial nerve (CN VII)

Geniculate ganglion

Internal acoustic meatus

Intermediate nerve

Internal carotid plexus
(on internal carotid artery)

Motor nucleus
of facial nerve

Greater petrosal nerve

Superior salivatory
nucleus

Deep petrosal nerve (from internal carotid plexus)

Solitary tract nucleus

Nerve (vidian) of pterygoid canal

Pterygopalatine
ganglion

Temporal branches

Zygomatic branches

Taste: anterior ⅔ of tongue

Buccal
branches

Occipital branch of
posterior auricular
nerve

Posterior auricular nerve

Nerve to stapedius muscle

Cervical branch

Stylomastoid foramen

Tympanic plexus

Sublingual
gland

Marginal
mandibular
branch

Glossopharyngeal nerve (IX)

Submandibular
ganglion

Digastric muscle (posterior belly)

Submandibular
gland

Stylohyoid muscle

Lingual nerve (from trigeminal nerve)

Chorda tympani nerve

—— **Efferent fibers**
—— **Afferent fibers**
······ **Parasympathetic fibers**
– – – **Sympathetic fibers**

Figure 2.13 FACIAL NERVE (CN VII)

2.14 VESTIBULOCOCHLEAR NERVE (CN VIII)

Like the facial nerve, CN VIII emerges from the brain at the medullary-pontine junction and travels through the internal acoustic meatus. The internal acoustic meatus connects the cranial cavity with the internal aspect of the temporal bone where components of the inner ear are located. CN VIII conducts special sensations for hearing and balance via its two divisions. Neurons from the vestibular apparatus of the inner ear form the **vestibular division of CN VIII** that conveys information for balance. The sensory cell bodies of these neurons are located in the **vestibular ganglion** in the internal acoustic meatus. Neurons conveying auditory information have cell bodies in one of the many **spiral ganglia** of the cochlea and their axons converge to form the **cochlear division of CN VIII.**

Clinical Focus

A **vestibular schwannoma** is a benign tumor that develops in the myelin sheath surrounding the vestibular division of CN VIII. These tumors are also called "acoustic neuromas" because they were thought to arise from the cochlear division of the nerve when they were first identified. Vestibular schwannomas compress the vestibulocochlear nerve and can cause symptoms such as hearing loss, dizziness, and loss of balance. If the tumor expands outside of the internal acoustic meatus, it can compress other cranial nerves, producing additional symptoms.

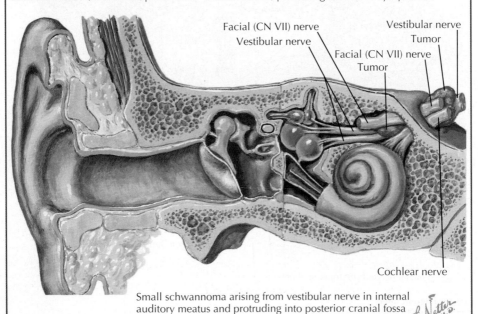

Facial (CN VII) nerve
Vestibular nerve
Vestibular nerve
Tumor
Facial (CN VII) nerve
Tumor
Cochlear nerve

Small schwannoma arising from vestibular nerve in internal auditory meatus and protruding into posterior cranial fossa

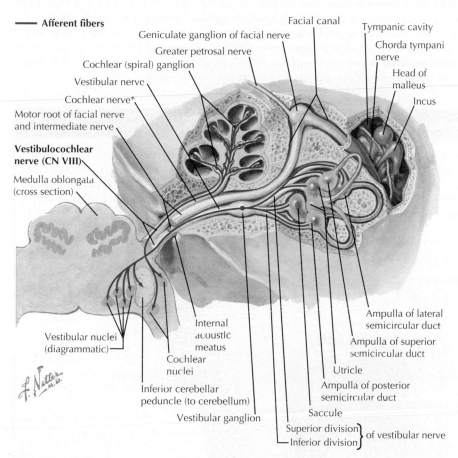

—— **Afferent fibers**

Facial canal

Tympanic cavity

Geniculate ganglion of facial nerve

Chorda tympani nerve

Greater petrosal nerve

Cochlear (spiral) ganglion

Head of malleus

Vestibular nerve

Cochlear nerve*

Incus

Motor root of facial nerve and intermediate nerve

Vestibulocochlear nerve (CN VIII)

Medulla oblongata (cross section)

Vestibular nuclei (diagrammatic)

Internal acoustic meatus

Ampulla of lateral semicircular duct

Ampulla of superior semicircular duct

Cochlear nuclei

Utricle

Inferior cerebellar peduncle (to cerebellum)

Ampulla of posterior semicircular duct

Vestibular ganglion

Saccule

Superior division ⎱ of vestibular nerve
Inferior division ⎰

*Note: The cochlear nerve also contains efferent fibers to the sensory epithelium.
These fibers are derived from the vestibular nerve while in the internal auditory meatus.*

Figure 2.14 VESTIBULOCOCHLEAR NERVE (CN VIII)

2.15 GLOSSOPHARYNGEAL NERVE (CN IX)

The ninth cranial nerve arises from the medulla and leaves the cranial cavity through the jugular foramen. It is primarily a sensory nerve, conveying afferent neurons from the tympanic cavity, pharynx and posterior one-third of the tongue via its **tympanic, pharyngeal, and lingual branches,** respectively. The afferent neurons in the lingual branch conduct both general sensation and special sensation for taste. CN IX also conveys information from chemoreceptors in the **carotid body** and baroreceptors in the **carotid sinus** that aids the maintenance of blood pressure and the chemical composition of the blood. CN IX has two sensory ganglia located within the vicinity of the jugular foramen. The somatic motor neurons in CN IX innervate the **stylopharyngeus muscle,** one of the longitudinal muscles of the pharynx. Finally, the glossopharyngeal nerve contains parasympathetic neurons that travel in the **lesser petrosal nerve** and synapse in the otic ganglion. Postganglionic parasympathetic neurons that arise in the otic ganglion innervate the parotid salivary gland.

Clinical Focus

During a cranial nerve exam, the integrity of CN IX is evaluated by testing the gag reflex with a tongue depressor. The gag reflex is a protective mechanism that causes contraction of the pharyngeal muscles when a foreign object touches the back of the throat or posterior part of the tongue. The glossopharyngeal nerve conveys the sensory neurons of the reflex, while the vagus nerve provides the motor neurons that innervate the pharyngeal musculature.

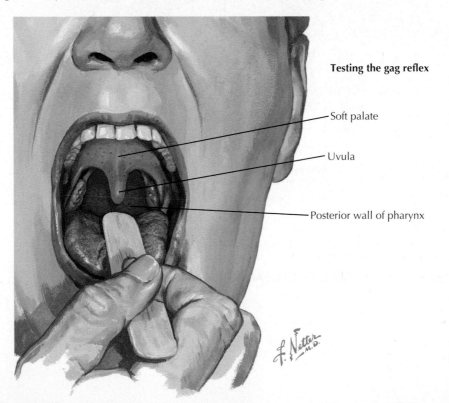

Testing the gag reflex

Soft palate

Uvula

Posterior wall of pharynx

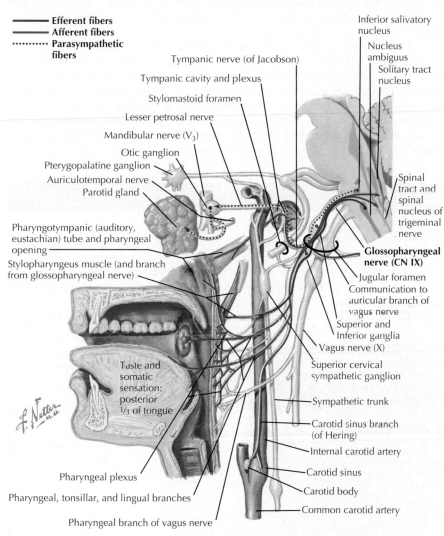

Efferent fibers
Afferent fibers
Parasympathetic fibers

Tympanic nerve (of Jacobson)

Tympanic cavity and plexus

Stylomastoid foramen

Lesser petrosal nerve

Mandibular nerve (V₃)

Otic ganglion

Pterygopalatine ganglion

Auriculotemporal nerve

Parotid gland

Pharyngotympanic (auditory, eustachian) tube and pharyngeal opening

Stylopharyngeus muscle (and branch from glossopharyngeal nerve)

Taste and somatic sensation: posterior ⅓ of tongue

Pharyngeal plexus

Pharyngeal, tonsillar, and lingual branches

Pharyngeal branch of vagus nerve

Inferior salivatory nucleus

Nucleus ambiguus

Solitary tract nucleus

Spinal tract and spinal nucleus of trigeminal nerve

Glossopharyngeal nerve (CN IX)

Jugular foramen

Communication to auricular branch of vagus nerve

Superior and Inferior ganglia

Vagus nerve (X)

Superior cervical sympathetic ganglion

Sympathetic trunk

Carotid sinus branch (of Hering)

Internal carotid artery

Carotid sinus

Carotid body

Common carotid artery

Figure 2.15 GLOSSOPHARYNGEAL NERVE (CN IX)

2.16 VAGUS NERVE (CN X)

The vagus nerve arises from the medulla as a collection of small rootlets that merge together and exit the skull through the jugular foramen. The word vagus means "wandering"; thus the name of the nerve reflects the fact that it has a wide distribution in the body. **Sensory neurons** in the vagus nerve convey sensations from the external acoustic meatus (ear canal), dura mater, laryngopharynx, interior of the larynx, and numerous visceral organs in the thorax and abdomen. Like the glossopharyngeal nerve, the vagus has two sensory ganglia near the jugular foramen. The superior ganglion contains cell bodies for somatic neurons, while the inferior ganglion houses cell bodies for visceral neurons. **Motor neurons** in vagal nerve branches of the head and neck innervate muscles of the palate, pharynx, larynx, and cervical part of the esophagus. The vagus nerve also contains **parasympathetic neurons** that are distributed to visceral organs in the thorax and abdomen as far distal as the splenic flexure of the colon.

Clinical Focus

Lesions of the vagus nerve cause problems with palatal elevation, swallowing, and speaking due to paralysis of the muscles that perform these functions. The integrity of the vagus nerve can be evaluated by examining the function of the soft palate. If both vagus nerves are intact, the uvula will remain in the midline when the soft palate elevates. In contrast, if one vagus nerve is damaged, the uvula will deviate away from the damaged side due to the pull of the muscles that are functioning. Unilateral vocal cord paralysis can also be observed via physical exam. Patients with this condition typically present with a hoarse voice and noisy breathing.

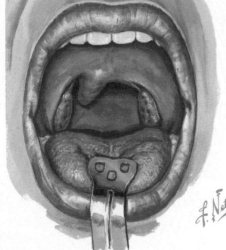

Uvular paralysis: uvula drawn to nonparalyzed side when patient says "A-AH"

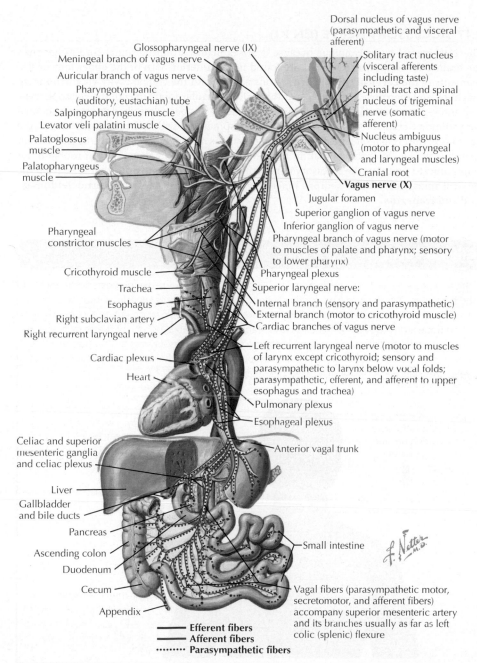

Dorsal nucleus of vagus nerve (parasympathetic and visceral afferent)

Solitary tract nucleus (visceral afferents including taste)

Spinal tract and spinal nucleus of trigeminal nerve (somatic afferent)

Nucleus ambiguus (motor to pharyngeal and laryngeal muscles)

Cranial root

Vagus nerve (X)

Glossopharyngeal nerve (IX)

Meningeal branch of vagus nerve

Auricular branch of vagus nerve

Pharyngotympanic (auditory, eustachian) tube

Salpingopharyngeus muscle

Levator veli palatini muscle

Palatoglossus muscle

Palatopharyngeus muscle

Jugular foramen

Superior ganglion of vagus nerve

Inferior ganglion of vagus nerve

Pharyngeal branch of vagus nerve (motor to muscles of palate and pharynx; sensory to lower pharynx)

Pharyngeal constrictor muscles

Pharyngeal plexus

Cricothyroid muscle

Trachea

Esophagus

Right subclavian artery

Right recurrent laryngeal nerve

Superior laryngeal nerve:

Internal branch (sensory and parasympathetic)

External branch (motor to cricothyroid muscle)

Cardiac branches of vagus nerve

Cardiac plexus

Heart

Left recurrent laryngeal nerve (motor to muscles of larynx except cricothyroid; sensory and parasympathetic to larynx below vocal folds; parasympathetic, efferent, and afferent to upper esophagus and trachea)

Pulmonary plexus

Esophageal plexus

Anterior vagal trunk

Celiac and superior mesenteric ganglia and celiac plexus

Liver

Gallbladder and bile ducts

Pancreas

Ascending colon

Duodenum

Cecum

Appendix

Small intestine

Vagal fibers (parasympathetic motor, secretomotor, and afferent fibers) accompany superior mesenteric artery and its branches usually as far as left colic (splenic) flexure

—— Efferent fibers
—— Afferent fibers
········ Parasympathetic fibers

Figure 2.16 VAGUS NERVE (CN X)

2.17 ACCESSORY NERVE (CN XI)

The 11th cranial nerve is unique because it arises mainly from the spinal cord rather than the brainstem. Neuronal cell bodies are found in the anterior horn of the upper four or five segments of the **cervical spinal cord.** Axons ascend into the cranial cavity via the foramen magnum, and then do a "U-turn" to exit through the jugular foramen with the glossopharyngeal and vagus nerves. Historically the accessory nerve has been described as having a cranial contribution ("cranial root") that briefly joins the spinal root within the jugular foramen. The neurons in the cranial root are distributed in the vagus nerve to muscles of the larynx. Recent anatomic studies have shown that, in most individuals, the spinal and cranial roots do not communicate, and thus the accessory nerve contains only motor neurons that arise from the cervical spinal cord. These neurons innervate two skeletal muscles, the **sternocleidomastoid** and **trapezius.**

Clinical Focus

The accessory nerve is most vulnerable to injury during procedures in the posterior triangle of the neck (e.g., lymph node biopsy, skin cancer excisions) due to its superficial location. The affected side exhibits shoulder droop and weakness in shoulder elevation due to loss of function of the trapezius muscle. The trapezius also stabilizes the medial border of the scapula against the chest wall especially during external rotation of the humerus. Loss of this support produces protrusion of the medial scapular border (scapular winging) when external rotation is tested against resistance—a clinical sign called the "scapular flip sign."

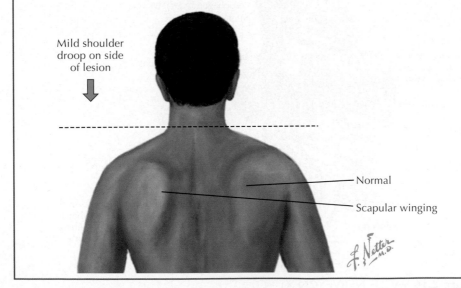

Mild shoulder droop on side of lesion

Normal

Scapular winging

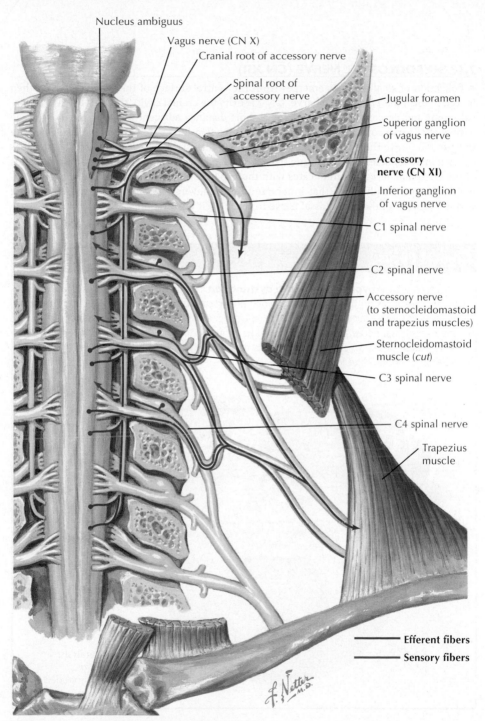

Figure 2.17 ACCESSORY NERVE (CN XI)

2.18 HYPOGLOSSAL NERVE (CN XII)

A collection of small rootlets emerges from the ventral surface of the medulla, which then merge to form the 12th cranial nerve. CN XII exits the cranial cavity through the **hypoglossal canal** and descends in the neck for a short distance adjacent to the vagus nerve. The hypoglossal nerve contains somatic motor neurons that innervate **extrinsic muscles of the tongue** that move the tongue as a whole (genioglossus, styloglossus, hyoglossus), as well as the **intrinsic muscles of the tongue** that alter its shape. For a short time the anterior ramus of the C1 spinal nerve communicates with the hypoglossal nerve. Some of the neurons arising in C1, specifically those that innervate the thyrohyoid and geniohyoid muscles, travel within branches of the hypoglossal nerve to reach their destination.

Clinical Focus

Common causes of **hypoglossal nerve dysfunction** include tumors, infections, trauma, and surgical procedures on the neck (e.g., carotid endarterectomy). A lesion of CN XII produces difficulty with tongue movements, chewing, speaking, and swallowing. To evaluate the integrity of the hypoglossal nerve, patients are asked to protrude their tongue. Unilateral lesions produce deviation of the tongue towards the damaged side, due to the unopposed genioglossus muscle on the side of the intact nerve.

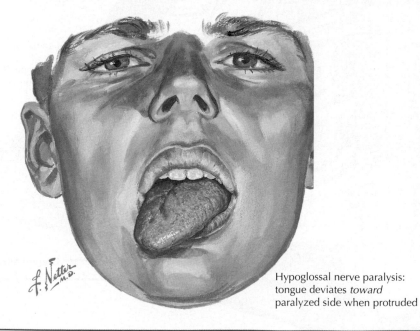

Hypoglossal nerve paralysis: tongue deviates *toward* paralyzed side when protruded

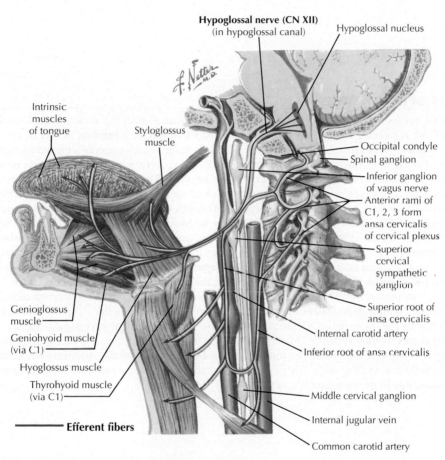

Figure 2.18 HYPOGLOSSAL NERVE (CN XII)

2.19 SPINAL NERVES

Spinal nerves emanate from the spinal cord and are named with the same regional names used for vertebrae. There are **8 cervical nerves, 12 thoracic, 5 lumbar, 5 sacral,** and **1 coccygeal.** Nerves are usually referred to by the first letter of each regional name and a number—for example, the 4th cervical nerve is the C4 spinal nerve, while the 8th thoracic nerve is the T8 spinal nerve. Spinal nerves develop in a segmental fashion and thus are attached to the spinal cord at regular intervals via collections of rootlets called **posterior** and **anterior roots.** The posterior root has a ganglion associated with it called the **spinal (posterior root) ganglion** that contains cell bodies for sensory neurons that travel in spinal nerves. Spinal nerves exit the vertebral column through gaps between vertebrae called **intervertebral foramina** (3.14); in the sacral region the openings in the sacrum are called **sacral foramina.** The cervical spinal nerves exit the vertebral column *superior* to their same numbered vertebra—for example, the C5 nerve passes through the intervertebral foramen between the C4 and C5 vertebrae. However, because there is an eighth cervical nerve but only seven cervical vertebrae, the C8 nerve passes inferior to the C7 vertebra and thus the T1 nerve must pass inferior to the T1 vertebra. Consequently, all the remaining spinal nerves pass *inferior* to their corresponding vertebra. Notice that because the spinal cord does not extend the entire length of the vertebral canal, the lumbar and sacral nerve roots travel inferiorly within the vertebral canal to their respective foramen. This collection of nerve roots is called the **cauda equina,** due to its resemblance to a "horse's tail."

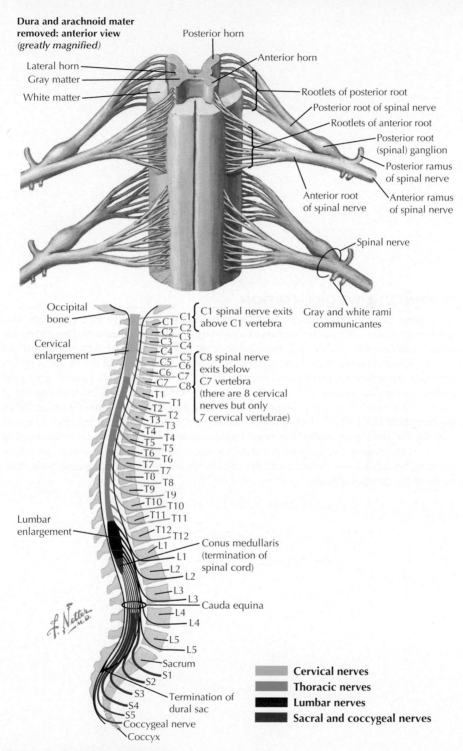

Dura and arachnoid mater removed: anterior view *(greatly magnified)*

Posterior horn

Anterior horn

Lateral horn

Gray matter

White matter

Rootlets of posterior root

Posterior root of spinal nerve

Rootlets of anterior root

Posterior root (spinal) ganglion

Posterior ramus of spinal nerve

Anterior root of spinal nerve

Anterior ramus of spinal nerve

Spinal nerve

Occipital bone

Cervical enlargement

C1 spinal nerve exits above C1 vertebra

Gray and white rami communicantes

C1
C2
C3
C4
C5
C6
C7
C8

C8 spinal nerve exits below C7 vertebra (there are 8 cervical nerves but only 7 cervical vertebrae)

T1
T2
T3
T4
T5
T6
T7
T8
T9
T10
T11
T12

Lumbar enlargement

Conus medullaris (termination of spinal cord)

L1
L2
L3
L4
L5

Cauda equina

Sacrum

S1
S2
S3
S4
S5

Termination of dural sac

Coccygeal nerve

Coccyx

Cervical nerves
Thoracic nerves
Lumbar nerves
Sacral and coccygeal nerves

Figure 2.19 SPINAL NERVES

2.20 SPINAL NERVE ORIENTATION

After passing through the intervertebral foramina, each spinal nerve bifurcates into two major branches, a smaller **posterior ramus** and a larger **anterior ramus.** Posterior rami are distributed to structures in the back and posterior part of the head and neck, while anterior rami innervate structures in the anterolateral neck, trunk, and limbs. In the thoracic region of the body, the anterior rami of spinal nerves travel around the trunk in parallel, giving off branches during their course; they are also known as intercostal nerves. In other regions of the body, the anterior rami intermingle to form nerve plexuses such as the plexuses shown in the bottom of Fig. 2.20 traveling to the lower extremity. Two additional branches of spinal nerves are the small **gray and white rami communicantes** that link the anterior rami to the sympathetic chains. The sympathetic chains are part of the autonomic system, and these connecting branches allow communication between spinal nerves and the sympathetic components of the nervous system.

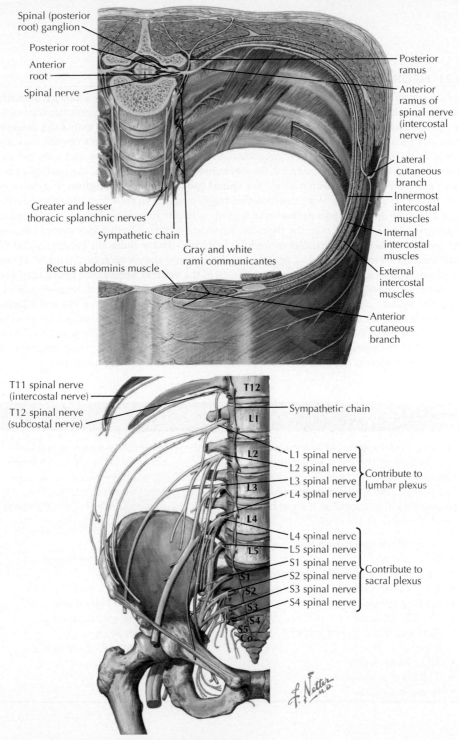

Figure 2.20 SPINAL NERVE ORIENTATION

2.21 NEURONS IN SPINAL NERVES

Spinal nerves contain the four main functional types of neurons (**somatic afferent, somatic efferent, visceral afferent, visceral efferent**). Somatic and visceral afferent neurons conveying information from structures in the limbs or body wall are located within the anterior rami and its branches. Likewise, afferent neurons conveying information from the back are found in the posterior rami. These neurons converge in the spinal nerve and then use the posterior root to reach the spinal cord; they terminate in the **dorsal horn.** The posterior root has a ganglion associated with it called the **spinal (posterior root) ganglion** that contains cell bodies for all of the sensory neurons that travel in spinal nerves. Somatic afferent neurons innervate the skin, and a **dermatome** is a region of skin innervated by a particular spinal nerve pair. The dermatomes in the thoracic region are arranged in uniform stripes because the anterior rami travel in parallel around the body wall. In the limbs the pattern is slightly distorted due to intermingling of neurons in plexuses and the rotation of the limbs during development. Somatic efferent neurons originate in the **ventral horn** of the spinal cord and use the anterior root to exit the spinal cord. These neurons innervate skeletal muscle and use both the anterior and posterior rami to reach their targets. The course of visceral efferent neurons is complex and will be discussed in Sections 2.22–2.24. Both spinal nerves and the anterior and posterior rami are "mixed" nerves because they contain both afferent and efferent neurons. In contrast, the roots of spinal nerves are not mixed, because the posterior root contains only afferent neurons and the anterior root contains only efferent neurons.

Clinical Focus

In clinical practice it is useful to know common dermatomes to identify lesions involving specific spinal nerves. There is overlap between skin territories supplied by particular spinal nerves; however, areas exist ("autonomous zones") that are exclusively supplied by one spinal nerve. For example, the autonomous zone of the C6 dermatome is the pad of the thumb. Thus, if a patient has lost sensation on the pad of their thumb, it indicates impairment of the C6 spinal nerve or one of its branches.

Levels of principal dermatomes
- C5 Clavicles
- C5, C6 Lateral sides of upper limbs
- C8, T1 Medial sides of upper limbs
- C6 Digit I (thumb)
- C6, C7, C8 Hand
- C8 Digits IV and V (ring and little fingers)
- T4 Level of nipples
- T10 Level of umbilicus
- L1 Inguinal region
- L1, L2, L3, L4 Anterior and inner surfaces of lower limbs
- L4, L5, S1 Foot
- L4 Medial side digit I (great toe)
- L5, S1, S2 Lateral and posterior surfaces of lower limbs
- S1 Lateral margin of foot and digit V (little toe)
- S2, S3, S4 Perineum

Schema of neurons within spinal nerves

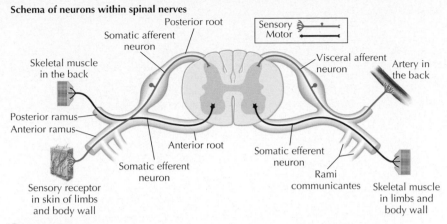

Dermatomes

Schematic demarcation of dermatomes (according to Keegan and Garrett) shown as distinct segments. There is actually considerable overlap between any two adjacent dermatomes. An alternative dermatome map is that provided by Foerster.

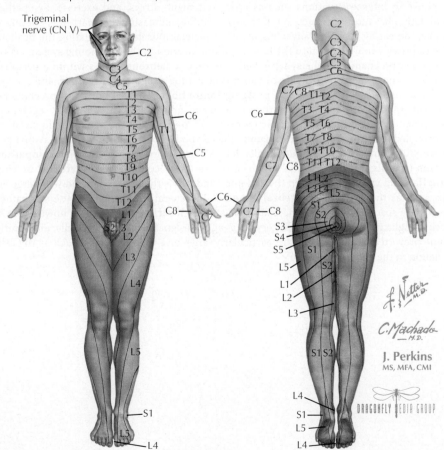

Figure 2.21 NEURONS IN SPINAL NERVES

2.22 SYMPATHETIC NERVOUS SYSTEM

The sympathetic nervous system consists of visceral neurons that modulate the body's response to intense situations such as fear, excitement, stress, and exercise. Sympathetic stimulation has multiple effects on the body, including increasing the heart rate, dilating the pupils, increasing sweating, diverting blood to skeletal muscles, and dilating the bronchial tree to provide more oxygen to the lungs. Communication in the autonomic system acts via a two-neuron chain, and the synapse between the two neurons occurs within a peripheral ganglion. Thus the axon of the first neuron is called the **preganglionic fiber,** and the axon of the second neuron is called the **postganglionic fiber.** The cell bodies of preganglionic sympathetic neurons are found in the thoracic and first two or three lumbar segments of the spinal cord, specifically in the lateral horn. For this reason, the sympathetic division is often called the **thoracolumbar division.** The cell bodies of the postganglionic sympathetic neurons are found in sympathetic ganglia that exist in two locations—in paired **sympathetic chains (trunks)** that extend the length of the vertebral column (**paravertebral or chain ganglia**), and within plexuses in the abdomen and pelvis that are associated with large vessels such as the aorta (**prevertebral ganglia**). In general, the ganglia of the sympathetic chains are spaced so there is one pair associated with each vertebral level; however, in the neck, ganglia merge to form three cervical ganglia designated superior, middle, and inferior. Some prevertebral ganglia that are particularly large have unique names, such as the celiac ganglion in the abdomen.

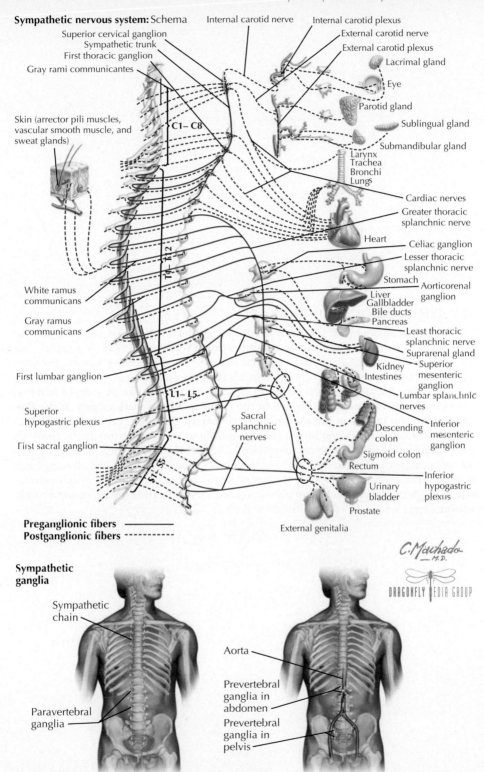

Sympathetic nervous system: Schema

Internal carotid nerve
Internal carotid plexus
External carotid nerve
External carotid plexus

Superior cervical ganglion
Sympathetic trunk
First thoracic ganglion
Gray rami communicantes

Lacrimal gland
Eye
Parotid gland
Sublingual gland
Submandibular gland

C1– C8

Skin (arrector pili muscles, vascular smooth muscle, and sweat glands)

Larynx
Trachea
Bronchi
Lungs

Cardiac nerves
Greater thoracic splanchnic nerve

Heart

Celiac ganglion
Lesser thoracic splanchnic nerve
Stomach
Aorticorenal ganglion

T1– T12

White ramus communicans

Liver
Gallbladder
Bile ducts
Pancreas

Gray ramus communicans

Least thoracic splanchnic nerve
Suprarenal gland
Superior mesenteric ganglion
Lumbar splanchnic nerves

Kidney
Intestines

First lumbar ganglion

L1– L5

Superior hypogastric plexus

Sacral splanchnic nerves

Descending colon
Inferior mesenteric ganglion

First sacral ganglion

S1– S5

Sigmoid colon
Rectum

Inferior hypogastric plexus

Urinary bladder
Prostate
External genitalia

Preganglionic fibers ————
Postganglionic fibers ---------

Sympathetic ganglia

Sympathetic chain

Paravertebral ganglia

Aorta

Prevertebral ganglia in abdomen

Prevertebral ganglia in pelvis

C. Machado
—M.D.

DRAGONFLY MEDIA GROUP

Figure 2.22 SYMPATHETIC NERVOUS SYSTEM

2.23 SYMPATHETIC NEURONS

All sympathetic neurons exit the spinal cord through the anterior root and pass into the sympathetic chain via a **white ramus communicans (WRC).** The WRC is a branch that connects the sympathetic chain to the anterior ramus of the spinal nerve. Once in the sympathetic chain, the course of the neurons depends on the intended target—where in the body they need to go. For simplicity, the targets of sympathetic neurons can be grouped into four categories: **targets in the head, targets in the limbs and body wall, targets in the thoracic cavity,** and **targets in the abdominopelvic cavity.** Drawings that illustrate the path of neurons, such as the figures on the facing page, show single axons for clarity. However, preganglionic axons in the autonomic system branch at their distal ends to synapse with multiple postganglionic neurons, thus creating a more widespread effect and allowing coordination of the sympathetic response at different levels. Additionally, postganglionic neurons have multiple swellings at their terminal ends called varicosities that release neurotransmitter over a large area in the effector tissue.

Route 1: Preganglionic sympathetic neurons that supply structures in the head proceed up the chain to synapse in the superior cervical ganglion. Postganglionic neurons leave the ganglion via branches that form plexuses on the internal and external carotid arteries. Neurons travel to their destination in these plexuses.

Route 2: The limbs and body wall contain blood vessels, sweat glands and arrector pili muscles that receive sympathetic innervation. Some preganglionic neurons that innervate these structures synapse in sympathetic chain ganglia at the level that they entered the chain; others travel up or down the chain first and synapse in a chain ganglion at the level of their target. Postganglionic neurons leave the sympathetic chain through the gray rami communicantes and proceed in branches of the posterior or anterior rami to their target.

Branches to external carotid plexus

Internal carotid nerve

Superior cervical ganglion

Vascular smooth muscle, sweat glands, and arrector pili muscles in skin

1   2
3   4

Posterior ramus

Anterior ramus

Gray ramus communicans

Sympathetic chain ganglion

Cardiac nerve

Splanchnic nerve

White ramus communicans

Sympathetic chain

Prevertebral sympathetic ganglion

Preganglionic sympathetic
Postganglionic sympathetic

Route 3: Structures in the thoracic cavity that receive sympathetic innervation include the heart, bronchial tree and blood vessels. Preganglionic neurons synapse in sympathetic chain ganglia and exit the chain within cardiac nerves, which arise from the anteromedial aspect of the sympathetic chain. The term "cardiac nerves" is misleading, because although they are distributed to the heart, they also supply other targets within the thorax.

Route 4: Preganglionic sympathetic neurons destined for structures in the abdominopelvic cavity exit the sympathetic chain without synapsing via splanchnic nerves. Neurons within splanchnic nerves synapse in the prevertebral ganglia that are associated with vessels in the abdomen and pelvis. Some of these ganglia have specific names—for example, the two ganglia that are adjacent to the celiac trunk are known as celiac ganglia. Many postganglionic neurons innervate the smooth muscle in blood vessels to regulate blood flow, while others follow branches of the major vessels to their target organ.

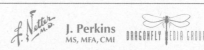
J. Netter M.D.   **J. Perkins**
MS, MFA, CMI   DRAGONFLY MEDIA GROUP

Figure 2.23 SYMPATHETIC NEURONS.

2.24 PARASYMPATHETIC NERVOUS SYSTEM

Neurons in the parasympathetic division are active when the body is at rest, and are associated with processes such as digestion, excretion, and reproduction. Effects of parasympathetic stimulation include decreasing the heart rate, constricting the pupils, increasing peristalsis and secretion of enzymes in the digestive tract, and contraction of the urinary bladder for voiding. The cell bodies of preganglionic parasympathetic neurons are found in two unique locations—in **nuclei in the brainstem** associated with certain cranial nerves, and in the lateral horn of the **2nd to 4th sacral segments** of the spinal cord. Thus the parasympathetic portion of the ANS is often called the **craniosacral division.** The preganglionic parasympathetic axons that exit the brainstem travel in four cranial nerves: **CN III, CN VII, CN IX, and CN X.** Those that emerge from the sacral spinal cord travel in branches of the anterior rami called **pelvic splanchnic nerves.** Preganglionic neurons synapse with postganglionic neurons in parasympathetic ganglia. Some parasympathetic ganglia in the head have specific names—the ciliary, pterygopalatine, submandibular, and otic ganglia—and the neurons that arise from these ganglia travel within branches of cranial nerves to their targets. Other parasympathetic ganglia are located in the wall of target organs, such as within the wall of the heart or the urinary bladder; thus postganglionic neurons from these ganglia are very short.

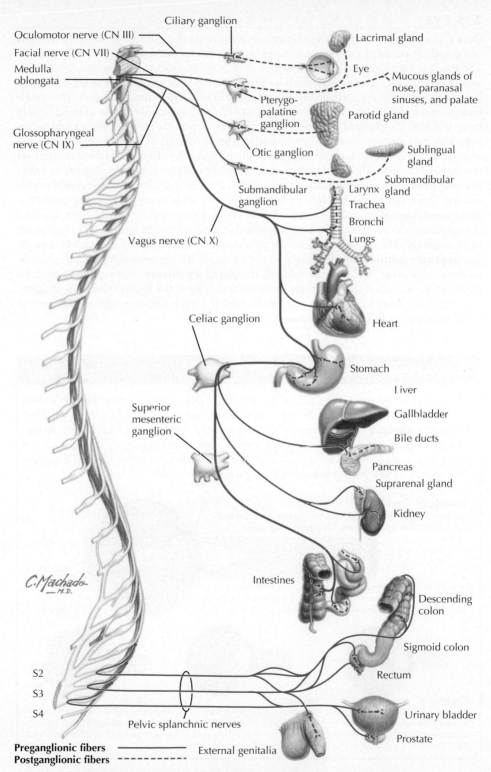

Figure 2.24 PARASYMPATHETIC NERVOUS SYSTEM

2.25 EYE

Only a small portion of the globe-shaped eye is visible on the exterior of the body. The **iris** and **pupil** are the most prominent features, surrounded by the sclera that is white in color. The **sclera** is the outermost layer of the eye that provides support and protection. It is continuous anteriorly with the **cornea,** which is the transparent layer anterior to the iris that allows light to pass into the eye through the pupil (i.e., the hole in the center of the iris). The middle layer of the eyeball is the **uvea,** which consists of three components: the choroid, ciliary body, and iris. The **choroid** is the posterior part of the uvea that contains vessels and nerves supplying the components of the eye. The **ciliary body** consists of a layer of epithelium that secretes aqueous humor (nourishing fluid in the eye) and the **ciliary muscle** that regulates the shape of the lens. The **lens** is attached to the ciliary body by suspensory ligaments called **zonular fibers.** The ciliary muscle is a sphincter; thus contraction releases tension on the zonular fibers and allows the lens to become rounder. This occurs during the process of **accommodation,** when the eye adjusts its focus from distant objects to near ones. The final component of the uveal layer, the **iris,** has cells that produce the pigment responsible for the color of the eye. The iris also contains two smooth muscles that regulate the size of the pupil. The **pupillary sphincter** decreases the size of the pupil; it is innervated by parasympathetic neurons originating in CN III. In contrast, the **pupillary dilator** increases the size of the pupil and is controlled by sympathetic neurons that arise in the superior cervical ganglion. The innermost layer of the eye is the **retina,** which contains photoreceptors that receive visual information from the environment.

Clinical Focus

Light that enters the eye is refracted by the cornea and lens before reaching the retina. With optimal vision, light is focused on the retina, but in many individuals the light is focused in front of the retina (**myopia** or nearsighted) or behind the retina (**hyperopia** or farsighted). **Astigmatism** is a condition where the curvature of the cornea or lens is irregular in shape, causing light to focus in multiple locations. Corrective lenses or refractive surgery (altering the shape of the cornea) can fix these problems so that light focuses on the retina.

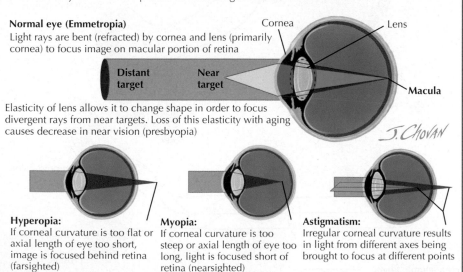

Normal eye (Emmetropia)
Light rays are bent (refracted) by cornea and lens (primarily cornea) to focus image on macular portion of retina

Cornea   Lens

Distant target   Near target

Macula

Elasticity of lens allows it to change shape in order to focus divergent rays from near targets. Loss of this elasticity with aging causes decrease in near vision (presbyopia)

J. CHOVAN

Hyperopia:
If corneal curvature is too flat or axial length of eye too short, image is focused behind retina (farsighted)

Myopia:
If corneal curvature is too steep or axial length of eye too long, light is focused short of retina (nearsighted)

Astigmatism:
Irregular corneal curvature results in light from different axes being brought to focus at different points

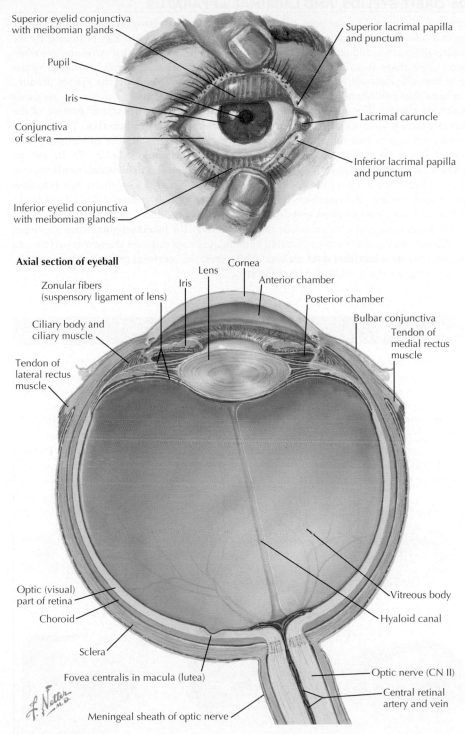

Superior eyelid conjunctiva with meibomian glands

Pupil

Iris

Conjunctiva of sclera

Inferior eyelid conjunctiva with meibomian glands

Superior lacrimal papilla and punctum

Lacrimal caruncle

Inferior lacrimal papilla and punctum

Axial section of eyeball

Zonular fibers (suspensory ligament of lens)

Ciliary body and ciliary muscle

Tendon of lateral rectus muscle

Iris

Lens

Cornea

Anterior chamber

Posterior chamber

Bulbar conjunctiva

Tendon of medial rectus muscle

Optic (visual) part of retina

Choroid

Sclera

Fovea centralis in macula (lutea)

Meningeal sheath of optic nerve

Vitreous body

Hyaloid canal

Optic nerve (CN II)

Central retinal artery and vein

Figure 2.25 EYE

2.26 ORBIT, EYELIDS, AND LACRIMAL APPARATUS

The eye is surrounded by the bony **orbit,** which serves a protective function and has openings that allow communication with the cranial cavity. The eyes are also protected by the eyelids, conjunctiva, and tear film. The **eyelids** are two folds of skin that cover the eye when closed. Their shape is maintained by **tarsal plates,** which are thick bands of connective tissue in the subcutaneous tissue of each eyelid. Glands associated with the eyelids produce secretions that contribute to the tear film (meibomian glands) and lubricate the eyelashes (sebaceous glands). The internal surface of the eyelid, as well as the scleral portion of the ocular surface, is lined with a thin layer of epithelium called the **conjunctiva.** The conjunctiva secretes mucus that lubricates the eye and participates in immune surveillance. Two muscles elevate the eyelid, the **levator palpebrae superioris** innervated by CN III and the **superior tarsal muscle** innervated by sympathetic neurons. The **orbicularis oculi** muscle, innervated by CN VII, closes the eyelids. The surface of the eye is kept moist by a **tear film** that protects the eye and nourishes the avascular cornea. It is composed of a lipid-based portion secreted by meibomian glands, an aqueous layer produced by the lacrimal glands, and a mucous layer produced mainly by the conjunctiva. The **lacrimal glands** are located in the orbit superolateral to each eye. During blinking, tears spread over the ocular surface and drain into the **nasolacrimal duct** via two small pores, the **lacrimal puncta.** The nasolacrimal duct empties into the inferior nasal meatus.

Clinical Focus

The ethmoid bone on the medial wall of the orbit is particularly thin; thus infections from the ethmoid sinuses can spread into the orbit through the bone. The conjunctiva is also prone to infection, and **conjunctivitis** ("pink eye") is a common inflammatory condition that is typically caused by bacteria, viruses, or allergies. A variety of conditions occur if the glands associated with the eyelids become infected or blocked. These include **blepharitis** (inflammation of the eyelids), **external stye** (infection of eyelash follicle), **chalazion** (swelling caused by a blocked meibomian gland), and **meibomianitis** (inflammation of meibomian glands). **Ptosis** (drooping of the lid) can be caused by loss of function of either the levator palpebrae superioris or superior tarsal muscle.

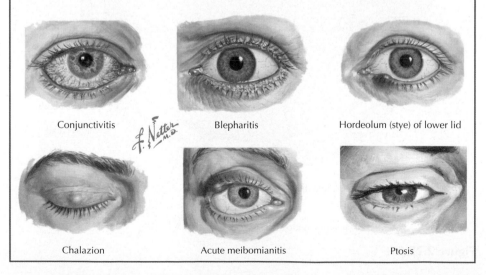

Conjunctivitis   Blepharitis   Hordeolum (stye) of lower lid

Chalazion   Acute meibomianitis   Ptosis

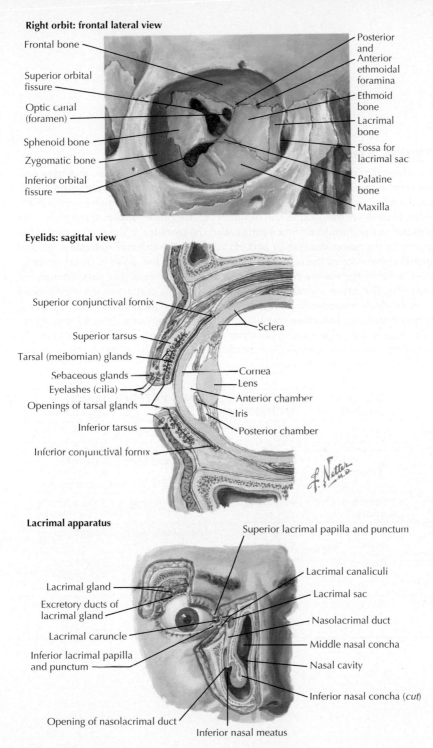

Right orbit: frontal lateral view

Frontal bone

Superior orbital fissure

Optic canal (foramen)

Sphenoid bone

Zygomatic bone

Inferior orbital fissure

Posterior and Anterior ethmoidal foramina

Ethmoid bone

Lacrimal bone

Fossa for lacrimal sac

Palatine bone

Maxilla

Eyelids: sagittal view

Superior conjunctival fornix

Superior tarsus

Tarsal (meibomian) glands

Sebaceous glands

Eyelashes (cilia)

Openings of tarsal glands

Inferior tarsus

Inferior conjunctival fornix

Sclera

Cornea

Lens

Anterior chamber

Iris

Posterior chamber

Lacrimal apparatus

Superior lacrimal papilla and punctum

Lacrimal gland

Excretory ducts of lacrimal gland

Lacrimal caruncle

Inferior lacrimal papilla and punctum

Opening of nasolacrimal duct

Inferior nasal meatus

Lacrimal canaliculi

Lacrimal sac

Nasolacrimal duct

Middle nasal concha

Nasal cavity

Inferior nasal concha (cut)

Figure 2.26 EYE

2.27 EXTRINSIC EYE MUSCLES

There are six extraocular muscles that move the eye. The four rectus muscles—**superior rectus, inferior rectus, medial rectus,** and **lateral rectus**—originate from a **common tendinous ring** in the posterior orbit. They insert into the anterior part of the globe, surrounding it on four sides. In contrast, the oblique muscles insert on the posterior part of the globe. The **superior oblique** passes through a fibrous sling called the **trochlea** in the medial part of the orbit and inserts on the posterior superior part of the globe. The **inferior oblique** originates from the anteromedial floor of the orbit and passes inferior to the globe to insert posterolaterally. Movements of the eye are rotations around imaginary axes that pass through the center of the globe. **Elevation** and **depression** are movements that cause the iris to move superiorly and inferiorly, respectively. Similarly, **abduction** and **adduction** cause the iris to move laterally and medially. **Intorsion** (medial rotation) and **extorsion** (lateral rotation) are rotational movements around the anteroposterior axis of the eyeball. Intorsion causes the superior part of the iris to rotate medially towards the nose; during extorsion the superior part of the iris rotates away from the nose.

MUSCLE	GENERAL ORIGIN	GENERAL INSERTION	INNERVATION	MAIN ACTIONS
Superior rectus	Common tendinous ring	Anterosuperior part of sclera	Oculomotor nerve	Elevates, adducts, and intorts the eye
Inferior rectus	Common tendinous ring	Anteroinferior part of sclera	Oculomotor nerve	Depresses, adducts, and extorts the eye
Medial rectus	Common tendinous ring	Anteromedial part of sclera	Oculomotor nerve	Adducts the eye
Lateral rectus	Common tendinous ring	Anterolateral part of sclera	Abducens nerve	Abducts the eye
Superior oblique	Posterior orbit near optic canal	Posterosuperior part of sclera, lateral portion	Trochlear nerve	Depresses, abducts, and intorts the eye
Inferior oblique	Anteromedial floor of the orbit	Posteroinferior part of sclera, lateral portion	Oculomotor nerve	Elevates, abducts, and extorts the eye

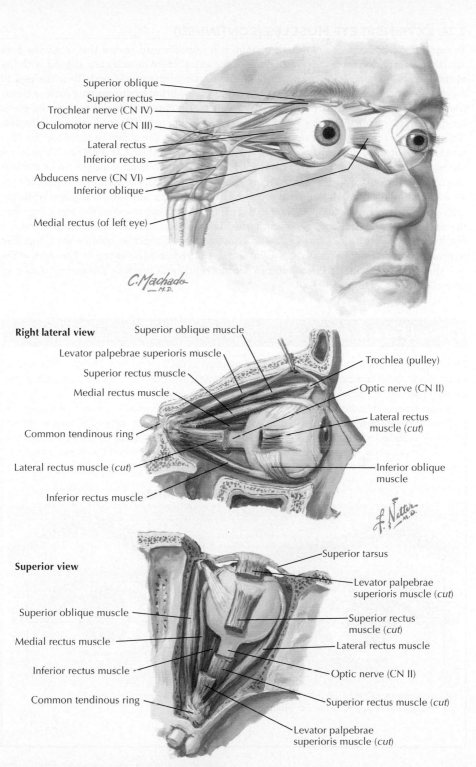

Superior oblique
Superior rectus
Trochlear nerve (CN IV)
Oculomotor nerve (CN III)
Lateral rectus
Inferior rectus
Abducens nerve (CN VI)
Inferior oblique

Medial rectus (of left eye)

C. Machado
_M.D.

Right lateral view   Superior oblique muscle

Levator palpebrae superioris muscle
Superior rectus muscle
Medial rectus muscle

Common tendinous ring

Lateral rectus muscle (*cut*)

Inferior rectus muscle

Trochlea (pulley)
Optic nerve (CN II)
Lateral rectus muscle (*cut*)
Inferior oblique muscle

f. Netter
M.D.

Superior view

Superior oblique muscle
Medial rectus muscle
Inferior rectus muscle
Common tendinous ring

Superior tarsus
Levator palpebrae superioris muscle (*cut*)
Superior rectus muscle (*cut*)
Lateral rectus muscle
Optic nerve (CN II)
Superior rectus muscle (*cut*)
Levator palpebrae superioris muscle (*cut*)

Figure 2.27 EXTRINSIC EYE MUSCLES

2.28 EXTRINSIC EYE MUSCLES *(CONTINUED)*

To understand how the eye muscles function, it is important to realize that when the eyes are facing forward (neutral position), none of the extraocular muscles are aligned with the **optical axis** (imaginary line drawn through the center of the pupil/lens). Thus the pull of most muscles on the eyeball causes torsion (rolling) in addition to movements such as elevation and depression. Compare the pull of the superior rectus on the globe when the eye is facing forward versus when the eye is abducted (Fig. 2.28, *top*). When the eye is abducted, the superior rectus can only elevate the eye—it no longer has the ability to cause torsion. The same is true for the oblique muscles when the eye is adducted (Fig. 2.28, *bottom*). To produce movements without torsion such as "pure" elevation or depression (straight up or straight down), muscles work in pairs to "cancel out" unwanted actions. For example, when the eyes are in a neutral position, the superior rectus elevates, adducts, and intorts the eye, while the inferior oblique elevates, abducts, and extorts the eye. If these two muscles work together, the actions of abduction/adduction and intorsion/extorsion counteract each other and the result is strictly elevation. Likewise, the inferior rectus and superior oblique work together to produce depression. Because the medial and lateral rectus muscles are on the sides of the eye, they do not produce torsion and can act individually to produce the desired action of adduction or abduction.

Clinical Focus

It is important during an eye exam to test the function of each extraocular muscle. The medial and lateral rectus muscles are easily evaluated by asking the patient to adduct and abduct the eyes. However, if a patient is asked to "look up" or "look down," two muscles are being tested because pairs of muscles produce these actions. To isolate each muscle, patients are asked to follow an **H-shaped pattern** with their eyes to align the optical axis with each muscle. When the eye is abducted the superior and inferior rectus can be evaluated by asking the patient to elevate (superior rectus) and depress (inferior rectus) the eye. When the eye is adducted, elevation tests the inferior oblique, while depression evaluates the superior oblique.

H-pattern used to test extraocular muscles

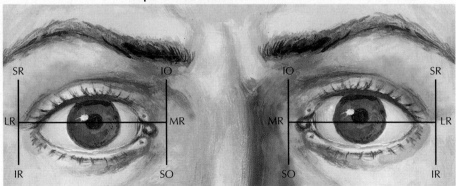

SR = superior rectus; IR = inferior rectus; MR = medial rectus; LR = lateral rectus;
SO = superior oblique; IO = inferior oblique

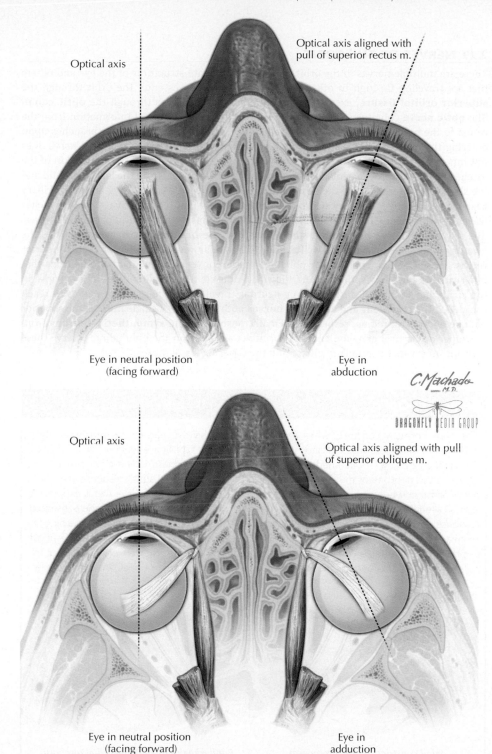

Optical axis

Optical axis aligned with pull of superior rectus m.

Eye in neutral position (facing forward)

Eye in abduction

Optical axis

Optical axis aligned with pull of superior oblique m.

Eye in neutral position (facing forward)

Eye in adduction

C. Machado M.D.

DRAGONFLY MEDIA GROUP

Figure 2.28 EXTRINSIC EYE MUSCLES (CONTINUED)

2.29 NERVES OF THE ORBIT

There are multiple nerves in the orbit, some that innervate structures of the eye and others that are traveling through to other destinations. Most nerves enter the orbit through the **superior orbital fissure,** except for the optic nerve that passes through the **optic canal.** The **optic nerve** contains special sensory neurons that convey visual information from the retina to the brain. The ophthalmic nerve (CN V$_1$) gives off its three major branches upon entering the orbit: the **frontal, lacrimal,** and **nasociliary nerves.** The frontal nerve does not innervate anything in the orbit; it conveys sensory neurons mainly from the skin of the forehead and scalp. The lacrimal nerve conveys sensory neurons from the lacrimal gland and the skin of the lateral part of the orbit. The nasociliary nerve gives off long and short ciliary branches that convey sensory neurons from the cornea and conjunctiva. Other branches leave the orbit to supply portions of the external nose, nasal cavities, and paranasal sinuses. The remaining nerves in the orbit supply muscles. The **oculomotor nerve** innervates the levator palpebrae superioris, as well as four extraocular muscles (superior rectus, inferior rectus, medial rectus, and inferior oblique). It also conveys parasympathetic neurons that innervate the pupillary sphincter and the ciliary muscle. Preganglionic neurons synapse in the ciliary ganglion, and postganglionic neurons travel in the short ciliary nerves to reach the globe. The **trochlear** and **abducens nerves** both innervate a single muscle, the superior oblique and lateral rectus, respectively. Finally, postganglionic **sympathetic neurons** from the superior cervical ganglion enter the orbit via a plexus on the ophthalmic artery. These neurons innervate the pupillary dilator and the superior tarsal muscle.

Clinical Focus

The pupil normally constricts when light is shined in the eye due to the **pupillary light reflex.** A normal response indicates that both CN II and CN III are functioning since CN II detects the light and CN III innervates the pupillary sphincter muscle. There are connections between the neurons of the reflex in the brain that produce a bilateral response (i.e., both pupils constrict when one eye is exposed to light). The response of the eye that is exposed to light is called the direct response, while the response of the other eye is called the consensual response. Another reflex associated with the eye is the **corneal (blink) reflex.** Touching the cornea (e.g., with a piece of cotton) normally causes the eye to blink—a protective response to prevent foreign bodies from entering the eye. CN V$_1$ conveys the sensory neurons of this reflex, while CN VII conducts the motor neurons that innervate the orbicularis oculi muscle.

Pupillary light reflex

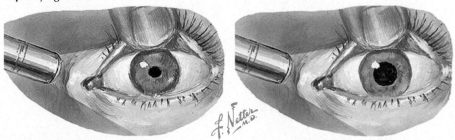

Pupil constricts (normal response)   *Pupil remains dilated (abnormal response)*

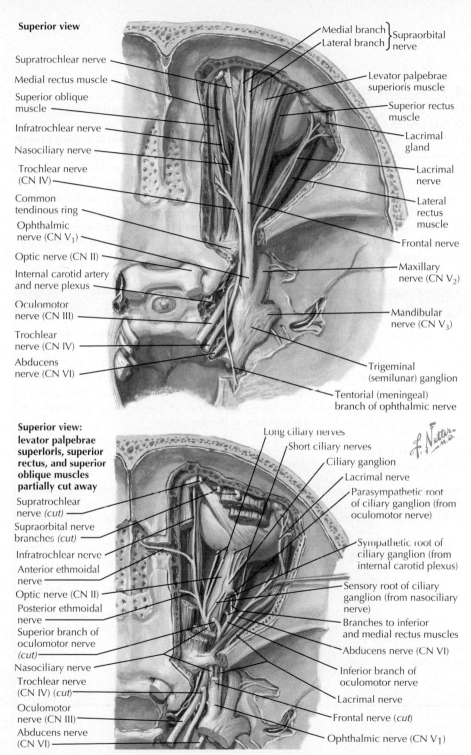

Superior view

Supratrochlear nerve

Medial rectus muscle

Superior oblique muscle

Infratrochlear nerve

Nasociliary nerve

Trochlear nerve (CN IV)

Common tendinous ring

Ophthalmic nerve (CN V₁)

Optic nerve (CN II)

Internal carotid artery and nerve plexus

Oculomotor nerve (CN III)

Trochlear nerve (CN IV)

Abducens nerve (CN VI)

Medial branch ⎱ Supraorbital
Lateral branch ⎰ nerve

Levator palpebrae superioris muscle

Superior rectus muscle

Lacrimal gland

Lacrimal nerve

Lateral rectus muscle

Frontal nerve

Maxillary nerve (CN V₂)

Mandibular nerve (CN V₃)

Trigeminal (semilunar) ganglion

Tentorial (meningeal) branch of ophthalmic nerve

Superior view: levator palpebrae superioris, superior rectus, and superior oblique muscles partially cut away

Supratrochlear nerve *(cut)*

Supraorbital nerve branches *(cut)*

Infratrochlear nerve

Anterior ethmoidal nerve

Optic nerve (CN II)

Posterior ethmoidal nerve

Superior branch of oculomotor nerve *(cut)*

Nasociliary nerve

Trochlear nerve (CN IV) *(cut)*

Oculomotor nerve (CN III)

Abducens nerve (CN VI)

Long ciliary nerves

Short ciliary nerves

Ciliary ganglion

Lacrimal nerve

Parasympathetic root of ciliary ganglion (from oculomotor nerve)

Sympathetic root of ciliary ganglion (from internal carotid plexus)

Sensory root of ciliary ganglion (from nasociliary nerve)

Branches to inferior and medial rectus muscles

Abducens nerve (CN VI)

Inferior branch of oculomotor nerve

Lacrimal nerve

Frontal nerve *(cut)*

Ophthalmic nerve (CN V₁)

Figure 2.29 NERVES OF THE ORBIT

2.30 VASCULATURE OF THE ORBIT

The blood supply to the structures in the orbit is provided by the **ophthalmic artery,** which is the first branch of the internal carotid artery. The ophthalmic artery enters the orbit with CN II through the optic canal and gives off multiple branches. The **central retinal branch** is particularly important because it supplies blood to the retina; obstruction of this vessel results in blindness. Posterior ciliary arteries pierce the sclera to travel within the choroid to supply structures of the globe such as the ciliary body and iris. Other branches, such as the supraorbital and supratrochlear arteries, pass through the orbit to supply the forehead and scalp. The veins draining the eye converge to form the **superior and inferior ophthalmic veins.** These exit the orbit through the superior orbital fissure and drain mainly into the cavernous sinus. Connections between the ophthalmic veins and other veins in the head (e.g., facial veins, pterygoid plexus) provide alternate drainage routes.

Clinical Focus

The health of the retina and optic nerve can be evaluated during a **funduscopic exam** (viewing the retina with an ophthalmoscope). The four major branches of the central retinal artery and vein are visualized, and their relative size is noted. Two common diseases that produce retinal changes are diabetes and hypertension. The high blood sugar levels associated with diabetes can damage the blood vessels in the retina, and this can be detected during exam. Hypertension can cause retinal hemorrhages that can also be found during fundoscopy and may provide information about the progression of the disease.

Right retinal vessels: funduscopic view

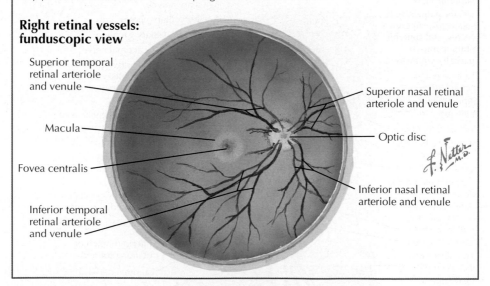

Superior temporal retinal arteriole and venule

Macula

Fovea centralis

Inferior temporal retinal arteriole and venule

Superior nasal retinal arteriole and venule

Optic disc

Inferior nasal retinal arteriole and venule

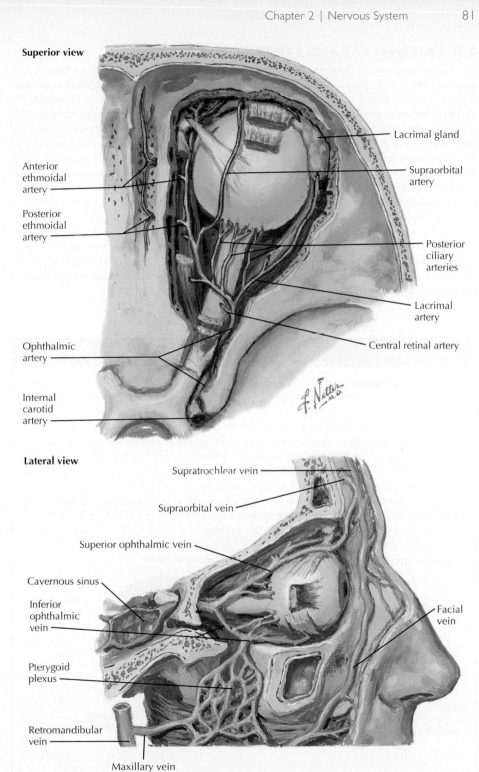

Superior view

Lacrimal gland

Anterior ethmoidal artery

Supraorbital artery

Posterior ethmoidal artery

Posterior ciliary arteries

Lacrimal artery

Ophthalmic artery

Central retinal artery

Internal carotid artery

Lateral view

Supratrochlear vein

Supraorbital vein

Superior ophthalmic vein

Cavernous sinus

Inferior ophthalmic vein

Facial vein

Pterygoid plexus

Retromandibular vein

Maxillary vein

Figure 2.30 VASCULATURE OF THE ORBIT

2.31 EXTERNAL EAR AND TYMPANIC MEMBRANE

The ear is composed of three regions designated external, middle, and internal (inner). The **external ear** has two parts, the auricle and external acoustic meatus. The **auricle** is an oval-shaped structure that consists of a core of elastic cartilage covered by skin. It surrounds the **external acoustic meatus** (ear canal), which is a curved passageway formed by cartilage (lateral part) and bone (medial part). The external acoustic meatus is lined with skin containing hair follicles and glands. The secretions of the glands, as well as dead skin cells, combine to form **cerumen** (earwax) that lubricates the skin and impedes the entry of foreign particles. At the medial end of the meatus is the semitransparent, oval-shaped **tympanic membrane,** which separates the external ear from the tympanic cavity of the middle ear. The tympanic cavity contains the ossicles (ear bones), and one of these, the malleus, has a handle that is attached to the internal surface of the tympanic membrane. This attachment puts slight tension on the membrane that produces a concavity on its external surface. The central part of the tympanic membrane where the tip of the handle is attached is called the **umbo.** Sounds waves collected by the external ear are transmitted to the ossicles of the middle ear via oscillations of the tympanic membrane. The components of the external ear receive sensory innervation from multiple nerves including CN V, CN VII, and CN X.

Clinical Focus

Acute otitis externa ("swimmer's ear") is inflammation of the ear canal that is typically caused by bacterial infection. Excessive exposure to water is the most common cause, because water can become trapped in the ear and create a moist environment for bacteria to flourish. Damage of the protective wax barrier, for example from cotton swab use, also creates an environment prone to infection. Viewing the tympanic membrane with an otoscope can provide clues to the health of the middle ear. When light hits the lateral side of the tympanic membrane, it normally produces a reflection at approximately 5 o'clock in the right ear and 7 o'clock in the left ear—the "light reflex" or "cone of light." Finding this reflection during otoscopy verifies that you have found the tympanic membrane. In a patient with an infection in the tympanic cavity **(otitis media)**, fluid can accumulate in the middle ear, causing the tympanic membrane to bulge out toward the ear canal.

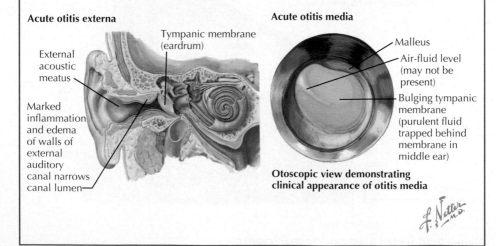

Acute otitis externa

External acoustic meatus

Tympanic membrane (eardrum)

Marked inflammation and edema of walls of external auditory canal narrows canal lumen

Acute otitis media

Malleus

Air-fluid level (may not be present)

Bulging tympanic membrane (purulent fluid trapped behind membrane in middle ear)

Otoscopic view demonstrating clinical appearance of otitis media

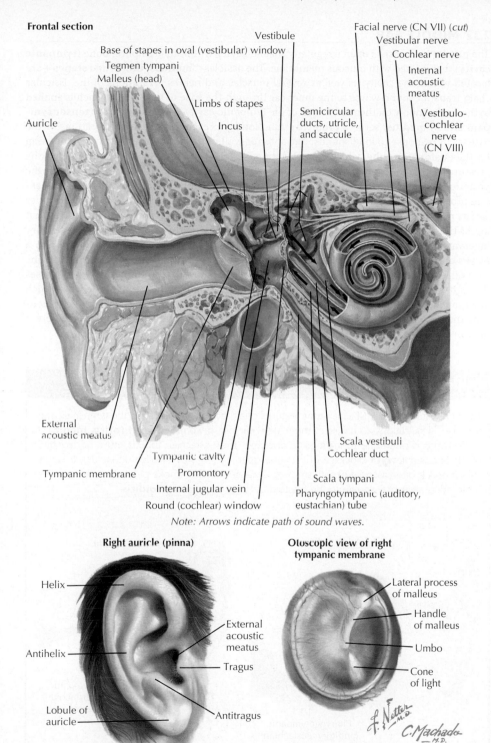

Frontal section

Vestibule

Base of stapes in oval (vestibular) window

Tegmen tympani
Malleus (head)

Limbs of stapes

Incus

Auricle

Semicircular
ducts, utricle,
and saccule

Facial nerve (CN VII) (*cut*)
Vestibular nerve
Cochlear nerve

Internal
acoustic
meatus

Vestibulo-
cochlear
nerve
(CN VIII)

External
acoustic meatus

Tympanic membrane

Tympanic cavity

Promontory

Internal jugular vein

Round (cochlear) window

Scala vestibuli
Cochlear duct

Scala tympani

Pharyngotympanic (auditory,
eustachian) tube

Note: Arrows indicate path of sound waves.

Right auricle (pinna)

Helix

Antihelix

Lobule of
auricle

External
acoustic
meatus

Tragus

Antitragus

**Otoscopic view of right
tympanic membrane**

Lateral process
of malleus

Handle
of malleus

Umbo

Cone
of light

f. Netter
M.D.

C. Machado
M.D.

Figure 2.31 EXTERNAL EAR AND TYMPANIC MEMBRANE.

2.32 MIDDLE EAR

The middle ear consists of an irregularly shaped cavity within the temporal bone (**tympanic cavity**) that is lined with mucous membrane. The ossicles—**malleus, incus,** and **stapes**—are located within the cavity, as well as several muscles and nerves. Vibrations of the ossicular chain transmit sound waves to the inner ear through the base of the stapes, which is applied to the oval window on the medial wall of the tympanic cavity. Two muscles, the **tensor tympani** and **stapedius,** serve a protective function by preventing excessive vibrations of the ossicles in response to loud sounds. The anterior wall of the tympanic cavity has an opening for the **eustachian tube,** which connects the middle ear to the nasopharynx and allows the pressure in the tympanic cavity to equalize with atmospheric pressure. An opening in the posterior wall, the **mastoid aditus,** is continuous with the mucosal-lined air cells in the mastoid process. The medial wall of the tympanic cavity separates the middle ear from the inner ear; its most important features are the **oval and round windows,** and the **promontory** that marks the position of the underlying cochlea. The mucosa of the middle ear receives sensory innervation from the **tympanic branch of the glossopharyngeal nerve,** which forms a plexus on the surface of the promontory. The **facial nerve** travels posterior to the tympanic cavity in the facial canal. It gives off two branches: the **chorda tympani nerve,** which passes through the middle ear between the malleus and incus; and the **nerve to stapedius,** which innervates the stapedius muscle. The chorda tympani nerve conveys parasympathetic neurons that innervate the submandibular and sublingual salivary glands, and special afferent neurons for taste from the anterior two-thirds of the tongue.

Clinical Focus

The epithelium of the eustachian tube features cilia that clear mucus from the tympanic cavity; however, if secretions accumulate, the middle ear can become inflamed (**otitis media**). In children this is often due to inadequate drainage (the eustachian tube is more horizontal in infants and toddlers) or blockage of the tube opening (e.g., by swollen adenoids). In adults, otitis media is often associated with smoking because tobacco smoke paralyzes cilia. Infections in the middle ear may spread to the mastoid air cells, causing **mastoiditis**.

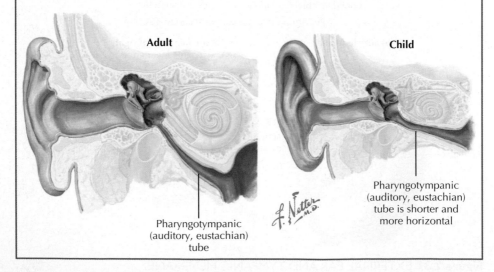

Adult

Child

Pharyngotympanic
(auditory, eustachian)
tube

Pharyngotympanic
(auditory, eustachian)
tube is shorter and
more horizontal

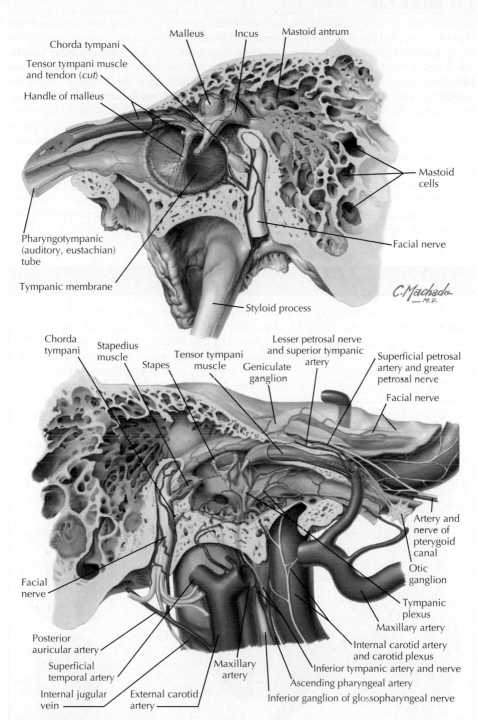

Malleus   Incus   Mastoid antrum

Chorda tympani

Tensor tympani muscle
and tendon (*cut*)

Handle of malleus

Mastoid
cells

Pharyngotympanic
(auditory, eustachian)
tube

Facial nerve

Tympanic membrane

C. Machado
—M.D.

Styloid process

Chorda
tympani   Stapedius
muscle
Stapes   Tensor tympani
muscle   Lesser petrosal nerve
and superior tympanic
artery
Geniculate
ganglion

Superficial petrosal
artery and greater
petrosal nerve

Facial nerve

Artery and
nerve of
pterygoid
canal

Otic
ganglion

Facial
nerve

Tympanic
plexus

Maxillary artery

Posterior
auricular artery

Internal carotid artery
and carotid plexus

Superficial
temporal artery

Maxillary
artery

Inferior tympanic artery and nerve

Internal jugular
vein   External carotid
artery

Ascending pharyngeal artery

Inferior ganglion of glossopharyngeal nerve

Figure 2.32 MIDDLE EAR

2.33 INNER EAR

The inner ear consists of multiple cavities within the petrous part of the temporal bone that contain the special sense organs for hearing and balance. These cavities, known collectively as the **bony labyrinth**, consist of the **cochlea, vestibule,** and three **semicircular canals.** The bony labyrinth is lined with a collection of sacs and ducts known as the **membranous labyrinth.** Specifically, the cochlea surrounds the **cochlear duct,** the vestibule houses the **utricle** and **saccule,** and the semicircular canals enclose the **semicircular ducts.** The membranous labyrinth is filled with a fluid called **endolymph,** while the space between the membranous and bony labyrinths is filled with **perilymph.** The cochlear duct contains the special sense organ for hearing (**organ of Corti**). The organs that convey information about balance (**maculae** and **cristae ampullares**) are located in the saccule, utricle, and the ampullae (dilated portions) of the semicircular ducts. The sensory receptors in these organs contain hair cells that are stimulated by fluid movement. Sound waves from the base of the stapes are transmitted through the perilymph and pass across the walls of the membranous labyrinth into the endolymph-filled cavities. Stimulation of hair cells generates action potentials in the cochlear and vestibular divisions of CN VIII.

Clinical Focus

There are three main types of hearing loss—conductive, sensorineural, and mixed. **Conductive hearing loss** occurs when an obstruction prevents sound waves from reaching the inner ear, such as excessive earwax or a tumor. Damage to hair cells of the inner ear or the vestibulocochlear nerve produces **sensorineural hearing loss.** The most common cause of this type is aging, and hearing aids are often an effective treatment unless the hearing loss is particularly severe. Cochlear implants are devices that convert sound waves into electrical signals, which can stimulate the vestibulocochlear nerve. These devices offer a treatment option for patients with severe hearing loss. Patients with **mixed hearing loss** have a combination of sensorineural and conductive hearing loss. One of the most common disorders of the vestibular system is **vertigo**—dizziness or the sensation that the surrounding environment is spinning. Vertigo is typically caused by accumulation of calcium carbonate crystals in the membranous labyrinth that interfere with fluid movement and cause abnormal stimulation of hair cells in the vestibular organs.

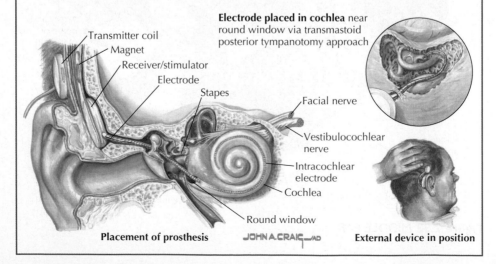

Electrode placed in cochlea near round window via transmastoid posterior tympanotomy approach

Transmitter coil
Magnet
Receiver/stimulator
Electrode
Stapes
Facial nerve
Vestibulocochlear nerve
Intracochlear electrode
Cochlea
Round window

Placement of prosthesis

JOHN A.CRAIG—AD

External device in position

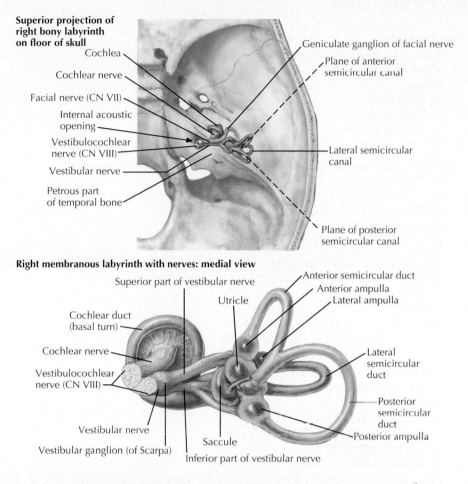

Superior projection of right bony labyrinth on floor of skull

Cochlea

Cochlear nerve

Facial nerve (CN VII)

Internal acoustic opening

Vestibulocochlear nerve (CN VIII)

Vestibular nerve

Petrous part of temporal bone

Geniculate ganglion of facial nerve

Plane of anterior semicircular canal

Lateral semicircular canal

Plane of posterior semicircular canal

Right membranous labyrinth with nerves: medial view

Superior part of vestibular nerve

Utricle

Cochlear duct (basal turn)

Cochlear nerve

Vestibulocochlear nerve (CN VIII)

Vestibular nerve

Vestibular ganglion (of Scarpa)

Saccule

Inferior part of vestibular nerve

Anterior semicircular duct

Anterior ampulla

Lateral ampulla

Lateral semicircular duct

Posterior semicircular duct

Posterior ampulla

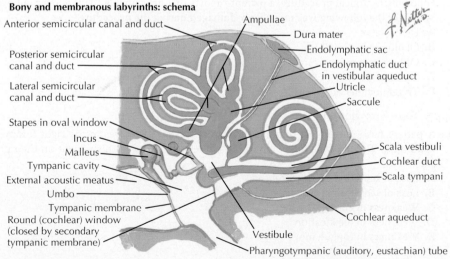

Bony and membranous labyrinths: schema

Anterior semicircular canal and duct

Posterior semicircular canal and duct

Lateral semicircular canal and duct

Stapes in oval window

Incus

Malleus

Tympanic cavity

External acoustic meatus

Umbo

Tympanic membrane

Round (cochlear) window (closed by secondary tympanic membrane)

Ampullae

Dura mater

Endolymphatic sac

Endolymphatic duct in vestibular aqueduct

Utricle

Saccule

Scala vestibuli

Cochlear duct

Scala tympani

Cochlear aqueduct

Vestibule

Pharyngotympanic (auditory, eustachian) tube

Figure 2.33 INNER EAR

REVIEW QUESTIONS

Test Your Recall

1. A physician needs to obtain a sample of cerebrospinal fluid (CSF) from a patient to screen them for meningitis. Where is the best location to insert a needle to obtain this sample?
   A. Dural sinus
   B. Epidural space
   C. Subarachnoid space
   D. Subdural space

2. Which cranial nerves leave the cranial cavity through the jugular foramen?
   A. CN VI, CN VII, and CN VIII
   B. CN VII and CN VIII
   C. CN VIII, CN IX, and CN X
   D. CN IX and CN X
   E. CN IX, CN X, and CN XI

3. A spectator at a baseball game fractured her cribriform plate after being hit in the face by a baseball. Which nerve was most likely damaged by the fracture?
   A. CN I
   B. CN II
   C. CN III
   D. CN IV
   E. CN VII

4. A blood cell is traveling within the straight sinus on its way to the internal jugular vein. Which sinus would it travel in next to reach its destination?
   A. Cavernous sinus
   B. Inferior petrosal sinus
   C. Superior sagittal sinus
   D. Superior petrosal sinus
   E. Transverse sinus

5. Following a surgical procedure, a patient reports that he is unable to close his right eye. Which of the following was most likely damaged during the procedure?
   A. Facial nerve
   B. Oculomotor nerve
   C. Ophthalmic nerve
   D. Optic nerve
   E. Trigeminal nerve

Apply Your Knowledge

6. A patient has a meningeal tumor that is compressing structures in the right foramen rotundum. Which of the following would you expect to see in this patient on the right side?
   A. Loss of sensation on the forehead
   B. Loss of sensation just inferior to the eye
   C. Weakness in closing the mouth
   D. Weakness in mastication
   E. Weakness in tongue movements

7. A middle ear adenoma (tumor derived from middle ear mucosa) is impeding the normal drainage of fluid from the tympanic cavity. Which wall of the tympanic cavity is this mass most likely located on?
   A. Anterior wall
   B. Posterior wall
   C. Medial wall
   D. Lateral wall
   E. Inferior wall (floor)
   F. Superior wall (roof)

8. A clot is compressing structures within the cavernous sinus ("cavernous sinus thrombosis"). Which of the following symptoms would you expect to see in this patient on the affected side?
   A. Fixed and dilated pupil
   B. Inability to abduct the eye
   C. Inability to adduct the eye
   D. Inability to elevate the eye
   E. Loss of sensation of the cornea

9. You are attempting to remove a small splinter from your finger with tweezers. Which of the following best describes the change in your lens that occurs when you focus on the splinter?
   A. Lens becomes round due to contraction of the ciliary muscle by parasympathetics.
   B. Lens becomes round due to contraction of the ciliary muscle by sympathetics.
   C. Lens becomes round due to relaxation of the ciliary muscle by parasympathetics.
   D. Lens becomes round due to relaxation of the ciliary muscle by sympathetics.
   E. Lens flattens due to contraction of the ciliary muscle by parasympathetics.
   F. Lens flattens due to contraction of the ciliary muscle by sympathetics.
   G. Lens flattens due to relaxation of the ciliary muscle by parasympathetics.
   H. Lens flattens due to relaxation of the ciliary muscle by sympathetics.

10. A man was brought to the emergency department after sustaining injuries in a motor vehicle accident. He exhibits slight ptosis and a constricted pupil. Which of the following was most likely injured in the accident?
    A. Ciliary ganglion
    B. Facial nerve (CN VII)
    C. Oculomotor nerve (CN III)
    D. Optic nerve (CN II)
    E. Superior cervical ganglion

See Appendix for answers.

CHAPTER 3

MUSCULOSKELETAL SYSTEM

3.1 THE MUSCULOSKELETAL SYSTEM

The **skeletal** and **muscular systems** are a natural pairing since they work together to support and move the body. The skeletal system consists of two major tissues, bone and cartilage, that together form the components of the axial and appendicular skeletons. **Bone** is a living tissue that can change in response to forces applied to it. Thus the various protuberances, ridges, and grooves that are seen on the surfaces of bones are typically associated with attachments of muscle tendons, ligaments, or structures traversing bones such as vessels and nerves. **Cartilage** covers the articular surfaces of bones to prevent friction at moveable joints and links bones together at joints designed for flexible strength. While there are three basic types of muscle in the muscular system, **skeletal muscle** is the only type that is associated with the skeleton to move the body. Skeletal muscle is also known as striated muscle because it has visible striations in its fibers, and voluntary muscle since it is under voluntary control. Skeletal muscle produces movement of the body by pulling on structures such as skin, bones, and connective tissue. Muscles cannot push—they can only pull by shortening the length of their fibers during contraction.

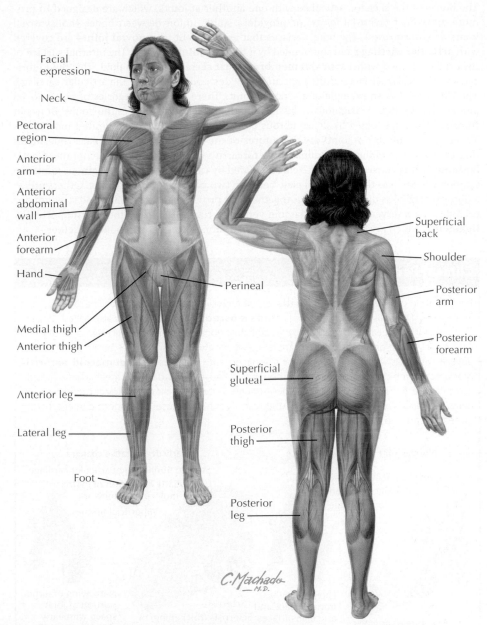

Figure 3.1 THE MUSCULOSKELETAL SYSTEM

3.2 JOINTS

The bones of the skeleton articulate with one another at joints, which are designed to promote movement (synovial joints) or provide a stable union between bones (nonsynovial joints or *synarthroses*). The bony surfaces that are adjacent in **synovial joints** are covered with **articular cartilage** and surrounded by a **fibrous joint capsule**. The internal surface of the capsule is lined with a **synovial membrane** that secretes synovial fluid. This fluid lubricates the articular surfaces of the joint and provides nourishment to the articular cartilage. The elbow joint is an example of a synovial joint. There are two categories of nonsynovial joints—fibrous and cartilaginous—classified by the material that unites the bones. Bones in **fibrous joints** are joined by dense fibrous connective tissue and have limited movement. Two examples of fibrous joints are the sutures of the skull and the radioulnar syndesmosis that connects the radius to the ulna in the forearm via an interosseous membrane. **Cartilaginous joints** consist of skeletal elements joined by cartilage. Some cartilaginous joints are temporary—such as the epiphyseal plate between two parts of a growing bone. Others utilize a fibrocartilaginous disc to link bones together that provides both flexibility and strength, for example, the intervertebral discs that join vertebrae together. Most joints are supported by **ligaments**, which are bands of connective tissue that connect parts of bones together.

Clinical Focus

Inflammation of a joint is called **arthritis**, and it typically produces pain, swelling, and stiffness in the joint. The most common type of arthritis is **osteoarthritis**, which is also called "degenerative arthritis" because it is caused by gradual deterioration of articular cartilage over time. In later stages of the disease, cartilage completely wears away, causing bone to rub against bone. Severe cases can be treated with a joint replacement (prosthesis). **Rheumatoid arthritis** is another common type of arthritis, although it is caused by a different mechanism—it is an autoimmune disorder. In this disease the immune system attacks the synovial membranes of joints, producing chronic inflammation that can eventually cause permanent damage to the bone and cartilage.

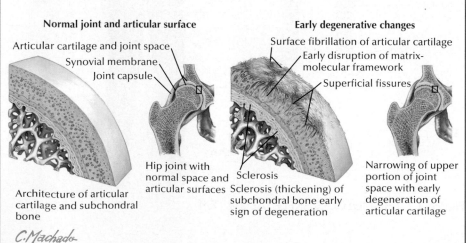

Normal joint and articular surface

Articular cartilage and joint space
Synovial membrane
Joint capsule

Architecture of articular cartilage and subchondral bone

Hip joint with normal space and articular surfaces

Early degenerative changes

Surface fibrillation of articular cartilage
Early disruption of matrix-molecular framework
Superficial fissures

Sclerosis
Sclerosis (thickening) of subchondral bone early sign of degeneration

Narrowing of upper portion of joint space with early degeneration of articular cartilage

C.Machado
—M.D.

Synovial joints

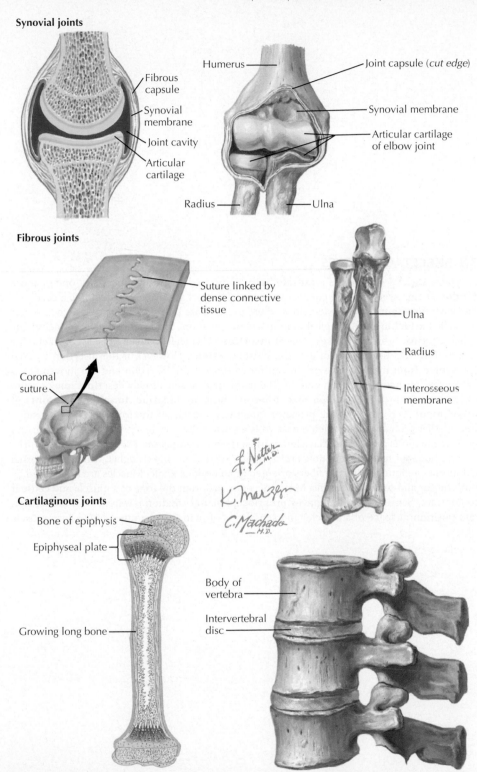

Fibrous capsule

Synovial membrane

Joint cavity

Articular cartilage

Humerus

Joint capsule (*cut edge*)

Synovial membrane

Articular cartilage of elbow joint

Radius

Ulna

Fibrous joints

Suture linked by dense connective tissue

Coronal suture

Ulna

Radius

Interosseous membrane

Cartilaginous joints

Bone of epiphysis

Epiphyseal plate

Growing long bone

Body of vertebra

Intervertebral disc

Figure 3.2 JOINTS

3.3 SKELETAL MUSCLES

A typical skeletal muscle has a **muscle belly** composed of muscle fibers and one or more **tendons** comprised of dense connective tissue. Tendons are usually shaped like a cord or a flat sheet (**aponeurosis**). The locations where muscles are linked to structures such as bones are called **attachments**. A typical muscle has one or more fixed (non-moving) attachments called **origins**. Movement takes place at **insertions**. Typically when a muscle contracts, the insertion moves toward the origin (the muscle **action**). However, if the insertion is fixed (prevented from moving), the origin can move toward the insertion and the movement is called the "reverse action" of a muscle. The name of a muscle usually describes one or more of its features, such as its **shape**, **size**, **fiber orientation**, **location**, **function,** or **points of attachment**. For example, the pronator quadratus muscle of the forearm is a four-sided muscle that pronates. Sternocleidomastoid is a muscle that originates from the sternum and clavicle (cleido is a word for clavicle) and inserts on the mastoid process of the skull. The muscle fibers of rectus abdominis are straight ("rectus" means straight), while the internal abdominal oblique has muscle fibers oriented at an oblique angle. Muscles are innervated by both motor and sensory neurons. Motor neurons maintain the tone of a muscle and cause it to contract. Sensory neurons convey proprioceptive information (awareness of the tension and position in space of a muscle) and sensations of pain, for example, due to torn muscle fibers.

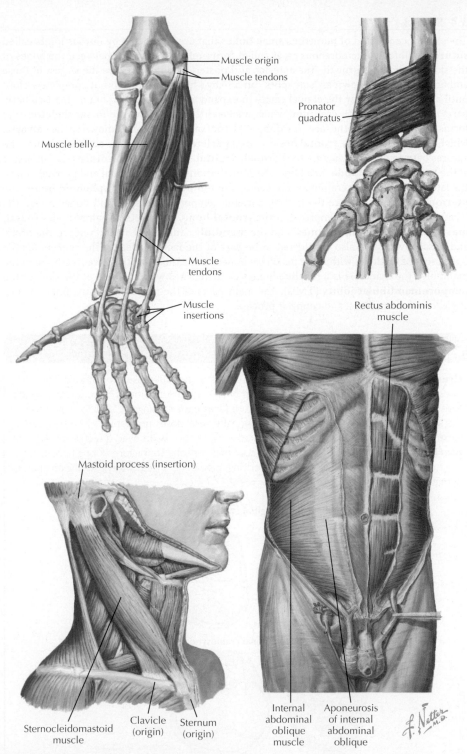

Muscle origin

Muscle tendons

Pronator quadratus

Muscle belly

Muscle tendons

Muscle insertions

Rectus abdominis muscle

Mastoid process (insertion)

Sternocleidomastoid muscle

Clavicle (origin)

Sternum (origin)

Internal abdominal oblique muscle

Aponeurosis of internal abdominal oblique

Figure 3.3 FEATURES OF SKELETAL MUSCLES

3.4 SKULL

The skull is comprised of numerous small bones that are connected by fibrous joints called **sutures**. In infants, membranous areas called **fontanelles** are present between the bones of the skull to allow for growth. The anterior and posterior fontanelles are the largest of these and are commonly known as "soft spots" on a baby's head. Sutures do not completely close until adulthood to allow the cranial cavity to expand with the growing brain. The two basic parts of the skull are the **cranium**, which encloses the brain, and the **facial skeleton** that forms the framework of the face. The dome-like roof of the cranium is known as the **calvaria**, which is comprised of the **frontal bone**, paired **parietal bones**, and the **occipital bone**. The sutures between these bones are the **coronal**, **sagittal**, and **lambdoid sutures** that intersect at the **bregma** and **lambda**. In addition to contributions from the frontal and parietal bones, the lateral aspect of the cranium is formed by the **temporal bone** and **sphenoid bone**. The **pterion** is the point where the frontal, parietal, temporal, and sphenoid bones meet. The facial skeleton is mainly comprised of the **frontal bone**, three sets of paired bones (**nasal, maxillary,** and **zygomatic bones**) and the **mandible**. Additional small bones in the orbits and nasal cavities are also considered to be part of the facial skeleton. The sockets for the upper row of teeth are within the maxillary bones, while those for the lower teeth are in the mandible. The mandible is a separate bone that articulates with the base of the skull at the **temporomandibular joints** (TMJs). The main parts of the mandible are the body, ramus, angle, coronoid process, and condylar process.

Clinical Focus

Craniosynostosis is a condition where the sutures of the skull close prematurely. This interferes with the normal growth of the skull and brain. The most common type of craniosynostosis is scaphocephaly, where the sagittal suture fuses early causing the skull to grow more at the anterior and posterior aspects. If the coronal suture closes prematurely, the skull cannot expand superiorly; thus it grows laterally producing a short, wide head (brachycephaly). The **pterion** is a particularly weak area of the skull that is prone to fracture during head trauma. Fractures in this area may damage the underlying middle meningeal artery, causing an epidural hematoma (see Clinical Focus 2.4).

Scaphocephaly due to sagittal craniosynostosis

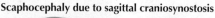

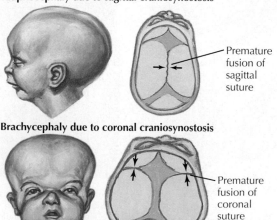

Premature fusion of sagittal suture

Brachycephaly due to coronal craniosynostosis

Premature fusion of coronal suture

JOHN A.CRAIG—AD

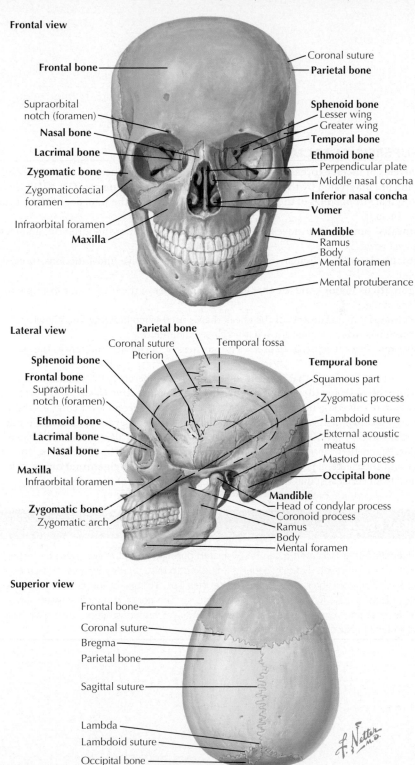

Frontal view

Frontal bone

Supraorbital
notch (foramen)

Nasal bone

Lacrimal bone

Zygomatic bone

Zygomaticofacial
foramen

Infraorbital foramen

Maxilla

Coronal suture

Parietal bone

Sphenoid bone
Lesser wing
Greater wing

Temporal bone

Ethmoid bone
Perpendicular plate
Middle nasal concha

Inferior nasal concha

Vomer

Mandible
Ramus
Body
Mental foramen

Mental protuberance

Lateral view

Sphenoid bone

Frontal bone
Supraorbital
notch (foramen)

Ethmoid bone

Lacrimal bone

Nasal bone

Maxilla
Infraorbital foramen

Zygomatic bone
Zygomatic arch

Parietal bone
Coronal suture
Pterion

Temporal fossa

Temporal bone

Squamous part

Zygomatic process

Lambdoid suture

External acoustic
meatus

Mastoid process

Occipital bone

Mandible
Head of condylar process
Coronoid process
Ramus
Body
Mental foramen

Superior view

Frontal bone

Coronal suture

Bregma

Parietal bone

Sagittal suture

Lambda

Lambdoid suture

Occipital bone

f. Netter
M.D.

Figure 3.4 THE SKULL

3.5 SUPERFICIAL FACIAL MUSCLES AND SCALP

The **muscles of facial expression** are located within the subcutaneous tissue of the face and neck, and are innervated by the terminal branches of the **facial nerve (CN VII)** (see 2.13). Most originate from bones of the skull or fascia and insert into the skin. Some of the primary muscles include:

- **Frontalis**—muscle that moves the scalp, wrinkles the skin of the forehead, and elevates the eyebrows.
- **Orbicularis oculi**—circular muscle that surrounds the eye and functions to close the eyelid.
- **Zygomaticus major**—muscle that elevates the corner of the mouth, for example to produce a smile.
- **Buccinator**—major muscle of the cheek that is used when blowing and chewing.
- **Orbicularis oris**—circular muscle that closes the mouth.
- **Platysma**—flat muscle that depresses the corners of the mouth and tenses the skin of the neck.

The scalp has five layers that can conveniently be remembered by the mnemonic "SCALP": **skin**, **connective tissue (dense)**, **aponeurosis**, **loose connective tissue**, and **pericranium** (periosteum of calvaria). The dense connective tissue of the second layer contains the vessels and nerves that supply the scalp. The aponeurosis in the third layer serves as the tendon for the frontalis muscle, as well as its counterpart on the posterior part of the skull, the occipitalis muscle; together these two muscle bellies form the occipitofrontalis muscle. The skin of the face and anterolateral part of the scalp are innervated by the **trigeminal nerve** (see 2.12). Branches from cervical spinal nerves supply the posterior part of the scalp.

Clinical Focus

The integrity of the facial nerve can be evaluated during a cranial nerve exam by testing the function of facial muscles. Typically patients are asked to raise their eyebrows, close their eyes tightly, smile, puff out their cheeks, and purse their lips. Lesions of the facial nerve produce deficits in facial muscle function (2.13 Clinical Focus). The dense connective tissue surrounding the arteries and veins of the scalp prevents significant vasoconstriction; thus scalp wounds typically bleed profusely.

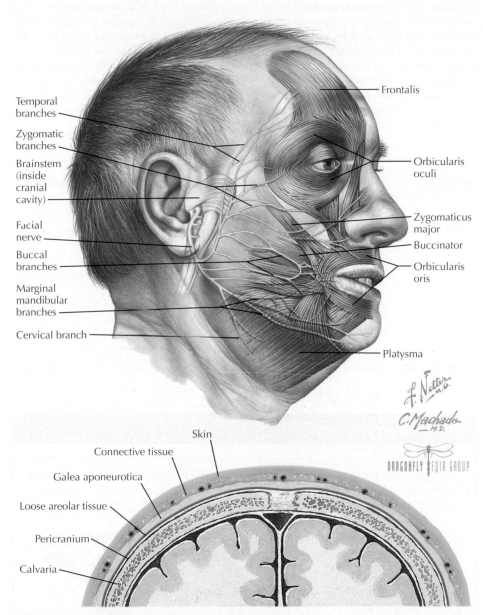

Frontalis

Temporal branches

Zygomatic branches

Brainstem (inside cranial cavity)

Orbicularis oculi

Facial nerve

Zygomaticus major

Buccal branches

Buccinator

Orbicularis oris

Marginal mandibular branches

Cervical branch

Platysma

Skin

Connective tissue

Galea aponeurotica

Loose areolar tissue

Pericranium

Calvaria

Figure 3.5 SUPERFICIAL FACIAL MUSCLES AND SCALP

3.6 DEEP FACIAL MUSCLES AND TEMPOROMANDIBULAR JOINT

The **temporomandibular joint** is formed by an articulation between the **condyle** of the mandible and the **mandibular fossa** of the temporal bone. There is an **articular disc** within the joint that separates the synovial cavity into two portions. The articular tubercle marks the anterior limit of the joint surface. There are four basic movements of the mandible at the TMJ: elevation, depression, protrusion (moving anteriorly), and retraction (moving posteriorly). Opening the jaw involves both depression and protrusion since the condyle of the mandible slides anteriorly onto the articular tubercle and undergoes downward rotation. The four **muscles of mastication** are the primary muscles that move the mandible. The complex movements that occur during chewing result from alternate contractions of muscles on the right and left side of the body.

MUSCLE	GENERAL ORIGIN	GENERAL INSERTION	INNERVATION	MAIN ACTIONS
Temporalis	Temporal fossa	Coronoid process of mandible	CN V_3	Elevates and retracts mandible
Masseter	Zygomatic arch	Ramus of mandible (lateral surface)	CN V_3	Elevates mandible
Medial pterygoid	Lateral pterygoid plate (medial surface)	Ramus of mandible (medial surface)	CN V_3	Elevates and protrudes mandible, side-to-side grinding
Lateral pterygoid	Sphenoid bone, Lateral pterygoid plate (lateral surface)	Articular disc/ capsule of TMJ, neck of mandible	CN V_3	Protrudes mandible, side-to-side grinding

The muscles of mastication are innervated by the mandibular division of the trigeminal nerve (CN V_3).

Clinical Focus

Dislocation of the TMJ can occur if the mouth is opened beyond the normal extent, or if structural changes alter the stability of the joint (e.g., due to arthritis). Dislocation typically occurs in an anterior direction when the condyle slides beyond the anterior tubercle and is unable to return to the mandibular fossa.

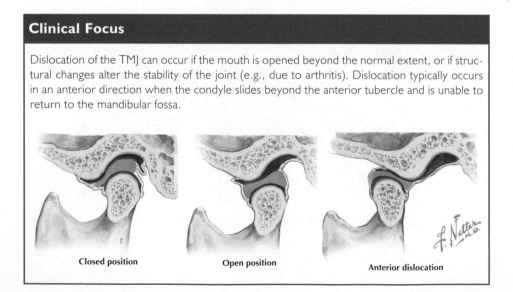

Closed position   **Open position**   **Anterior dislocation**

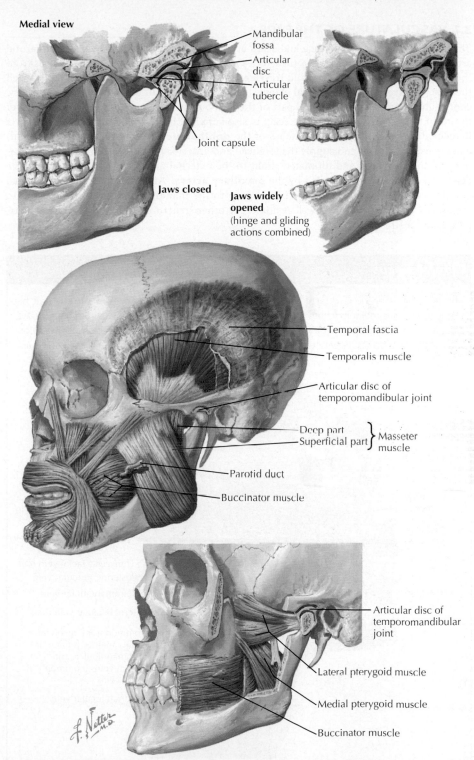

Medial view

Mandibular fossa

Articular disc

Articular tubercle

Joint capsule

Jaws closed

Jaws widely opened
(hinge and gliding actions combined)

Temporal fascia

Temporalis muscle

Articular disc of temporomandibular joint

Deep part
Superficial part } Masseter muscle

Parotid duct

Buccinator muscle

Articular disc of temporomandibular joint

Lateral pterygoid muscle

Medial pterygoid muscle

Buccinator muscle

Figure 3.6 DEEP FACIAL MUSCLES AND TEMPOROMANDIBULAR JOINT

3.7 VASCULATURE OF THE FACE

The arteries that supply the face and scalp are primarily branches of the external carotid arteries; however the internal carotid arteries also contribute. The **facial artery** arises from the external carotid in the neck and traverses the inferior border of the mandible to reach the face. The **superficial temporal artery**, a terminal branch of the external carotid artery, contributes branches to the lateral part of the face but mainly supplies the lateral aspect of the scalp. The posterior part of the scalp is also supplied by the external carotid artery via its occipital branch. Terminal branches of the **ophthalmic artery** (from internal carotid) emerge from the orbit and supply the forehead and anterior part of the scalp. Veins accompany all these arteries and ultimately drain to the external and internal jugular veins. The deep part of the face is supplied by the **maxillary artery**. After arising from the external carotid artery, the maxillary artery travels deep to the mandible and gives off branches to the muscles of mastication, as well as numerous other structures including the nasal cavity, palate, and teeth.

Clinical Focus

The deep veins of the face form an extensive plexus called the **pterygoid plexus** that has connections with multiple veins including those of the orbit, nasal cavities, and oral cavity. Additionally, small veins connect the plexus to the cavernous sinus. Thus infections from regions such as the face or nasal cavity can spread via the venous system to the cranial cavity (see also 2.6 Clinical Focus).

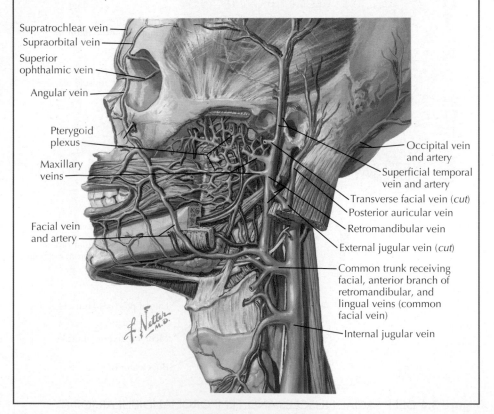

Supratrochlear vein
Supraorbital vein
Superior ophthalmic vein
Angular vein
Pterygoid plexus
Maxillary veins
Facial vein and artery

Occipital vein and artery
Superficial temporal vein and artery
Transverse facial vein (*cut*)
Posterior auricular vein
Retromandibular vein
External jugular vein (*cut*)
Common trunk receiving facial, anterior branch of retromandibular, and lingual veins (common facial vein)
Internal jugular vein

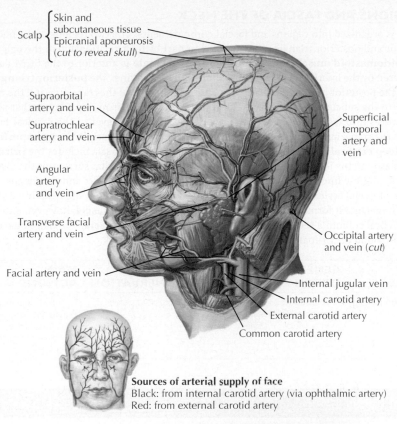

Scalp {
Skin and subcutaneous tissue
Epicranial aponeurosis (*cut to reveal skull*)
}

Supraorbital artery and vein

Supratrochlear artery and vein

Angular artery and vein

Transverse facial artery and vein

Facial artery and vein

Superficial temporal artery and vein

Occipital artery and vein (*cut*)

Internal jugular vein
Internal carotid artery
External carotid artery
Common carotid artery

Sources of arterial supply of face
Black: from internal carotid artery (via ophthalmic artery)
Red: from external carotid artery

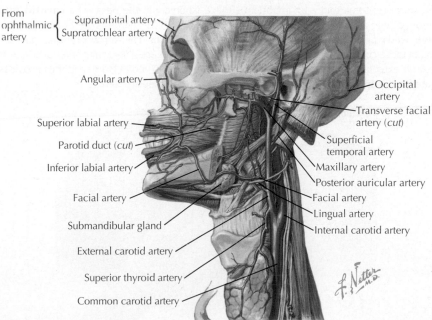

From ophthalmic artery {
Supraorbital artery
Supratrochlear artery
}

Angular artery

Superior labial artery

Parotid duct (*cut*)

Inferior labial artery

Facial artery

Submandibular gland

External carotid artery

Superior thyroid artery

Common carotid artery

Occipital artery
Transverse facial artery (*cut*)
Superficial temporal artery
Maxillary artery
Posterior auricular artery
Facial artery
Lingual artery
Internal carotid artery

Figure 3.7 VASCULATURE OF THE FACE

3.8 REGIONS AND FASCIA OF THE NECK

The **neck** is organized into regions and fascial compartments. The two regions of the neck—the anterior and posterior triangles—are defined in part by their relationship to the palpable **sternocleidomastoid muscle (SCM)**. The **anterior triangle** is anterior to the SCM and is also bordered by the inferior edge of the mandible and the midline. The **posterior triangle** is bound by the posterior border of the SCM, the anterior border of the trapezius, and the clavicle. Deep to the subcutaneous tissue, the deep cervical fascia has multiple layers that separate structures into fascial compartments. The most superficial layer of the cervical fascia surrounds the trapezius and SCM muscles and is known by the descriptive term **superficial layer of deep cervical fascia**. The middle layer of deep cervical fascia includes the **infrahyoid fascia** around the infrahyoid muscles, the **pretracheal fascia** that surrounds the viscera of the neck, and the **buccopharyngeal fascia** posterior to the pharynx and esophagus. The deep layer of deep cervical fascia surrounds the cervical vertebrae and the deep muscles of the neck. In general it forms a single layer called the **prevertebral fascia**; however, anterior to the vertebral column a second layer is recognized, called **alar fascia**. The paired **carotid sheaths** surround the primary neurovascular structures in the neck.

MUSCLE	GENERAL ORIGIN	GENERAL INSERTION	INNERVATION	MAIN ACTIONS
Sternocleidomastoid	Manubrium of sternum and medial 1/3 of clavicle	Mastoid process of temporal bone	Accessory nerve	Laterally flexes neck, causing the chin to point toward the contralateral side of the body

Clinical Focus

The sternocleidomastoid is an important surface landmark in the neck. The **carotid pulse** can be located anterior to the superior half of the SCM, while the posterior border is used to guide needle placement for **cervical plexus nerve blocks**. The retropharyngeal space is an area of loose connective tissue posterior to the buccopharyngeal fascia and anterior to the alar fascia. It extends from the base of the skull to the superior mediastinum, and thus provides a route for the **spread of infection** from the neck to the mediastinum.

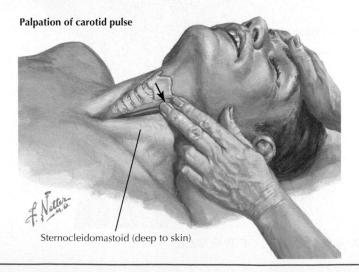

Palpation of carotid pulse

Sternocleidomastoid (deep to skin)

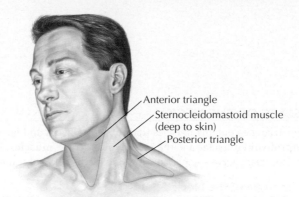

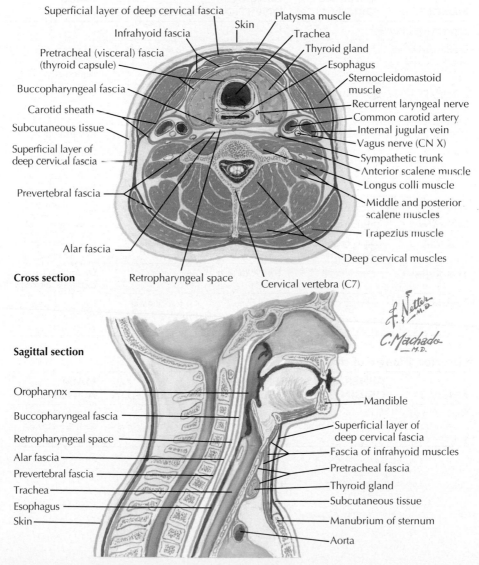

Figure 3.8 FASCIA AND REGIONS OF THE NECK

3.9 MUSCLES OF THE NECK

The anterior triangle contains muscles that move the hyoid and laryngeal skeleton, specifically the **suprahyoid muscles** and the **infrahyoid "strap" muscles**. In contrast, the muscles in the posterior triangle are associated with moving the cervical spine and aiding respiration.

Anterior Triangle of the Neck

MUSCLE	GENERAL ORIGIN	GENERAL INSERTION	INNERVATION	MAIN ACTIONS
Suprahyoid Muscles				
Digastric, anterior belly	Mandible	Hyoid bone via intermediate tendon	N. to mylohyoid (CN V$_3$)	Elevates and stabilizes hyoid, depresses mandible if hyoid is fixed
Digastric, posterior belly	Mastoid process (medial side)	Hyoid bone via intermediate tendon	Facial nerve	
Stylohyoid	Styloid process	Hyoid bone	Facial nerve	Elevates hyoid
Mylohyoid	Mandible	Midline raphe, hyoid	N. to mylohyoid (CN V3)	Elevates hyoid, floor of the mouth, and tongue (e.g., during swallowing)
Infrahyoid Muscles				
Sternohyoid	Manubrium	Hyoid bone	Ansa cervicalis	Depresses hyoid
Omohyoid	Superior border of the scapula	Hyoid bone	Ansa cervicalis	Depresses hyoid
Sternothyroid	Manubrium	Thyroid cartilage	Ansa cervicalis	Depresses thyroid cartilage and larynx
Thyrohyoid	Thyroid cartilage	Hyoid bone	C1 traveling with hypoglossal nerve	Depresses hyoid; elevates larynx when hyoid is fixed

Posterior Triangle of the Neck

MUSCLE	GENERAL ORIGIN	GENERAL INSERTION	INNERVATION	MAIN ACTIONS
Anterior, middle and posterior scalenes	Transverse processes of cervical vertebrae	1st and 2nd ribs	Anterior rami of cervical spinal nerves	Laterally flexes neck, elevates 1st and 2nd ribs

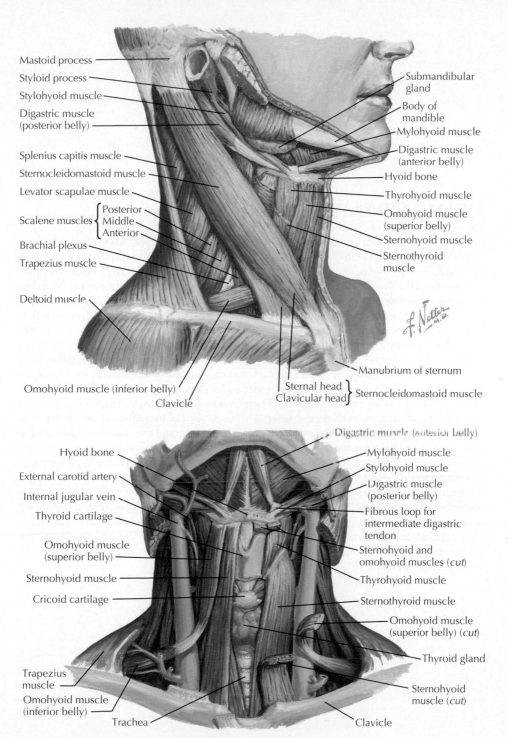

Mastoid process

Styloid process

Stylohyoid muscle

Digastric muscle
(posterior belly)

Splenius capitis muscle

Sternocleidomastoid muscle

Levator scapulae muscle

Scalene muscles { Posterior
Middle
Anterior

Brachial plexus

Trapezius muscle

Deltoid muscle

Omohyoid muscle (inferior belly)

Clavicle

Submandibular
gland

Body of
mandible

Mylohyoid muscle

Digastric muscle
(anterior belly)

Hyoid bone

Thyrohyoid muscle

Omohyoid muscle
(superior belly)

Sternohyoid muscle

Sternothyroid
muscle

Manubrium of sternum

Sternal head }
Clavicular head } Sternocleidomastoid muscle

Digastric muscle (anterior belly)

Hyoid bone

External carotid artery

Internal jugular vein

Thyroid cartilage

Omohyoid muscle
(superior belly)

Sternohyoid muscle

Cricoid cartilage

Trapezius
muscle

Omohyoid muscle
(inferior belly)

Trachea

Mylohyoid muscle

Stylohyoid muscle

Digastric muscle
(posterior belly)

Fibrous loop for
intermediate digastric
tendon

Sternohyoid and
omohyoid muscles (cut)

Thyrohyoid muscle

Sternothyroid muscle

Omohyoid muscle
(superior belly) (cut)

Thyroid gland

Sternohyoid
muscle (cut)

Clavicle

Figure 3.9 MUSCLES OF THE NECK

3.10 VASCULATURE AND NERVES OF THE NECK

The **carotid** sheath contains important neurovascular structures that pass through the superior part of the anterior triangle. The right **common carotid artery** arises from the brachiocephalic trunk, while the left is a branch of the aortic arch. Both ascend in the neck and bifurcate into the external and internal carotid arteries at approximately the level of the superior border of the thyroid cartilage. The **internal carotid artery** does not have any branches in the neck; however its proximal dilated part (**carotid sinus**) contains baroreceptors that are sensitive to changes in arterial blood pressure. The **carotid body**, a chemoreceptor that detects oxygen content in the blood, is also located near the carotid bifurcation. The **external carotid artery** gives rise to several branches in the neck before ascending to the head, most notably the superior thyroid, lingual and facial arteries. The **internal jugular vein** receives venous blood from the head and neck and lies adjacent to the carotid vessels within the carotid sheath. The **vagus nerve** is the other major structure within the carotid sheath; it travels posterior to the vessels and gives off branches to the pharynx, larynx, and heart while in the neck. Other nerves within the anterior triangle are the **hypoglossal nerve** that traverses the carotid vessels near the posterior digastric muscle, and the **ansa cervicalis** on the anterior surface of the carotid sheath that gives off branches to the infrahyoid muscles. The posterior triangle contains the proximal portions of the **brachial plexus**. The large nerves of this plexus travel between the anterior and middle scalene muscles on their way to the upper extremity. The **accessory nerve** innervates the sternocleidomastoid and then traverses the posterior triangle to reach its other target—the trapezius. Finally, the posterior triangle also contains the proximal portions of the **cutaneous nerves of the neck** (great auricular, transverse cervical, supraclavicular, and lesser occipital nerves). These nerves are branches of the cervical plexus (C1–C4 anterior rami) that emerge from the posterior border of the SCM and innervate the skin.

Superficial view

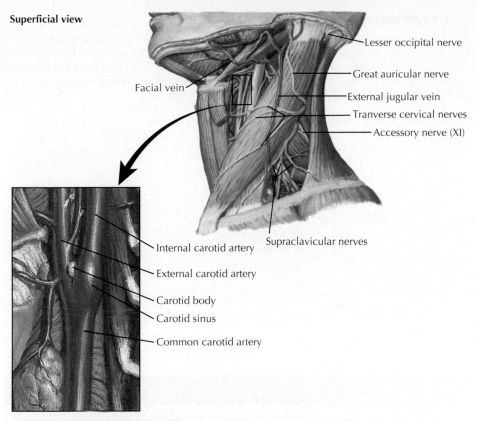

Lesser occipital nerve

Great auricular nerve

Facial vein

External jugular vein

Tranverse cervical nerves

Accessory nerve (XI)

Internal carotid artery

Supraclavicular nerves

External carotid artery

Carotid body

Carotid sinus

Common carotid artery

Deep view: sternocleidomastoid reflected

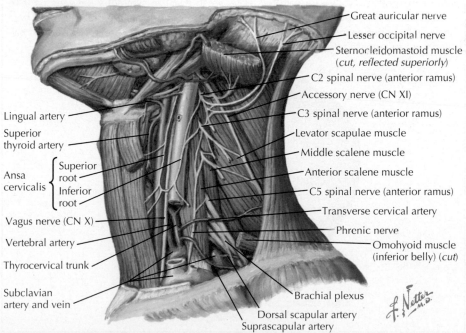

Great auricular nerve

Lesser occipital nerve

Sternocleidomastoid muscle
(*cut, reflected superiorly*)

C2 spinal nerve (anterior ramus)

Accessory nerve (CN XI)

Lingual artery

C3 spinal nerve (anterior ramus)

Superior
thyroid artery

Levator scapulae muscle

Middle scalene muscle

Ansa
cervicalis

Superior
root

Anterior scalene muscle

Inferior
root

C5 spinal nerve (anterior ramus)

Transverse cervical artery

Vagus nerve (CN X)

Phrenic nerve

Vertebral artery

Omohyoid muscle
(inferior belly) (*cut*)

Thyrocervical trunk

Subclavian
artery and vein

Brachial plexus

Dorsal scapular artery

Suprascapular artery

Figure 3.10 VESSELS AND NERVES OF THE NECK

3.11 LYMPHATICS OF THE HEAD AND NECK

The lymph nodes of the head and neck are organized into superficial and deep groups. The superficial nodes are found in a variety of locations, while the deep nodes are located within the carotid sheath adjacent to the internal jugular vein. All lymph from the head and neck eventually passes through these **deep cervical lymph nodes** and enters the circulation via the **thoracic duct** (left side) or **right lymphatic duct** (right side).

Major Groups of Lymph Nodes in the Head and Neck

NODES	LOCATION
Occipital	Base of posterior skull
Postauricular (mastoid)	Posterior to the ear
Preauricular (parotid)	Anterior to the ear
Tonsillar (jugulodigastric)	Adjacent to the angle of the mandible
Submandibular	Along the inferior border of the mandible
Submental	Floor of the mouth
Superficial cervical	Superficial to sternocleidomastoid, adjacent to external jugular vein
Deep cervical	Within carotid sheath, adjacent to internal jugular vein
Supraclavicular	Superior to clavicle in the supraclavicular fossa

Clinical Focus

Lymph node examination in the head and neck is performed to identify infections, inflammation, or malignancy. Nodes are palpated bilaterally to evaluate symmetry between the two sides. Nodes in the head are commonly examined from posterior to anterior, beginning with the occipital nodes and ending with the submental nodes. Nodes in the neck are often palpated from superior to inferior.

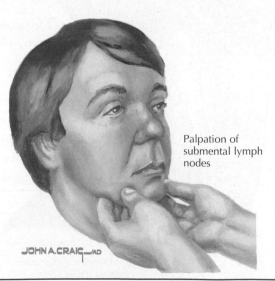

Palpation of submental lymph nodes

JOHN A.CRAIG—AD

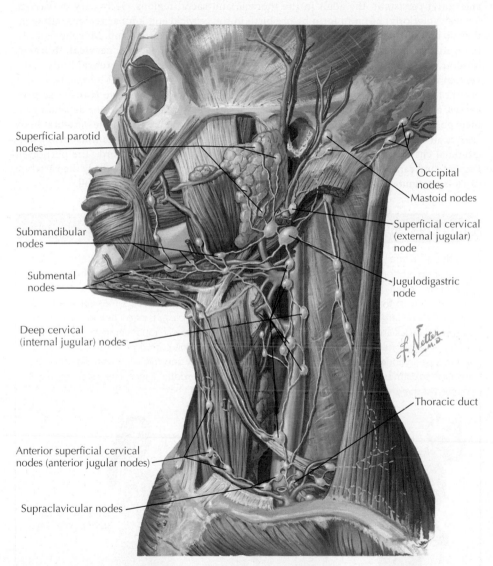

Figure 3.11 LYMPHATICS OF THE HEAD AND NECK

3.12 VERTEBRAL COLUMN

The **vertebral column** protects the spinal cord and supports the weight of the head and trunk. It is comprised of 33 vertebrae that are either separated by intervertebral discs or fused into named structures (**sacrum, coccyx**). The vertebral column is not straight, rather it curves in the sagittal plane. The primary curvature that was present in the fetus (concave anteriorly) persists in the adult in the thoracic and sacral regions. Secondary curvatures (convex anteriorly) begin to form before birth in the cervical and lumbar regions, although they do not fully develop until a baby holds its head up and learns to stand. Morphologically, there are five regional types of vertebrae that form the vertebral column: **cervical, thoracic, lumbar, sacral**, and **coccygeal**. A typical vertebra is comprised of a **vertebral body** and a **vertebral arch.** The arch is formed by two **pedicles** and two **laminae**. Multiple processes project from the vertebral arch including a midline **spinous process**, two **transverse processes**, and four **articular processes** that are designated superior or inferior depending on their position relative to the arch. The fusion of the vertebral arch with the vertebral body creates an opening called the **vertebral foramen**. Successive vertebral foramina form a longitudinal channel named the **vertebral canal** that houses the spinal cord. The portion of the vertebral canal that extends into the sacrum is the **sacral canal**. Superiorly the vertebral canal is continuous with the cranial cavity via the foramen magnum of the skull.

Clinical Focus

Alterations in the shape of individual vertebrae or forces exerted on the vertebral column can produce abnormal curvatures. Exaggerated thoracic curvature is called **kyphosis**. This is frequently caused by reduction of bone mass in the anterior portions of vertebral bodies due to osteoporosis. **Scoliosis** is lateral curvature of the spine that often becomes apparent when adolescents undergo a growth spurt before puberty. The etiology is often unknown; however congenital issues are one cause, for example, if the vertebrae do not develop in a symmetrical fashion. Exaggerated lumbar curvature is called **lordosis**. One common cause is obesity since an increase in abdominal weight shifts the center of gravity and this is compensated for by a postural adjustment. Pregnant women usually adopt a lordotic stance late in pregnancy to counteract the weight of the fetus.

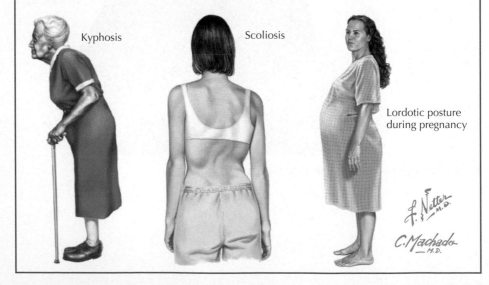

Kyphosis

Scoliosis

Lordotic posture during pregnancy

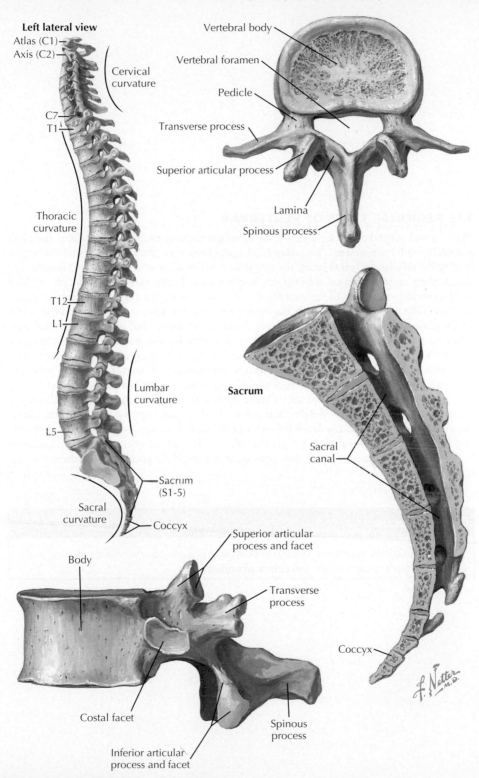

Left lateral view

Atlas (C1)
Axis (C2)
Cervical curvature
C7
T1
Thoracic curvature
T12
L1
Lumbar curvature
L5
Sacrum (S1-5)
Sacral curvature
Coccyx

Vertebral body
Vertebral foramen
Pedicle
Transverse process
Superior articular process
Lamina
Spinous process

Sacrum

Sacral canal

Coccyx

Body
Superior articular process and facet
Transverse process
Costal facet
Inferior articular process and facet
Spinous process

Figure 3.12 VERTEBRAL COLUMN

3.13 REGIONAL TYPES OF VERTEBRAE

The first and second cervical vertebrae have unique features designed to support the skull and facilitate its movement. The **atlas** (C1) articulates with the occipital condyles of the skull at the **atlantooccipital joint**; the movement at this joint is flexion and extension, e.g., the nodding motion used to indicate yes with your head. The **axis** (C2) looks more like a typical cervical vertebra with the exception of the large tooth-like superior projection called the **dens**. The dens articulates with the anterior arch of the atlas at the **atlantoaxial joint**, which allows rotation of the head, for example when indicating "no." A typical **cervical vertebra** exhibits a **bifid spinous process** and a **transverse foramen** in each of the transverse processes. In all but C7, the transverse foramen conducts the paired vertebral arteries that are traveling superiorly to the brain. **Thoracic vertebrae** have **costal facets** for articulation with ribs, and long sloping spinous processes. **Lumbar vertebrae** are characterized by large, sturdy vertebral bodies and short, blunt spinous processes. Their large size reflects the fact that they support more weight than the cervical and thoracic vertebrae. In the sacral region, the five vertebrae are fused into a single structure known as the **sacrum**. Anterior and posterior **sacral foramina** are present that allow passage of spinal nerve roots (see 2.19). The **coccyx** is a small bone that consists of three to four coccygeal vertebrae that are typically fused.

Clinical Focus

C7 has a particularly prominent spinous process that is easily palpable during physical exam; thus this vertebra is often called "**vertebra prominens.**"

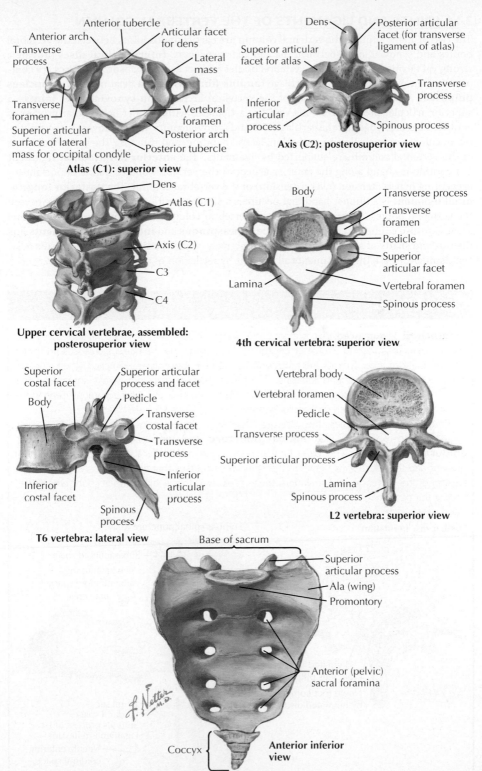

Atlas (C1): superior view

Anterior tubercle
Anterior arch
Transverse process
Articular facet for dens
Lateral mass
Transverse foramen
Vertebral foramen
Superior articular surface of lateral mass for occipital condyle
Posterior arch
Posterior tubercle

Axis (C2): posterosuperior view

Dens
Superior articular facet for atlas
Posterior articular facet (for transverse ligament of atlas)
Inferior articular process
Transverse process
Spinous process

Upper cervical vertebrae, assembled: posterosuperior view

Dens
Atlas (C1)
Axis (C2)
C3
C4

4th cervical vertebra: superior view

Body
Lamina
Transverse process
Transverse foramen
Pedicle
Superior articular facet
Vertebral foramen
Spinous process

T6 vertebra: lateral view

Superior costal facet
Body
Inferior costal facet
Superior articular process and facet
Pedicle
Transverse costal facet
Transverse process
Inferior articular process
Spinous process

L2 vertebra: superior view

Vertebral body
Vertebral foramen
Pedicle
Transverse process
Superior articular process
Lamina
Spinous process

Anterior inferior view

Base of sacrum
Superior articular process
Ala (wing)
Promontory
Anterior (pelvic) sacral foramina
Coccyx

Figure 3.13 REGIONAL TYPES OF VERTEBRAE

3.14 JOINTS AND LIGAMENTS OF THE VERTEBRAL COLUMN

The two primary joints of the vertebral column are cartilaginous joints between the vertebral bodies and synovial joints between the articular processes. **Intervertebral discs** provide a strong yet flexible union between vertebral bodies and act as shock absorbers. Discs are comprised of an outer layer of fibrocartilage (**anulus fibrosus**) and a gelatinous core (**nucleus pulposus**). The articular processes of the vertebral arches form **synovial facet joints**—a superior articular process from one vertebra articulates with an inferior articular process of another vertebra. Together the cartilaginous and synovial joints permit movement of the vertebral column, namely flexion, extension, lateral bending, and rotation. The bones and joints of the vertebral column are supported by ligaments. The **anterior longitudinal ligament** is a continuous band along the anterior aspect of the vertebral bodies that is important for preventing hyperextension (over extension) of the vertebral column. The **posterior longitudinal ligament** is a thinner band that occupies a similar position on the posterior aspect of the vertebral bodies; it limits flexion of the vertebral column. Components of the vertebral arches are also connected by ligaments: the **supraspinous** and **interspinous ligaments** link the tips and shafts of spinous processes, respectively, while the **ligamenta flava** spans adjacent laminae. These three ligaments all prevent hyperflexion of the vertebral column.

Clinical Focus

A **herniated** or **ruptured disc** is a common source of back pain. In this condition, the anulus fibrosus tears (e.g., due to trauma or degenerative changes) and the nucleus pulposus protrudes through the torn area. Typically the protrusion occurs in a posterolateral direction where support from the longitudinal ligaments is lacking. The prolapsed nucleus pulposus may compress spinal nerve roots or the spinal cord causing back pain. Herniated discs are most commonly seen in the lumbar region; approximately 95% occur between L4 and L5 or L5 and S1.

Physicians need to access the vertebral canal for a variety of reasons including obtaining a sample of cerebrospinal fluid (**lumbar puncture**) and administration of anesthesia (e.g. **epidural anesthesia**). The lower lumbar region is favorable because the spinal cord is not present and there are gaps between the spinous processes that allow access with a needle. Flexion of the vertebral column widens these gaps; thus this is taken into account when positioning the patient.

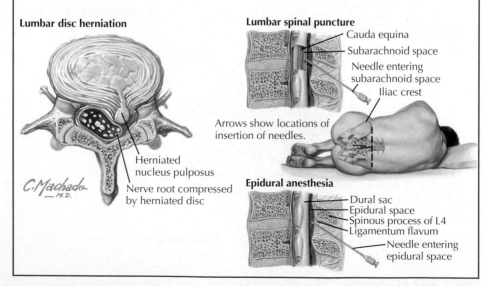

Lumbar disc herniation

Herniated nucleus pulposus

Nerve root compressed by herniated disc

C. Machado —M.D.

Lumbar spinal puncture

Cauda equina

Subarachnoid space

Needle entering subarachnoid space

Iliac crest

Arrows show locations of insertion of needles.

Epidural anesthesia

Dural sac

Epidural space

Spinous process of L4

Ligamentum flavum

Needle entering epidural space

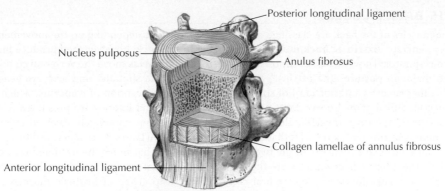

Posterior longitudinal ligament

Nucleus pulposus

Anulus fibrosus

Collagen lamellae of annulus fibrosus

Anterior longitudinal ligament

Intervertebral disc composed of central nuclear zone of collagen and hydrated proteoglycans surrounded by concentric lamellae of collagen fibers

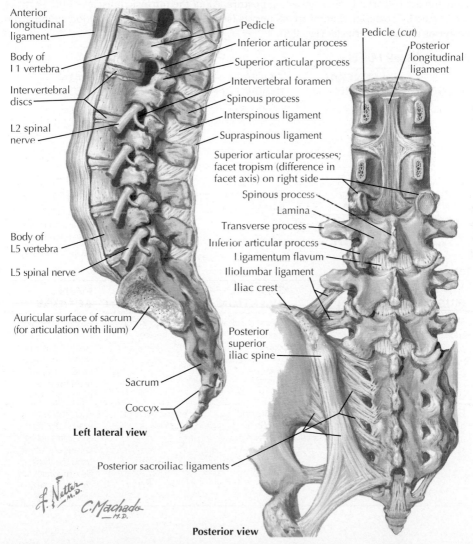

Anterior longitudinal ligament

Body of L1 vertebra

Intervertebral discs

L2 spinal nerve

Pedicle

Inferior articular process

Superior articular process

Intervertebral foramen

Spinous process

Interspinous ligament

Supraspinous ligament

Pedicle (*cut*)

Posterior longitudinal ligament

Superior articular processes; facet tropism (difference in facet axis) on right side

Spinous process

Lamina

Transverse process

Inferior articular process

Ligamentum flavum

Iliolumbar ligament

Iliac crest

Body of L5 vertebra

L5 spinal nerve

Auricular surface of sacrum (for articulation with ilium)

Sacrum

Coccyx

Left lateral view

Posterior superior iliac spine

Posterior sacroiliac ligaments

Posterior view

Figure 3.14 JOINTS AND LIGAMENTS OF THE VERTEBRAL COLUMN

3.15 BACK MUSCLES

The muscles of the back are classified as extrinsic or intrinsic depending on the movements they generate. **Extrinsic back muscles** are located in the back; however they produce limb and respiratory movements. In contrast, **intrinsic back muscles** move the vertebral column and maintain posture. The extrinsic muscles that move the shoulder and arm are generally innervated by anterior rami of spinal nerves, with the exception of trapezius, which is innervated by a cranial nerve. Serratus posterior superior and inferior are presumed to be accessory respiratory muscles, although their function is not completely clear. There are numerous intrinsic back muscles that are classified into three layers from superficial to deep. The superficial layer consists of the two **splenius muscles** that move the head and cervical spine. The intermediate muscles are the **erector spinae** that are the primary muscles that extend and laterally bend the vertebral column. The deep group of intrinsic muscles are collectively known as the **transversospinal muscles** because their fibers extend between the transverse and spinous processes. These muscles extend and stabilize the vertebral column and are important for maintaining posture. All of the intrinsic muscles of the back are innervated by posterior rami of spinal nerves (see Fig. 2.20) and receive blood supply from posterior intercostal arteries (Fig. 2.5).

Extrinsic Back Muscles

MUSCLE	GENERAL ORIGIN	GENERAL INSERTION	INNERVATION	MAIN ACTIONS
Trapezius	Occipital bone, spinous processes of C7–T12	Lateral 1/3 of clavicle, acromion, spine of scapula	Accessory nerve	Elevates, retracts, laterally rotates, and depresses scapula
Latissimus dorsi	Spinous processes of T7–L5, iliac crest, sacrum	Intertubercular groove of humerus	Thoracodorsal nerve	Extends, adducts, and medially rotates humerus
Levator scapulae	Transverse processes of C1–C4	Superior angle of scapula	Dorsal scapular nerve	Elevates and medially rotates scapula
Rhomboid major and minor	Spinous processes of C7–T5	Medial border of scapula	Dorsal scapular nerve	Retracts and medially rotates scapula

Intrinsic Back Muscles

MUSCLE	GENERAL ORIGIN	GENERAL INSERTION	INNERVATION	MAIN ACTIONS
Splenius capitis and cervicis	Spinous processes of C7–T6	Capitis: occipital bone and mastoid process Cervicis: transverse processes of C1–C3	Posterior rami of spinal nerves	Acting bilaterally, extend the head and neck; acting unilaterally, rotate head and laterally bend the neck to the ipsilateral side
Erector spinae	Sacrum, iliac crest, spinous processes of lumbar and sacral vertebrae	Spinous and transverse processes of vertebrae, ribs, skull	Posterior rami of spinal nerves	Acting bilaterally, extend the head and trunk; acting unilaterally, laterally bend the trunk; also important for controlling flexion against gravity

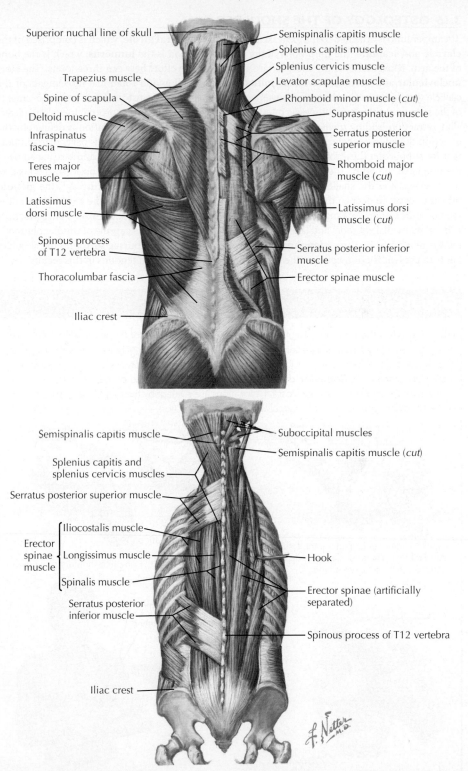

Figure 3.15 BACK MUSCLES

3.16 OSTEOLOGY OF THE SHOULDER

The upper limb is attached to the axial skeleton via the **pectoral girdle**, which is comprised of the **clavicle** and **scapula**. The third bone of the shoulder region is the **humerus**, which is the bone of the arm. Movements of the shoulder are a collaborative effort between three joints. The **sternoclavicular** and **acromioclavicular joints** facilitate gliding and rotational movements of the clavicle that result in simultaneous movements of the scapula against the chest wall. Movements of the scapula at this scapulothoracic interface are elevation, depression, protraction (sliding laterally), retraction (sliding medially), medial rotation, and lateral rotation (rotation is defined by the direction the inferior angle moves). The strong **coracoclavicular ligament** is particularly important for supporting these joints by holding the clavicle and scapula together and bearing some of the weight of the limb. The **glenohumeral joint** is a ball-and-socket joint between the head of the humerus and the shallow glenoid fossa of the scapula. A ring of fibrocartilage, the **glenoid labrum**, serves to deepen the fossa to more effectively hold the humerus. The architecture of the joint permits significant range of motion of the humerus, specifically flexion, extension, abduction, adduction, medial rotation, and lateral rotation (Fig. 1.4). The fibrous capsule of the glenohumeral joint is reinforced by three **glenohumeral ligaments**. Numerous bursae surround the shoulder joints to prevent friction between the various bones, ligaments, and tendons in this region.

Clinical Focus

Force applied to the tip of the shoulder may rupture the ligaments of the acromioclavicular joint, producing an injury called "**shoulder separation**." In a complete separation, the loss of ligament integrity causes the scapula and clavicle to widely separate since the clavicle is no longer supporting the weight of the limb. **Shoulder dislocations** occur when the head of the humerus moves out of its normal position in the glenoid fossa. Dislocations are evident by the loss of the normal contour of the shoulder, and they typically happen in an anterior direction.

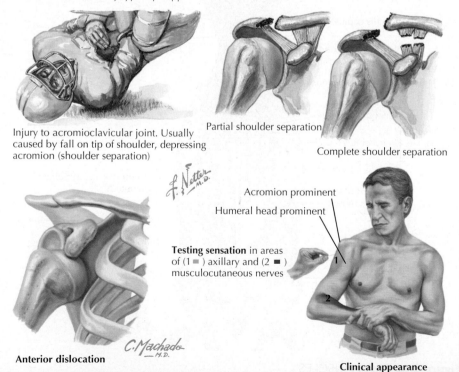

Injury to acromioclavicular joint. Usually caused by fall on tip of shoulder, depressing acromion (shoulder separation)

Partial shoulder separation

Complete shoulder separation

Acromion prominent

Humeral head prominent

Testing sensation in areas of (1 ■) axillary and (2 ■) musculocutaneous nerves

Anterior dislocation

Clinical appearance

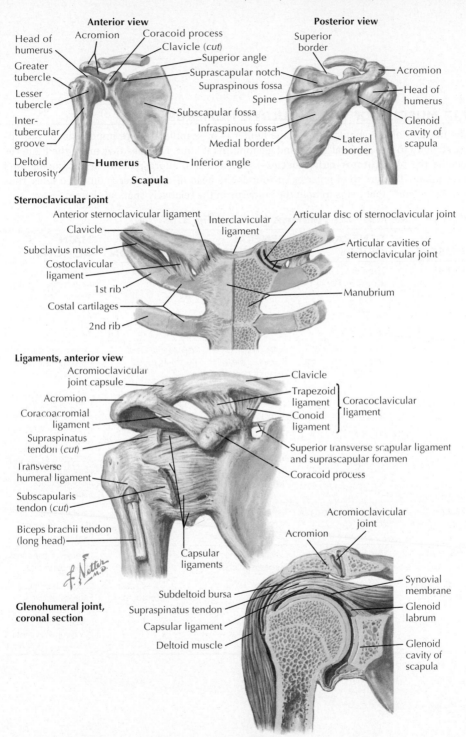

Anterior view

Head of humerus
Acromion
Coracoid process
Clavicle (*cut*)
Superior angle
Suprascapular notch
Supraspinous fossa
Greater tubercle
Lesser tubercle
Spine
Subscapular fossa
Inter-tubercular groove
Infraspinous fossa
Medial border
Deltoid tuberosity
Humerus
Inferior angle
Scapula

Posterior view

Superior border
Acromion
Head of humerus
Glenoid cavity of scapula
Lateral border

Sternoclavicular joint

Anterior sternoclavicular ligament
Interclavicular ligament
Articular disc of sternoclavicular joint
Clavicle
Subclavius muscle
Articular cavities of sternoclavicular joint
Costoclavicular ligament
1st rib
Manubrium
Costal cartilages
2nd rib

Ligaments, anterior view

Acromioclavicular joint capsule
Clavicle
Trapezoid ligament
Conoid ligament
} Coracoclavicular ligament
Acromion
Coracoacromial ligament
Supraspinatus tendon (*cut*)
Superior transverse scapular ligament and suprascapular foramen
Transverse humeral ligament
Coracoid process
Subscapularis tendon (*cut*)
Acromioclavicular joint
Biceps brachii tendon (long head)
Acromion
Capsular ligaments

Glenohumeral joint, coronal section

Synovial membrane
Subdeltoid bursa
Supraspinatus tendon
Glenoid labrum
Capsular ligament
Deltoid muscle
Glenoid cavity of scapula

Figure 3.16 OSTEOLOGY OF THE SHOULDER

3.17 MUSCLES OF THE SHOULDER: HUMERUS

The muscles of the shoulder move the humerus or scapula and are important for providing stability to the pectoral girdle and glenohumeral joint. Muscles that move the humerus include the four **rotator cuff muscles**—subscapularis, supraspinatus, infraspinatus, and teres minor. This group of muscles surrounds the head of the humerus on three sides, thus forming a "cuff" that helps to hold the humerus in the relatively shallow glenoid fossa.

Muscles That Move the Humerus (see also Fig. 3.18)

MUSCLE	GENERAL ORIGIN	GENERAL INSERTION	INNERVATION	MAIN ACTIONS
Deltoid	Spine of the scapula, acromion, lateral 1/3 of clavicle	Deltoid tuberosity of humerus	Axillary nerve	Abducts arm at glenohumeral joint; anterior fibers can flex arm, posterior fibers can extend arm
Pectoralis major	Clavicle, sternum and upper six costal cartilages	Anterior side of humerus (lateral lip of intertubercular groove)	Medial and lateral pectoral nerves	Flexes, adducts, and medially rotates arm at glenohumeral joint
Subscapularis	Subscapular fossa of scapula	Lesser tubercle of humerus	Upper and lower subscapular nerves	Adducts and medially rotates arm at glenohumeral joint
Supraspinatus	Supraspinous fossa of scapula	Greater tubercle of humerus (superior part)	Suprascapular nerve	Abducts arm at glenohumeral joint; responsible for initiating abduction
Infraspinatus	Infraspinous fossa of scapula	Greater tubercle of humerus (middle part)	Suprascapular nerve	Laterally rotates arm at glenohumeral joint
Teres minor	Lateral border of scapula (upper part)	Greater tubercle of humerus (inferior part)	Axillary nerve	Laterally rotates arm at glenohumeral joint
Teres major	Lateral border of scapula (lower part)	Anterior side of humerus (medial lip of intertubercular groove)	Lower subscapular nerve	Extends, adducts, and medially rotates arm at glenohumeral joint

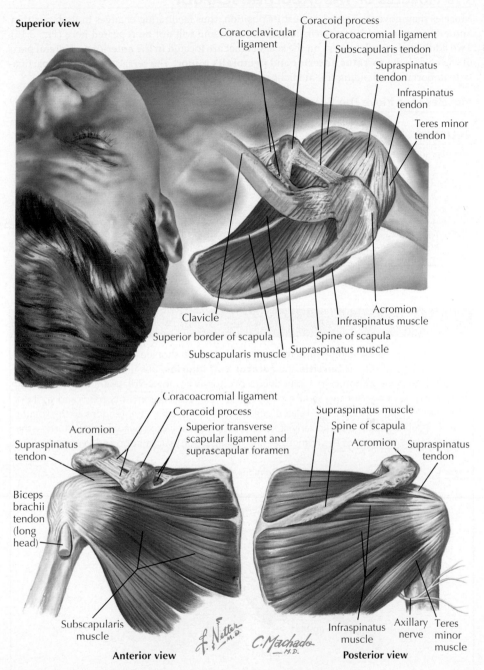

Superior view

Coracoclavicular ligament

Coracoid process

Coracoacromial ligament

Subscapularis tendon

Supraspinatus tendon

Infraspinatus tendon

Teres minor tendon

Clavicle

Superior border of scapula

Subscapularis muscle

Supraspinatus muscle

Spine of scapula

Infraspinatus muscle

Acromion

Coracoacromial ligament

Coracoid process

Superior transverse scapular ligament and suprascapular foramen

Acromion

Supraspinatus tendon

Biceps brachii tendon (long head)

Subscapularis muscle

Anterior view

Supraspinatus muscle

Spine of scapula

Acromion

Supraspinatus tendon

Infraspinatus muscle

Axillary nerve

Teres minor muscle

Posterior view

Figure 3.17 MUSCLES OF THE SHOULDER: ROTATOR CUFF

3.18 MUSCLES OF THE SHOULDER: SCAPULA

Muscles that move the scapula adjust its position, thus facilitating changes in limb position. Some of these muscles are extrinsic back muscles and will not be repeated here (Fig. 3.15). Two additional muscles insert on the scapula that are located in the anterior and lateral parts of the chest—the **serratus anterior** and **pectoralis minor**. The serratus anterior is particularly important for holding the medial part of the scapula against the chest wall.

Muscles that Move the Scapula (see also 3.15)

MUSCLE	GENERAL ORIGIN	GENERAL INSERTION	INNERVATION	MAIN ACTIONS
Serratus anterior	Ribs 1–8	Medial border of the scapula (anterior side)	Long thoracic nerve	Protracts and laterally rotates scapula; important for holding the scapula against the chest wall
Pectoralis minor	Ribs 3–5	Coracoid process of scapula	Medial pectoral nerve	Depresses scapula and assists with protraction

Clinical Focus

Individuals that perform repetitive movements with their shoulder (e.g., baseball pitchers, carpenters) are at risk for **bursitis** and **rotator cuff injuries**. Bursitis is inflammation of the bursae around the glenohumeral joint due to overuse of the joint. Treatment involves resting the joint and interventions to reduce swelling (e.g., ice, anti-inflammatory medications). Loss of integrity of the bursae or age-related degeneration can weaken the tendons of the rotator cuff. The supraspinatus is particularly at risk since it passes between two bony structures—the acromion and the head of the humerus—and thus may rub against bone and eventually tear.

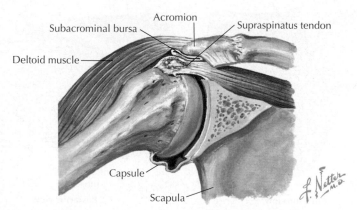

Abduction of arm causes repeated impingement of greater tubercle of humerus on acromion, leading to degeneration and inflammation of supraspinatus tendon, secondary inflammation of bursa, and pain on abduction of arm. Calcific deposits in the supraspinatus tendon may progress to acute calcific tendinitis and sudden onset of severe pain.

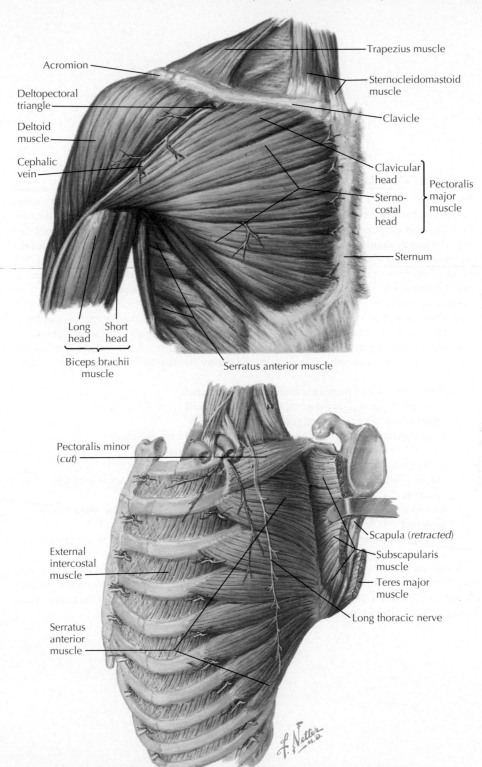

Figure 3.18 MUSCLES OF THE SHOULDER: ANTERIOR AND LATERAL VIEWS

3.19 VASCULATURE OF THE SHOULDER AND AXILLA

The shoulder region receives blood supply from branches of the subclavian and axillary arteries. Since these arteries are on the anterior side of the shoulder, branches to the posterior shoulder must pass between muscles or around the edges of the scapula to reach their targets. The **quadrangular space**, bordered by the humerus, teres major, teres minor, and the long head of triceps brachii, is an example of such a passageway for vessels and nerves. The primary branches of the **subclavian artery** that supply the shoulder region are the suprascapular and dorsal scapular arteries. The **suprascapular artery** passes over the transverse scapular ligament as it enters the supraspinous fossa to supply mainly the supraspinatus and infraspinatus muscles. The **dorsal scapular artery** travels along the medial border of the scapula and furnishes branches to the posterior shoulder region. The subclavian artery becomes the **axillary artery** when it passes the inferior border of the 1st rib. The axillary artery is described as having three parts based on its relationship to the pectoralis minor muscle:

- **1st part** (proximal to pectoralis minor) has **one** branch
  o   superior thoracic artery that supplies the chest wall
- **2nd part** (deep to pectoralis minor) has **two** branches
  o   thoracoacromial trunk that gives off four branches to the shoulder
  o   lateral thoracic artery that travels along the lateral chest wall
- **3rd part** (distal to pectoralis minor) has **three** branches
  o   anterior circumflex humeral artery that passes around the anterior side of the humerus
  o   posterior circumflex humeral artery that traverses the quadrangular space to the posterior side of the humerus
  o   subscapular artery that bifurcates into the circumflex scapular and thoracodorsal arteries

Anastomoses between branches of the suprascapular, dorsal scapular, and circumflex scapular arteries provide collateral circulation to the shoulder region, supplemented by small connections between the circumflex humeral arteries and the thoracoacromial trunk. Veins accompany the arteries and ultimately drain to the superior vena cava.

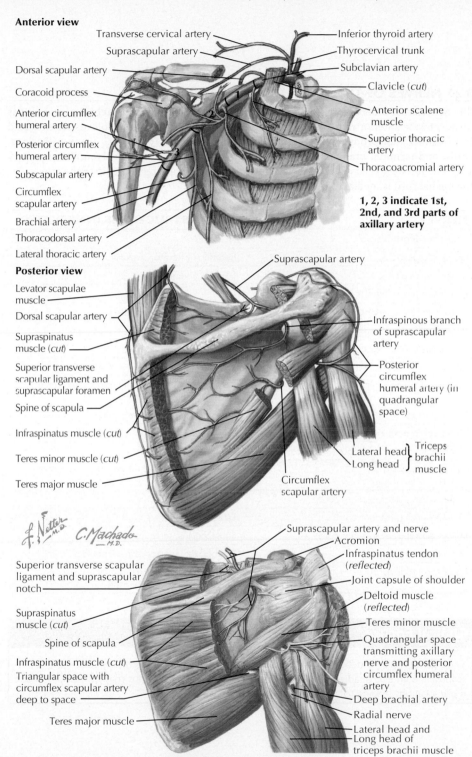

Anterior view

Transverse cervical artery
Suprascapular artery
Dorsal scapular artery
Coracoid process
Anterior circumflex humeral artery
Posterior circumflex humeral artery
Subscapular artery
Circumflex scapular artery
Brachial artery
Thoracodorsal artery
Lateral thoracic artery

Inferior thyroid artery
Thyrocervical trunk
Subclavian artery
Clavicle (*cut*)
Anterior scalene muscle
Superior thoracic artery
Thoracoacromial artery

1, 2, 3 indicate 1st, 2nd, and 3rd parts of axillary artery

Posterior view

Levator scapulae muscle
Dorsal scapular artery
Supraspinatus muscle (*cut*)
Superior transverse scapular ligament and suprascapular foramen
Spine of scapula
Infraspinatus muscle (*cut*)
Teres minor muscle (*cut*)
Teres major muscle

Suprascapular artery
Infraspinous branch of suprascapular artery
Posterior circumflex humeral artery (in quadrangular space)
Lateral head } Triceps
Long head } brachii muscle
Circumflex scapular artery

Superior transverse scapular ligament and suprascapular notch
Supraspinatus muscle (*cut*)
Spine of scapula
Infraspinatus muscle (*cut*)
Triangular space with circumflex scapular artery deep to space
Teres major muscle

Suprascapular artery and nerve
Acromion
Infraspinatus tendon (*reflected*)
Joint capsule of shoulder
Deltoid muscle (*reflected*)
Teres minor muscle
Quadrangular space transmitting axillary nerve and posterior circumflex humeral artery
Deep brachial artery
Radial nerve
Lateral head and Long head of triceps brachii muscle

Figure 3.19 ARTERIES OF THE SHOULDER AND AXILLA

3.20 NERVES OF THE SHOULDER AND AXILLA

The **nerves** that innervate the shoulder muscles are branches of the **brachial plexus** that is formed by the anterior rami of the C5–T1 spinal nerves. The rami of the plexus are entwined in a manner that produces five descriptive divisions: roots (the rami), trunks, divisions, cords, and terminal branches. In the axilla the cords of the plexus surround the axillary artery within the axillary sheath; their names derive from their relationship to the artery (i.e., the medial cord is medial to the artery).

NERVE	MAJOR STRUCTURES INNERVATED
Branches from Roots	
Dorsal scapular (C5)	Rhomboids, levator scapulae
Long thoracic (C5, C6, C7)	Serratus anterior
Branches from Trunks	
Suprascapular (superior trunk)	Supraspinatus, infraspinatus
Branches from Cords	
Lateral pectoral (lateral cord)	Pectoralis major
Musculocutaneous (lateral cord)	Anterior arm muscles, skin of lateral forearm
Median (lateral and medial cords)	Anterior forearm and hand muscles, skin of the hand
Medial pectoral (medial cord)	Pectoralis major, pectoralis minor
Medial brachial cutaneous (medial cord)	Skin of medial arm
Medial antebrachial cutaneous (medial cord)	Skin of medial forearm
Ulnar (medial cord)	Anterior forearm and hand muscles, skin of the hand
Upper subscapular (posterior cord)	Subscapularis
Thoracodorsal (posterior cord)	Latissimus dorsi
Lower subscapular (posterior cord)	Subscapularis, teres major
Axillary (posterior cord)	Deltoid, teres minor, skin of shoulder
Radial (posterior cord)	Posterior arm and forearm muscles; skin of posterior arm, forearm, hand

Clinical Focus

The suprascapular and axillary nerves both pass through small anatomical spaces—the suprascapular notch and quadrangular space, respectively (Fig. 3.19)—thus may be compressed in these locations leading to loss of function.

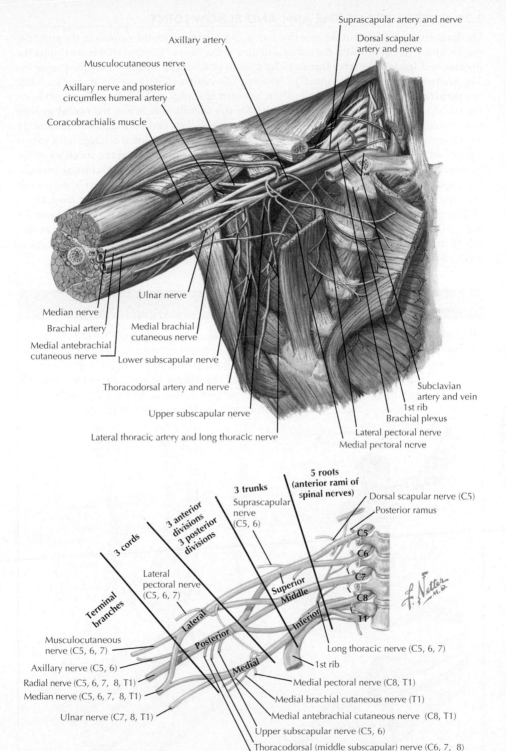

Figure 3.20 NERVES OF THE SHOULDER AND AXILLA

3.21 OSTEOLOGY OF THE ARM AND ELBOW JOINT

The **humerus** is the bone of the arm that has an articulation with the scapula in the shoulder region, and articulations with the radius and ulna at the elbow. The proximal end exhibits the **greater** and **lesser tubercles** that serve as sites of attachment for the rotator cuff muscles. The **anatomical neck** is the junction between the head and neck of the humerus, while the **surgical neck** occurs at the transition between the neck and the shaft. Landmarks on the midshaft include the **deltoid tuberosity** for the deltoid muscle and the **radial groove** that conveys the radial nerve. The **epicondyles** at the distal end are palpable landmarks where numerous muscles of the forearm originate. The **elbow joint** is a hinge joint that is comprised of two articulations: the sturdy **humeroulnar joint** between the **trochlea** of the humerus and **trochlear notch** of the ulna, and the less stable **humeroradial joint** between the **capitulum** of the humerus and the head of the **radius**. A fibrous capsule surrounds the joint and **collateral ligaments** provide support medially and laterally for movements of flexion and extension. The elbow region contains a third articulation that is between the radial head and the radial notch on the ulna. This forms the **proximal radioulnar joint** that is held together by the **anular ligament**. The radial head pivots within the anular ligament to produce pronation and supination of the forearm (see 3.25).

Clinical Focus

Radial head subluxation (RHS) is a condition where the radial head partially or completely slides out of the anular ligament, causing the ligament to tear or become trapped between the radius and capitulum. RHS most commonly occurs in young children when traction is applied to an extended forearm. **Dislocation of the elbow** typically occurs with a fall on an outstretched hand or during a motor vehicle accident. Posterior dislocations are the most common and are easily recognized by a prominent bulge from the displaced olecranon.

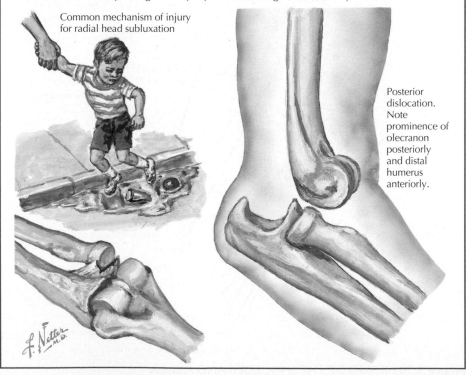

Common mechanism of injury for radial head subluxation

Posterior dislocation. Note prominence of olecranon posteriorly and distal humerus anteriorly.

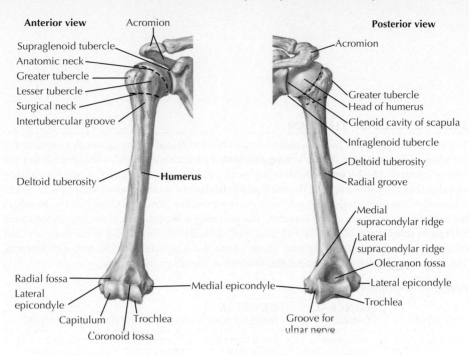

Anterior view   Acromion

Supraglenoid tubercle
Anatomic neck
Greater tubercle
Lesser tubercle
Surgical neck
Intertubercular groove

Deltoid tuberosity   **Humerus**

Radial fossa
Lateral
epicondyle
Capitulum   Trochlea
Coronoid fossa
Medial epicondyle

Posterior view

Acromion

Greater tubercle
Head of humerus
Glenoid cavity of scapula
Infraglenoid tubercle
Deltoid tuberosity
Radial groove

Medial
supracondylar ridge
Lateral
supracondylar ridge
Olecranon fossa
Lateral epicondyle
Trochlea
Groove for
ulnar nerve

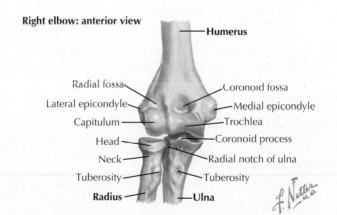

Right elbow: anterior view

Humerus

Radial fossa
Lateral epicondyle
Capitulum
Head
Neck
Tuberosity
Radius

Coronoid fossa
Medial epicondyle
Trochlea
Coronoid process
Radial notch of ulna
Tuberosity
Ulna

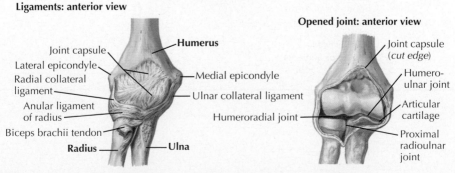

Ligaments: anterior view

Joint capsule
Lateral epicondyle
Radial collateral
ligament
Anular ligament
of radius
Biceps brachii tendon
Radius   **Ulna**

Humerus

Medial epicondyle
Ulnar collateral ligament

Opened joint: anterior view

Joint capsule
(*cut edge*)
Humero-
ulnar joint
Articular
cartilage
Proximal
radioulnar
joint

Humeroradial joint

Figure 3.21 OSTEOLOGY OF THE ARM AND ELBOW JOINT

3.22 MUSCLES OF THE ARM

The arm (brachium) has two muscular compartments created by intermuscular septa of the deep fascia. The **anterior (flexor) compartment** contains three muscles that mainly flex the arm or forearm. The **biceps brachii** is the most superficial muscle and has two heads (long and short) as the name implies. The **coracobrachialis** is a shorter muscle that inserts on the midshaft of the humerus; thus it acts only on the shoulder joint. The third muscle, **brachialis,** is the strongest flexor of the forearm. The posterior compartment of the arm contains the **triceps brachii** that has long, lateral, and medial heads. The long head is the only one that crosses both the shoulder and elbow joints—thus it can extend both the arm and forearm. The lateral and medial heads extend the forearm at the elbow joint.

Anterior Compartment of Arm

MUSCLE	GENERAL ORIGIN	GENERAL INSERTION	INNERVATION	MAIN ACTIONS
Biceps brachii	Short head: coracoid process of scapula Long head: supraglenoid tubercle of scapula	Radial tuberosity, antebrachial fascia via bicipital aponeurosis	Musculocutaneous nerve	Supinates forearm at radioulnar joints, flexes forearm at elbow joint
Coracobrachialis	Coracoid process of scapula	Medial surface of humerus (midway)	Musculocutaneous nerve	Adducts and flexes arm at glenohumeral joint
Brachialis	Anterior surface of the humerus (distal half)	Ulnar tuberosity	Musculocutaneous nerve	Flexes forearm at elbow joint

Posterior Compartment of Arm

MUSCLE	GENERAL ORIGIN	GENERAL INSERTION	INNERVATION	MAIN ACTIONS
Triceps brachii	Long head: infraglenoid tubercle of scapula Lateral head: posterior humerus superior to radial groove Medial head: posterior humerus inferior to radial groove	Olecranon of ulna	Radial nerve	Extends forearm at elbow joint

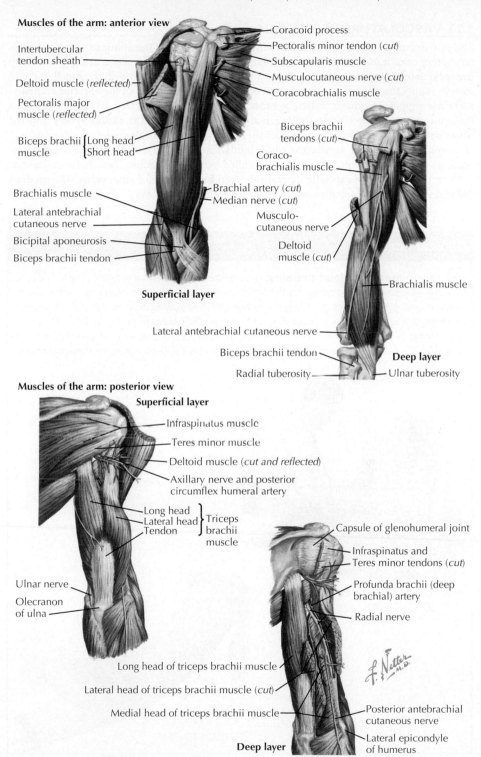

Muscles of the arm: anterior view

Intertubercular tendon sheath

Deltoid muscle (*reflected*)

Pectoralis major muscle (*reflected*)

Biceps brachii muscle { Long head / Short head

Brachialis muscle

Lateral antebrachial cutaneous nerve

Bicipital aponeurosis

Biceps brachii tendon

Superficial layer

Coracoid process

Pectoralis minor tendon (*cut*)

Subscapularis muscle

Musculocutaneous nerve (*cut*)

Coracobrachialis muscle

Biceps brachii tendons (*cut*)

Coraco-brachialis muscle

Brachial artery (*cut*)

Median nerve (*cut*)

Musculo-cutaneous nerve

Deltoid muscle (*cut*)

Brachialis muscle

Lateral antebrachial cutaneous nerve

Biceps brachii tendon

Radial tuberosity

Deep layer

Ulnar tuberosity

Muscles of the arm: posterior view

Superficial layer

Infraspinatus muscle

Teres minor muscle

Deltoid muscle (*cut and reflected*)

Axillary nerve and posterior circumflex humeral artery

Long head / Lateral head / Tendon } Triceps brachii muscle

Ulnar nerve

Olecranon of ulna

Capsule of glenohumeral joint

Infraspinatus and Teres minor tendons (*cut*)

Profunda brachii (deep brachial) artery

Radial nerve

Long head of triceps brachii muscle

Lateral head of triceps brachii muscle (*cut*)

Medial head of triceps brachii muscle

Posterior antebrachial cutaneous nerve

Lateral epicondyle of humerus

Deep layer

Figure 3.22 MUSCLES OF THE ARM

3.23 VASCULATURE OF THE ARM

The primary artery of the arm is the **brachial artery,** which is the continuation of the axillary artery once it leaves the axilla. The first major branch of the brachial artery is the **deep brachial artery** (profunda brachii) that travels around the humerus with the radial nerve to mainly supply the posterior compartment of the arm. The muscles of the anterior compartment are supplied by direct muscular branches of the brachial artery. In the cubital fossa (anterior aspect of the elbow), the brachial artery divides into the **radial artery** and the **ulnar artery**. Multiple branches connect these two arteries with the brachial artery to provide collateral circulation around the elbow joint. The veins that accompany the major arteries (e.g., brachial vein) often exist in pairs called venae comitantes. Two major superficial veins in the arm are the **cephalic** (lateral side) and **basilic** (medial side) **veins**. The **median cubital vein** links the cephalic and basilic veins in the cubital fossa.

Clinical Focus

One way to **measure blood pressure** is to utilize a sphygmomanometer. The cuff of this device is inflated with air to compress the brachial artery and eliminate blood flow. Air is slowly released and eventually the pressure inside the artery is greater than in the cuff. When this happens, blood flow resumes, producing a noise (systolic pressure measurement). When the sound fades away the measurement on the device indicates the diastolic pressure. The median cubital vein is usually prominent in the cubital fossa and is frequently used for **venipuncture**.

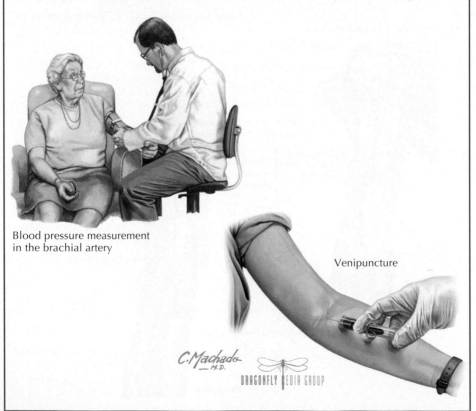

Blood pressure measurement
in the brachial artery

Venipuncture

C. Machado
—M.D.

DRAGONFLY MEDIA GROUP

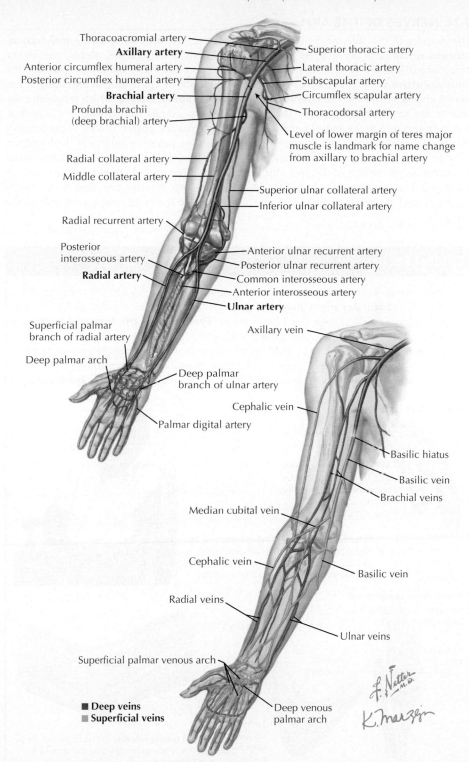

Thoracoacromial artery
Axillary artery
Anterior circumflex humeral artery
Posterior circumflex humeral artery
Brachial artery
Profunda brachii (deep brachial) artery
Radial collateral artery
Middle collateral artery
Radial recurrent artery
Posterior interosseous artery
Radial artery

Superior thoracic artery
Lateral thoracic artery
Subscapular artery
Circumflex scapular artery
Thoracodorsal artery
Level of lower margin of teres major muscle is landmark for name change from axillary to brachial artery
Superior ulnar collateral artery
Inferior ulnar collateral artery
Anterior ulnar recurrent artery
Posterior ulnar recurrent artery
Common interosseous artery
Anterior interosseous artery
Ulnar artery

Superficial palmar branch of radial artery
Deep palmar arch
Deep palmar branch of ulnar artery
Palmar digital artery

Axillary vein
Cephalic vein
Basilic hiatus
Basilic vein
Brachial veins
Median cubital vein
Cephalic vein
Basilic vein
Radial veins
Ulnar veins
Superficial palmar venous arch
Deep venous palmar arch

■ **Deep veins**
■ **Superficial veins**

Figure 3.23 VESSELS OF THE ARM

3.24 NERVES OF THE ARM

The muscles in the anterior compartment of the arm are innervated by the **musculocutaneous nerve**. This nerve arises from the lateral cord of the brachial plexus, pierces the coracobrachialis, and then travels between the biceps brachii and brachialis muscles. The musculocutaneous nerve becomes superficial lateral to the biceps tendon in the cubital fossa; here it changes names to the **lateral antebrachial cutaneous nerve**, which innervates the skin of the anterolateral forearm. The muscle of the posterior compartment, triceps brachii, is innervated by the **radial nerve.** After arising from the posterior cord of the brachial plexus, the radial nerve travels in the radial groove on the posterior surface of the humerus. In addition to providing muscular branches to the triceps, the radial nerve furnishes cutaneous branches to the skin of the posterior arm. The **median** and **ulnar nerves** also travel in the arm but have no branches until they reach the forearm. Notably, the ulnar nerve travels on the posterior surface of the medial epicondyle, where it can be compressed against the bone.

Clinical Focus

The radial nerve is prone to compression in the arm where it lies against the humerus in the radial groove (**Saturday night palsy**). The subsequent loss of innervation to forearm extensors produces a clinical sign called "wrist drop." **Fractures of the humeral shaft** may injure the nerve and the accompanying deep brachial artery. The ulnar nerve can be transiently compressed against the medial epicondyle of the humerus producing pain and tingling distal to the elbow ("bumping your funny bone"). These sensations can also be recurring if the nerve becomes trapped or chronically compressed in this location (**cubital tunnel syndrome**).

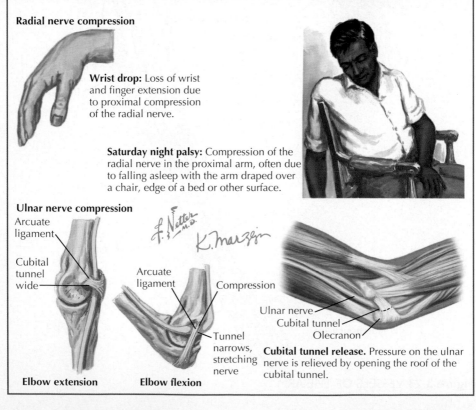

Radial nerve compression

Wrist drop: Loss of wrist and finger extension due to proximal compression of the radial nerve.

Saturday night palsy: Compression of the radial nerve in the proximal arm, often due to falling asleep with the arm draped over a chair, edge of a bed or other surface.

Ulnar nerve compression

Arcuate ligament

Cubital tunnel wide

Elbow extension

Arcuate ligament

Tunnel narrows, stretching nerve

Elbow flexion

Compression

Ulnar nerve

Cubital tunnel

Olecranon

Cubital tunnel release. Pressure on the ulnar nerve is relieved by opening the roof of the cubital tunnel.

Musculocutaneous nerve: anterior view

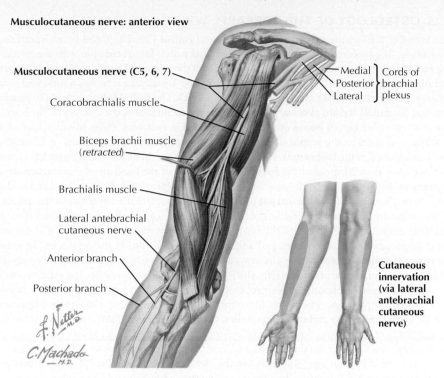

Musculocutaneous nerve (C5, 6, 7)

Coracobrachialis muscle

Biceps brachii muscle (*retracted*)

Brachialis muscle

Lateral antebrachial cutaneous nerve

Anterior branch

Posterior branch

Medial
Posterior } Cords of brachial
Lateral } plexus

Cutaneous innervation (via lateral antebrachial cutaneous nerve)

Radial nerve: posterior view

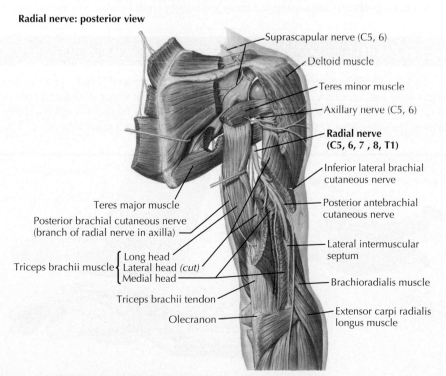

Suprascapular nerve (C5, 6)

Deltoid muscle

Teres minor muscle

Axillary nerve (C5, 6)

Radial nerve (C5, 6, 7 , 8, T1)

Inferior lateral brachial cutaneous nerve

Posterior antebrachial cutaneous nerve

Lateral intermuscular septum

Brachioradialis muscle

Extensor carpi radialis longus muscle

Teres major muscle

Posterior brachial cutaneous nerve (branch of radial nerve in axilla)

Triceps brachii muscle { Long head
Lateral head *(cut)*
Medial head

Triceps brachii tendon

Olecranon

Figure 3.24 NERVES OF THE ARM

3.25 OSTEOLOGY OF THE FOREARM, WRIST, AND HAND

The bones of the forearm are the **ulna** (medial) and **radius** (lateral), joined by an interosseous membrane. The proximal ulna features the **trochlear notch** for articulation with the humerus; the **radial notch** for articulation with the radius; and the **coronoid process, ulnar tuberosity**, and **olecranon** that serve as sites of muscle attachment. Distally the ulna has a head and styloid process. Landmarks on the radius include the **head, neck**, and **radial tuberosity** at the proximal end, and the **radial styloid process** and **carpal articular surface** at the distal end. The bones of the wrist are called **carpal bones** and they are arranged in two rows. From lateral to medial, the proximal row contains the **scaphoid, lunate, triquetrum**, and **pisiform** bones, while the distal row is comprised of the **trapezium, trapezoid, capitate**, and **hamate**. The hamate has an anterior hook-like projection called the **hamulus**. The bones of the hand are the **metacarpals** and **phalanges**. Note that the thumb only has two phalanges (proximal and distal), while the digits have three. The wrist joint (**radiocarpal joint**) consists of an articulation between the distal end of the radius and the scaphoid and lunate; a fibrocartilaginous articular disc separates the other proximal carpals from the head of the ulna. Four main movements are permitted at the wrist joint: flexion, extension, abduction, and adduction (Fig. 1.4). Also in the region of the wrist is the **distal radioulnar joint** that works in synergy with the proximal radioulnar joint to produce pronation and supination of the forearm. During pronation, the radius pivots and crosses over the ulna. Supination is the opposite movement that returns the limb to anatomical position. Numerous ligaments support the wrist joint, including the palmar and dorsal **radiocarpal ligaments** and the **radial and ulnar collateral ligaments**. **Carpometacarpal (CMC) joints** exist between the distal row of carpals and the metacarpals. For digits 2 to 5, small gliding movements occur at these joints. The CMC of the thumb has a unique "saddle" shape that allows flexion, extension, adduction, and abduction. The joints between the metacarpals and proximal phalanges (**metacarpophalangeal or MCP joints**) allow flexion, extension, adduction, and abduction. In contrast, the **interphalangeal (IP) joints** are typical hinge joints that permit flexion and extension only.

Clinical Focus

The wrist is commonly injured by a **fall on an outstretched hand**. Elderly patients with osteoporosis are particularly at risk for **fractures**, and the most frequently injured bone is the radius. A distal radius fracture with dorsal displacement of the fragment is called a Colles fracture. The other bone typically fractured in this type of injury is the scaphoid.

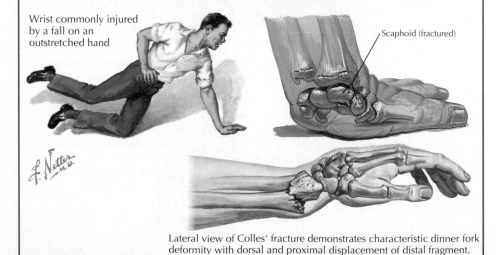

Wrist commonly injured by a fall on an outstretched hand

Scaphoid (fractured)

Lateral view of Colles' fracture demonstrates characteristic dinner fork deformity with dorsal and proximal displacement of distal fragment.

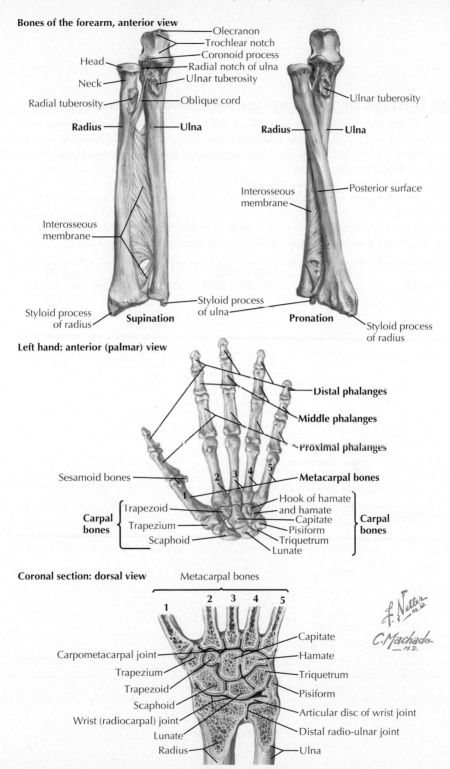

Bones of the forearm, anterior view

Olecranon
Trochlear notch
Coronoid process
Radial notch of ulna
Ulnar tuberosity
Head
Neck
Radial tuberosity
Oblique cord
Radius
Ulna

Ulnar tuberosity
Radius
Ulna

Interosseous membrane
Posterior surface

Interosseous membrane

Styloid process of radius
Supination
Styloid process of ulna
Pronation
Styloid process of radius

Left hand: anterior (palmar) view

Distal phalanges

Middle phalanges

Proximal phalanges

Sesamoid bones
Metacarpal bones

Trapezoid
Hook of hamate and hamate
Capitate
Pisiform
Triquetrum
Lunate
Carpal bones
Trapezium
Scaphoid
Carpal bones

Coronal section: dorsal view
Metacarpal bones

Capitate
Hamate
Triquetrum
Pisiform
Articular disc of wrist joint
Distal radio-ulnar joint
Ulna

Carpometacarpal joint
Trapezium
Trapezoid
Scaphoid
Wrist (radiocarpal) joint
Lunate
Radius

Figure 3.25 OSTEOLOGY OF THE FOREARM, WRIST, AND HAND

3.26 MUSCLES OF THE FOREARM: ANTERIOR COMPARTMENT

Similar to the arm, the forearm is separated into anterior and posterior compartments by intermuscular septa. The **anterior compartment** contains flexor and pronator muscles that are arranged in three layers. There are **four superficial muscles**, **one intermediate muscle**, and **three deep muscles**. All of these muscles are innervated by the **median nerve**, with the exception of the flexor carpi ulnaris and the medial half of the flexor digitorum profundus, which are innervated by the **ulnar nerve**. Of note is the unique arrangement of the flexor digitorum tendons with respect to their insertions. Since the flexor digitorum superficialis tendon inserts on the middle phalanx, it must split into two parts to allow the tendon of the flexor digitorum profundus to pass through to the distal phalanx (see 3.28).

MUSCLE	GENERAL ORIGIN	GENERAL INSERTION	INNERVATION	MAIN ACTIONS
Superficial Muscles				
Pronator teres	Medial epicondyle of humerus	Radius, mid-shaft	Median nerve	Pronates forearm at radioulnar joints
Flexor carpi radialis	Medial epicondyle of humerus	2nd metacarpal	Median nerve	Flexes and abducts hand at wrist joint
Palmaris longus	Medial epicondyle of humerus	Palmar aponeurosis	Median nerve	Flexes hand at wrist joint
Flexor carpi ulnaris	Medial epicondyle of humerus, ulna	Pisiform, hamate, 5th metacarpal	Ulnar nerve	Flexes and adducts hand at wrist joint
Intermediate Muscle				
Flexor digitorum superficialis	Medial epicondyle of humerus, radius	Middle phalanges of digits 2–5	Median nerve	Flexes hand at wrist joint, flexes digits 2–5 at MCP/PIP joints
Deep Muscles				
Flexor pollicis longus	Radius (anterior surface), interosseous membrane	Distal phalanx of thumb	Median nerve (anterior interosseous branch)	Flexes thumb at MCP/IP joints
Flexor digitorum profundus	Ulna (anterior surface), interosseous membrane	Distal phalanges of digits 2–5	Median nerve (lateral half), ulnar nerve (medial half)	Flexes digits 2–5 at MCP/IP joints
Pronator quadratus	Ulna, distal shaft	Radius, distal shaft	Median nerve (anterior interosseous branch)	Pronates forearm at radioulnar joints

IP, interphalangeal joint; MP, metacarpophalangeal joint; PIP, proximal interphalangeal joint.

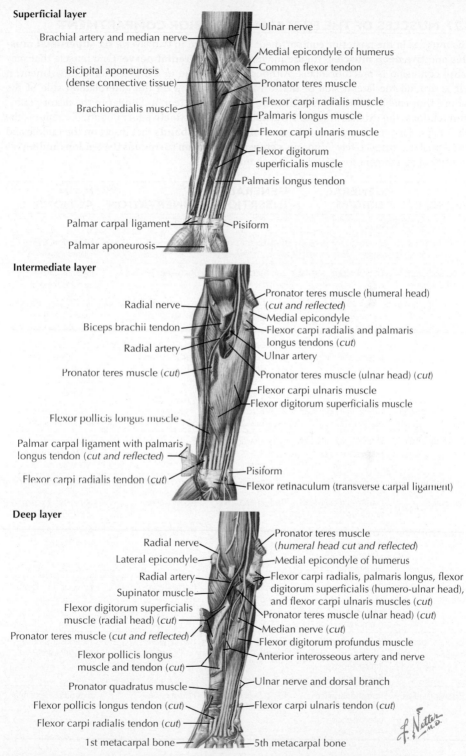

Superficial layer

Brachial artery and median nerve
Bicipital aponeurosis (dense connective tissue)
Brachioradialis muscle

Ulnar nerve
Medial epicondyle of humerus
Common flexor tendon
Pronator teres muscle
Flexor carpi radialis muscle
Palmaris longus muscle
Flexor carpi ulnaris muscle
Flexor digitorum superficialis muscle
Palmaris longus tendon

Palmar carpal ligament
Palmar aponeurosis
Pisiform

Intermediate layer

Radial nerve
Biceps brachii tendon
Radial artery
Pronator teres muscle (cut)
Flexor pollicis longus muscle
Palmar carpal ligament with palmaris longus tendon (cut and reflected)
Flexor carpi radialis tendon (cut)

Pronator teres muscle (humeral head) (cut and reflected)
Medial epicondyle
Flexor carpi radialis and palmaris longus tendons (cut)
Ulnar artery
Pronator teres muscle (ulnar head) (cut)
Flexor carpi ulnaris muscle
Flexor digitorum superficialis muscle
Pisiform
Flexor retinaculum (transverse carpal ligament)

Deep layer

Radial nerve
Lateral epicondyle
Radial artery
Supinator muscle
Flexor digitorum superficialis muscle (radial head) (cut)
Pronator teres muscle (cut and reflected)
Flexor pollicis longus muscle and tendon (cut)
Pronator quadratus muscle
Flexor pollicis longus tendon (cut)
Flexor carpi radialis tendon (cut)
1st metacarpal bone

Pronator teres muscle (humeral head cut and reflected)
Medial epicondyle of humerus
Flexor carpi radialis, palmaris longus, flexor digitorum superficialis (humero-ulnar head), and flexor carpi ulnaris muscles (cut)
Pronator teres muscle (ulnar head) (cut)
Median nerve (cut)
Flexor digitorum profundus muscle
Anterior interosseous artery and nerve
Ulnar nerve and dorsal branch
Flexor carpi ulnaris tendon (cut)
5th metacarpal bone

Figure 3.26 MUSCLES OF THE FOREARM: ANTERIOR COMPARTMENT

3.27 MUSCLES OF THE FOREARM: POSTERIOR COMPARTMENT

The muscles in the posterior compartment are arranged in two layers, **six superficial muscles** and **five deep muscles**. All are innervated by the **radial nerve**. One muscle that may cause confusion is brachioradialis. Although it is located in the posterior compartment, it winds around the lateral side of the forearm and inserts on the anterolateral side of the radius, thus enabling it to flex the forearm rather than extend it. Similar to the flexor digitorum tendons, the extensor digitorum tendons have a distinctive form of attachment on the phalanges. Each tendon gives rise to **central** and **lateral bands** that insert on the middle and distal phalanx, respectively. A fibrous **extensor expansion** surrounds the tendons and serves as a site of attachment for muscles of the hand.

MUSCLE	GENERAL ORIGIN	GENERAL INSERTION	INNERVATION	MAIN ACTIONS
Superficial Muscles				
Brachioradialis	Lateral supracondylar ridge	Radius, distal end	Radial nerve	Flexes forearm at elbow joint
Extensor carpi radialis longus	Lateral supracondylar ridge	2nd metacarpal	Radial nerve	Extends and abducts hand at wrist joint
Extensor carpi radialis brevis	Lateral epicondyle of humerus	3rd metacarpal	Radial nerve	Extends and abducts hand at wrist joint
Extensor digitorum	Lateral epicondyle of humerus	Digits 2–5 via extensor expansion	Radial nerve	Extends hand at wrist joint, extends digits 2–5 at MCP/IP joints
Extensor digiti minimi	Lateral epicondyle of humerus	Digit 5 via extensor expansion	Radial nerve	Extends little finger at MCP/IP joints
Extensor carpi ulnaris	Lateral epicondyle of humerus	5th metacarpal	Radial nerve	Extends and adducts hand at wrist joint
Deep Muscles				
Supinator	Lateral epicondyle of humerus	Radius, proximal 1/3	Radial nerve	Supinates forearm at radioulnar joints
Abductor pollicis longus	Posterior surface of ulna, radius, and interosseous membrane	1st metacarpal	Radial nerve	Abducts thumb at CMC joint
Extensor pollicis brevis	Posterior surface of radius and interosseous membrane	Proximal phalanx of thumb	Radial nerve	Extends thumb at CMC joint
Extensor pollicis longus	Posterior surface of ulna and interosseous membrane	Distal phalanx of thumb	Radial nerve	Extends thumb at MCP/IP joints
Extensor indicis	Posterior surface of ulna and interosseous membrane	Digit 2 via extensor expansion	Radial nerve	Extends index finger at MCP/IP joints

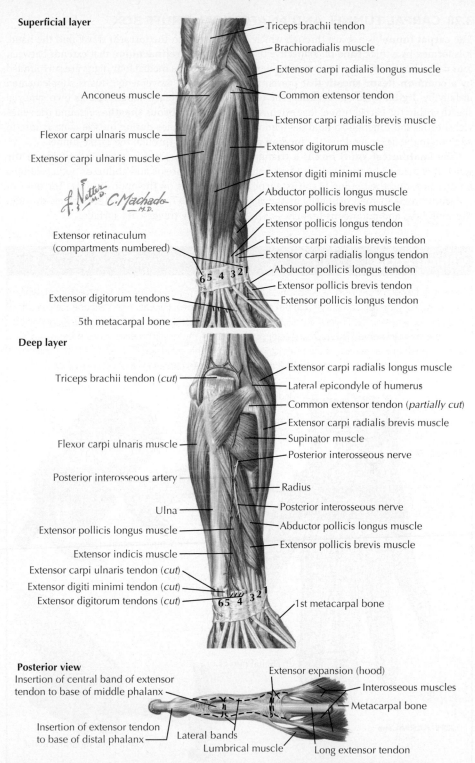

Superficial layer

- Triceps brachii tendon
- Brachioradialis muscle
- Extensor carpi radialis longus muscle
- Common extensor tendon
- Anconeus muscle
- Extensor carpi radialis brevis muscle
- Flexor carpi ulnaris muscle
- Extensor digitorum muscle
- Extensor carpi ulnaris muscle
- Extensor digiti minimi muscle
- Abductor pollicis longus muscle
- Extensor pollicis brevis muscle
- Extensor pollicis longus tendon
- Extensor retinaculum (compartments numbered)
- Extensor carpi radialis brevis tendon
- Extensor carpi radialis longus tendon
- Abductor pollicis longus tendon
- 6 5 4 3 2 1
- Extensor pollicis brevis tendon
- Extensor digitorum tendons
- Extensor pollicis longus tendon
- 5th metacarpal bone

Deep layer

- Triceps brachii tendon (*cut*)
- Extensor carpi radialis longus muscle
- Lateral epicondyle of humerus
- Common extensor tendon (*partially cut*)
- Extensor carpi radialis brevis muscle
- Flexor carpi ulnaris muscle
- Supinator muscle
- Posterior interosseous nerve
- Posterior interosseous artery
- Radius
- Ulna
- Posterior interosseous nerve
- Extensor pollicis longus muscle
- Abductor pollicis longus muscle
- Extensor pollicis brevis muscle
- Extensor indicis muscle
- Extensor carpi ulnaris tendon (*cut*)
- Extensor digiti minimi tendon (*cut*)
- Extensor digitorum tendons (*cut*)
- 6 5 4 3 2 1
- 1st metacarpal bone

Posterior view

- Insertion of central band of extensor tendon to base of middle phalanx
- Extensor expansion (hood)
- Interosseous muscles
- Metacarpal bone
- Insertion of extensor tendon to base of distal phalanx
- Lateral bands
- Lumbrical muscle
- Long extensor tendon

Figure 3.27 MUSCLES OF THE FOREARM: POSTERIOR COMPARTMENT

3.28 CARPAL TUNNEL AND ANATOMICAL SNUFF BOX

The **carpal tunnel** is a space through which structures from the forearm travel into the hand. It is formed by a thick band of connective tissue, the **flexor retinaculum**, that extends between four carpal bones. Within the tunnel, the flexor tendons of the medial four digits are surrounded by a **common flexor sheath** that prevents friction during movements; this is supplemented distally by **digital synovial sheaths**. The tendon of flexor pollicis longus has its own synovial sheath within the carpal tunnel that extends into the digit. **Fibrous sheaths** surround the synovial sheaths and function to hold the tendons against the bones during muscle contraction. In addition to the flexor tendons, the **median nerve** also travels through the carpal tunnel.

The **anatomical snuff box** is a triangular-shaped depression on the radial side of the wrist. It is defined by the tendons of the extensor pollicis brevis and abductor pollicis longus on one side, and the tendon of the extensor pollicis longus on the opposite side. The floor of the snuff box is formed primarily by the **scaphoid bone**. The **radial artery** travels through the snuff box, and cutaneous branches of the radial nerve traverse its surface.

Clinical Focus

Repetitive flexion of the wrist or digits can cause inflammation and swelling in the carpal tunnel, which may compress the median nerve (**carpal tunnel syndrome**). Patients often experience pain, tingling, or numbness in the fingers, apart from the little finger that does not receive sensory innervation from the median nerve. The palmar cutaneous branch of the median nerve arises proximal to the carpal tunnel; thus sensation of the palm is not affected in this condition. Tenderness in the anatomical snuff box is indicative of a **scaphoid fracture**, which can damage the radial artery (see 3.25).

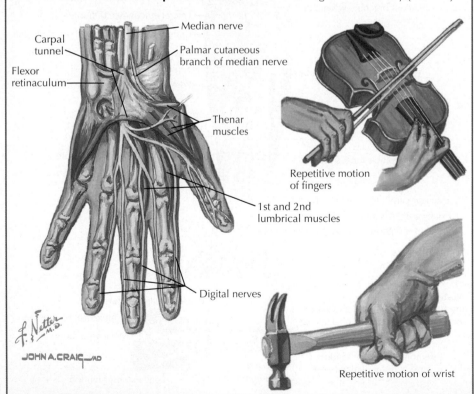

Carpal tunnel

Flexor retinaculum

Median nerve

Palmar cutaneous branch of median nerve

Thenar muscles

Repetitive motion of fingers

1st and 2nd lumbrical muscles

Digital nerves

JOHN A. CRAIG—MD

Repetitive motion of wrist

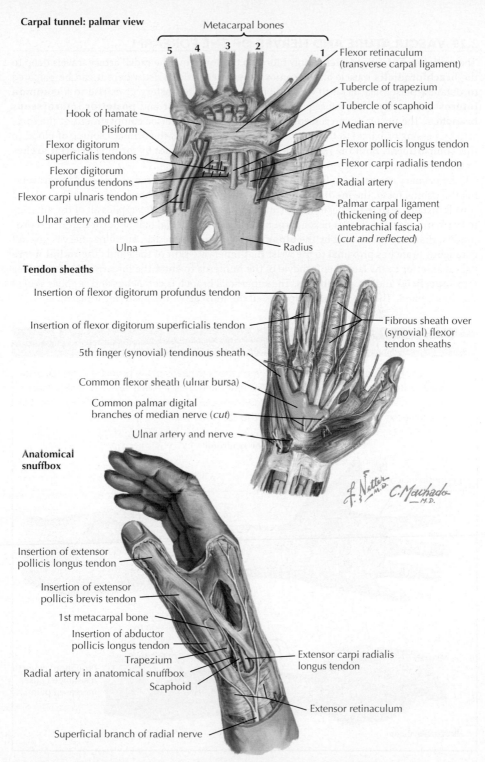

Figure 3.28 CARPAL TUNNEL AND ANATOMICAL SNUFF BOX

3.29 VASCULATURE AND NERVES OF THE FOREARM

The **radial** and **ulnar arteries** supply blood to the forearm. The radial artery travels deep to the **brachioradialis** muscle and becomes superficial at the wrist, where it can be palpated to obtain a pulse. Just distal to the cubital fossa, the ulnar artery gives rise to a **common interosseous artery** that subsequently divides into **anterior** and **posterior interosseous branches.** The posterior interosseous artery enters the posterior compartment of the forearm by passing proximal to the interosseous membrane; it is the primary source of blood to this compartment. Both the radial and ulnar arteries terminate by forming **arterial arches** in the hand.

The primary nerves of the forearm are the median, ulnar, and radial nerves. After traversing the cubital fossa, the **median nerve** passes between the two heads of pronator teres and travels distally deep to the flexor digitorum superficialis muscle. It supplies all of the anterior forearm muscles, apart from flexor carpi ulnaris and the medial half of flexor digitorum profundus; these are innervated by the **ulnar nerve**. Both the median and ulnar nerves give off cutaneous branches proximal to the wrist that innervate skin of the hand. The **radial nerve** passes anterior to the lateral epicondyle of the humerus to enter the forearm. Here it divides into **superficial** and **deep branches**. The superficial branch is cutaneous and supplies skin of the dorsal hand. The deep branch supplies all the muscles of the posterior forearm.

Clinical Focus

The median nerve may be compressed between the two heads of the pronator teres (**pronator syndrome**) producing pain, loss of sensation, and muscle weakness. Loss of sensation on the palm distinguishes pronator syndrome from carpal tunnel syndrome (3.28) since the palmar cutaneous branch arises proximal to the carpal tunnel.

Pronator syndrome

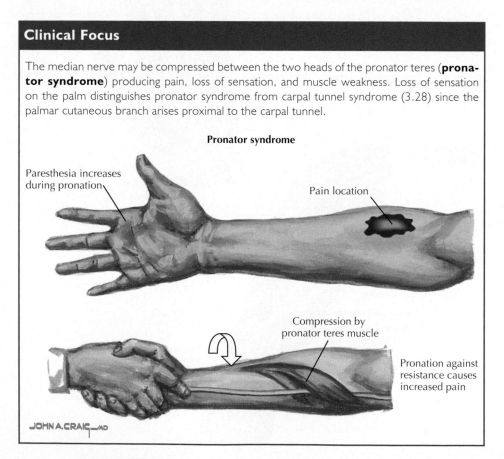

Paresthesia increases during pronation

Pain location

Compression by pronator teres muscle

Pronation against resistance causes increased pain

JOHN A. CRAIG—AD

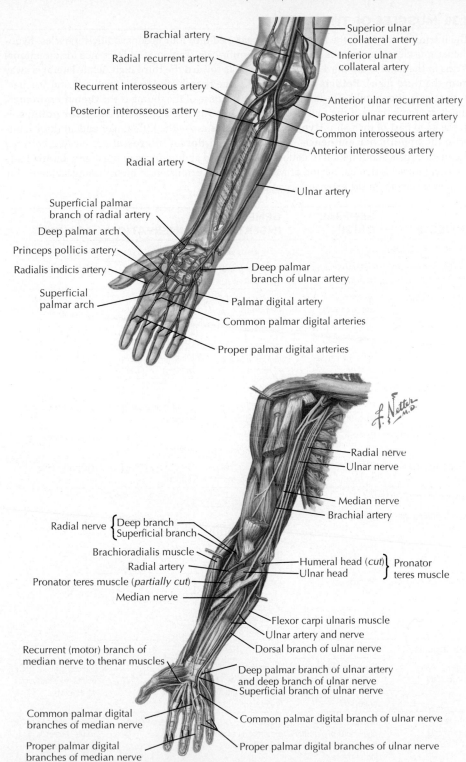

Figure 3.29 VESSELS AND NERVES OF THE FOREARM

3.30 MUSCLES OF THE HAND

The intrinsic muscles of the hand can be organized into four groups: pollicis muscles, hypothenar muscles, interosseous muscles, and lumbricals. The point of reference for directional terms in the hand is the third digit (i.e., medial is toward the third digit, while lateral is away from the third digit). **Pollicis muscles** act on the thumb (the terms "pollicis" and "thenar" both refer to the thumb). The fleshy mound at the base of the thumb is the **thenar eminence**, and it contains three of the four pollicis muscles. The fourth muscle, **adductor pollicis**, is in the deep part of the palm. **Hypothenar muscles** move the little finger and all three comprise the **hypothenar eminence**. The **palmar** and **dorsal interossei** are located between the metacarpals and function to adduct (palmar) and abduct (dorsal) the digits. **Lumbricals** are small muscles that aid flexion of MCP joints and extension of interphalangeal joints due to their insertion on the extensor expansions.

MUSCLE	GENERAL ORIGIN	GENERAL INSERTION	INNERVATION	MAIN ACTIONS
Pollicis Muscles				
Flexor pollicis brevis	Flexor retinaculum, trapezium	Proximal phalanx of thumb	Median nerve (recurrent branch)	Flexes thumb
Abductor pollicis brevis	Flexor retinaculum, lateral carpals	Proximal phalanx of thumb	Median nerve (recurrent branch)	Abducts thumb
Opponens pollicis	Flexor retinaculum, lateral carpals	1st metacarpal	Median nerve (recurrent branch)	Opposes thumb
Adductor pollicis	3rd metacarpal, capitate	Proximal phalanx of thumb	Ulnar nerve (deep branch)	Adducts thumb
Hypothenar Muscles				
Flexor digiti minimi brevis	Flexor retinaculum, hamate	Proximal phalanx of little finger	Ulnar nerve (deep branch)	Flexes little finger
Abductor digiti minimi	Pisiform	Proximal phalanx of little finger	Ulnar nerve (deep branch)	Abducts little finger
Opponens digiti minimi	Flexor retinaculum, hamate	5th metacarpal	Ulnar nerve (deep branch)	Opposes little finger
Interosseous Muscles				
Dorsal interossei	Metacarpals	Extensor expansions and proximal phalanges of digits 2–4	Ulnar nerve (deep branch)	Abducts digits 2–4
Palmar interossei	Metacarpals	Extensor expansions and proximal phalanges of digits 2, 4, and 5	Ulnar nerve (deep branch)	Adducts digits 2, 4, 5
Lumbricals				
Lateral two lumbricals	Tendons of flexor digitorum profundus for index and middle fingers	Extensor expansions of index and middle fingers	Median nerve	Flexes digits at MCP joints, extends digits at IP joints
Medial two lumbricals	Tendons of flexor digitorum profundus for middle, ring and little fingers	Extensor expansions of ring and little fingers	Ulnar nerve (deep branch)	Flexes digits at MCP joints, extends digits at IP joints

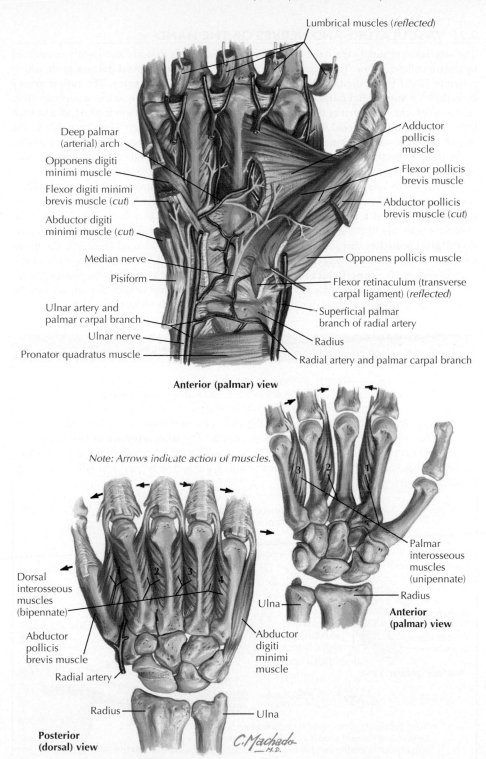

Lumbrical muscles (*reflected*)

Deep palmar (arterial) arch

Opponens digiti minimi muscle

Flexor digiti minimi brevis muscle (*cut*)

Abductor digiti minimi muscle (*cut*)

Median nerve

Pisiform

Ulnar artery and palmar carpal branch

Ulnar nerve

Pronator quadratus muscle

Adductor pollicis muscle

Flexor pollicis brevis muscle

Abductor pollicis brevis muscle (*cut*)

Opponens pollicis muscle

Flexor retinaculum (transverse carpal ligament) (*reflected*)

Superficial palmar branch of radial artery

Radius

Radial artery and palmar carpal branch

Anterior (palmar) view

Note: Arrows indicate action of muscles.

3   2   1

Palmar interosseous muscles (unipennate)

Radius

Ulna

Anterior (palmar) view

Dorsal interosseous muscles (bipennate)

1   2   3   4

Abductor pollicis brevis muscle

Radial artery

Abductor digiti minimi muscle

Ulna

Radius

Ulna

Posterior (dorsal) view

C. Machado
M.D.

Figure 3.30 MUSCLES OF THE HAND

3.31 VASCULATURE AND NERVES OF THE HAND

The arteries that supply the hand form two vascular arches that are sufficiently connected to ensure collateral flow. The **ulnar artery** gives rise to the **superficial palmar arch**, which provides blood to the digits via **common** and **proper digital arteries.** The **radial artery** contributes a **superficial palmar branch** that forms the lateral side of the superficial arch. At the wrist, the radial artery traverses the anatomical snuff box where it gives off a branch that forms the **dorsal carpal arch** on the dorsum of the hand. It then issues branches to the thumb and index finger (**princeps pollicis** and **radialis indicis,** respectively) and continues as the **deep palmar arch**. Connections between the ulnar artery and deep arch are provided by metacarpal branches and the deep palmar branch of the ulnar artery.

The nerves that supply the hand are mainly the median and ulnar, with a small contribution provided by the radial nerve. The **median nerve** enters the hand through the carpal tunnel and gives off a **recurrent branch** that innervates the thenar muscles. It provides muscular branches to the lateral two lumbricals then divides into **common** and **proper palmar digital branches** that supply the skin of the distal palm and lateral 3½ digits. The **ulnar nerve** traverses the wrist lateral to the pisiform bone, and then bifurcates into superficial and deep branches. The **superficial branch** gives off common and proper digital nerves to supply the skin of the medial 1½ digits. The **deep branch** is a motor branch that innervates the hypothenar muscles, interossei, medial two lumbricals, and the adductor pollicis.

Clinical Focus

Cutaneous innervation between individuals is variable, although some areas of skin are reliably innervated by a particular nerve. These areas are called **autogenous zones**, and they can be utilized to test the integrity of nerves. The autogenous zone for the median nerve is the pad of the index finger; for the ulnar nerve it is the pad of the little finger; and for the radial nerve it is the skin over the first dorsal interosseous muscle. The **dermatomes of the hand** are also useful to remember since they can be used to evaluate the function of spinal nerves. **C6** is the dermatome for the thumb, **C7** for the index and middle fingers, and **C8** for the ring and little fingers.

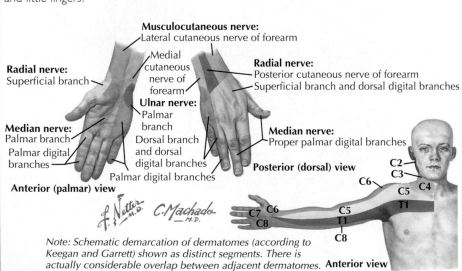

Radial nerve:
Superficial branch

Musculocutaneous nerve:
Lateral cutaneous nerve of forearm

Medial cutaneous nerve of forearm

Radial nerve:
Posterior cutaneous nerve of forearm
Superficial branch and dorsal digital branches

Ulnar nerve:
Palmar branch
Dorsal branch and dorsal digital branches
Palmar digital branches

Median nerve:
Palmar branch
Palmar digital branches

Anterior (palmar) view

Median nerve:
Proper palmar digital branches

Posterior (dorsal) view

Anterior view

Note: Schematic demarcation of dermatomes (according to Keegan and Garrett) shown as distinct segments. There is actually considerable overlap between adjacent dermatomes.

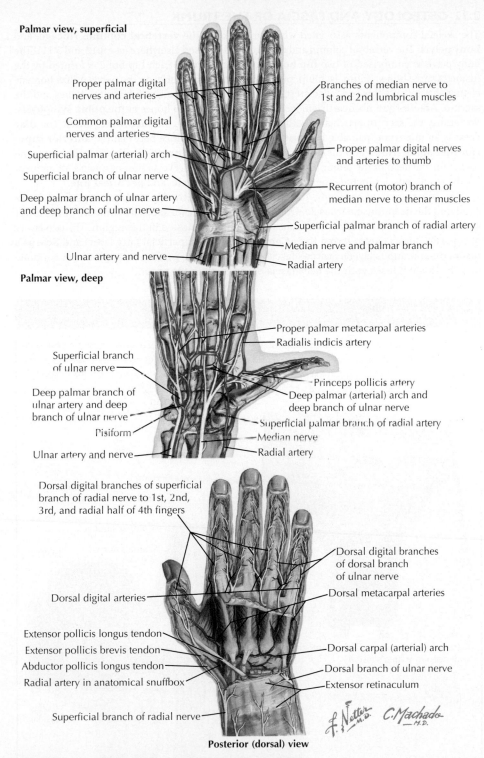

Palmar view, superficial

Proper palmar digital nerves and arteries

Common palmar digital nerves and arteries

Superficial palmar (arterial) arch

Superficial branch of ulnar nerve

Deep palmar branch of ulnar artery and deep branch of ulnar nerve

Ulnar artery and nerve

Branches of median nerve to 1st and 2nd lumbrical muscles

Proper palmar digital nerves and arteries to thumb

Recurrent (motor) branch of median nerve to thenar muscles

Superficial palmar branch of radial artery

Median nerve and palmar branch

Radial artery

Palmar view, deep

Superficial branch of ulnar nerve

Deep palmar branch of ulnar artery and deep branch of ulnar nerve

Pisiform

Ulnar artery and nerve

Proper palmar metacarpal arteries

Radialis indicis artery

Princeps pollicis artery

Deep palmar (arterial) arch and deep branch of ulnar nerve

Superficial palmar branch of radial artery

Median nerve

Radial artery

Dorsal digital branches of superficial branch of radial nerve to 1st, 2nd, 3rd, and radial half of 4th fingers

Dorsal digital arteries

Extensor pollicis longus tendon

Extensor pollicis brevis tendon

Abductor pollicis longus tendon

Radial artery in anatomical snuffbox

Superficial branch of radial nerve

Dorsal digital branches of dorsal branch of ulnar nerve

Dorsal metacarpal arteries

Dorsal carpal (arterial) arch

Dorsal branch of ulnar nerve

Extensor retinaculum

J. Netter M.D.   C. Machado M.D.

Posterior (dorsal) view

Figure 3.31 VESSELS AND NERVES OF THE HAND

3.32 OSTEOLOGY AND FASCIA OF THE TRUNK

The skeletal components associated with the trunk are the **vertebral column**, **ribcage**, and **bony pelvis**. The vertebral column and ribcage are discussed elsewhere (see 3.12 and 5.11). The bony pelvis is comprised of two **hip bones** and the **sacrum**. Each hip bone is formed by the fusion of three bones (ilium, ischium, pubis) and many landmarks on the pelvis utilize nomenclature that reflects this (e.g., iliac crest, ischial spine). Three joints link the hip bones and the sacrum. Anteriorly, a fibrocartilaginous disc joins the two hip bones at the **pubic symphysis**. Posteriorly the sacrum articulates with the two hip bones at the **sacroiliac joints**. The **iliac crest** is an important palpable landmark that spans the distance between the **anterior superior iliac spine** (ASIS) and the **posterior superior iliac spine** (PSIS). The **acetabulum** is the socket for the head of the femur (3.38). Other features that serve as sites of muscle attachment for the trunk muscles include the **pubic crest**, **pubic tubercle**, and **pectineal line**.

Like other areas of the body, the trunk is covered with skin and has superficial fascia overlying the deep muscular fascia. Due to the propensity for fat to accumulate in the lower abdomen, a denser layer of membranous fascia can be identified in this region. The two layers of superficial fascia are referred to as **Camper's fascia** (superficial fatty layer) and **Scarpa's fascia** (membranous layer). Scarpa's fascia extends into the perineum but does not continue into the thigh; it fuses with the deep fascia of the thigh in the groin.

Clinical Focus

The continuity of Scarpa's fascia into the perineum has clinical significance. Trauma to the perineum can result in urethral rupture or tearing of erectile tissue. With this type of injury, urine and blood can spread superiorly into the abdominal wall deep to Scarpa's fascia. In contrast, fluid cannot spread into the thigh due to the fusion of Scarpa's fascia to the deep fascia of the thigh.

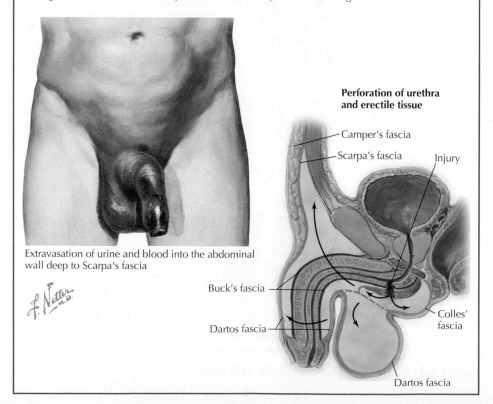

Extravasation of urine and blood into the abdominal wall deep to Scarpa's fascia

Perforation of urethra and erectile tissue

Camper's fascia

Scarpa's fascia

Injury

Buck's fascia

Dartos fascia

Colles' fascia

Dartos fascia

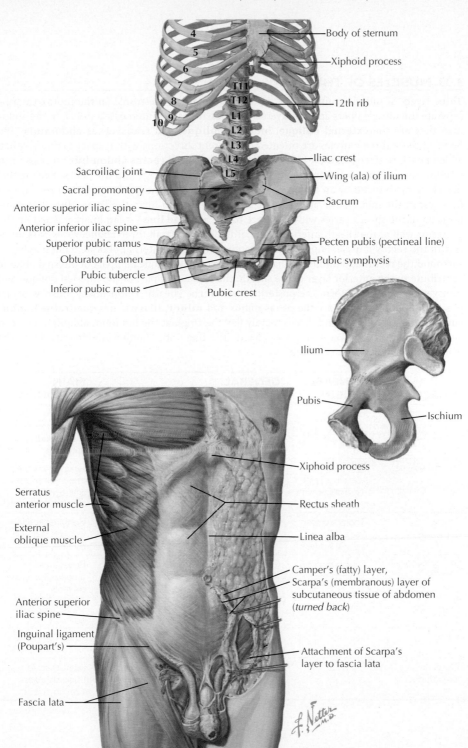

Figure 3.32 OSTEOLOGY AND FASCIA OF THE TRUNK

3.33 MUSCLES OF THE TRUNK

Three layers of muscle comprise the anterolateral part of the trunk. In the thorax the ribs separate the muscle fibers and the layered muscles are called intercostals (5.11). In the abdomen they are the **external oblique**, **internal oblique**, and **transversus abdominis**. The fibers of these three muscles are oriented in different directions with respect to one another, which provides strength to the abdominal wall. The paired **rectus abdominis** muscles form a supportive column between the inferior margin of the ribcage and the pelvis. Each rectus muscle is surrounded by an aponeurotic sheath formed by the tendons of the three-layered muscles; in the midline the aponeuroses come together to form the **linea alba**. The composition of the sheath varies with reference to the **arcuate line**—a landmark created on the posterior wall of the sheath inferior to the umbilicus when all three aponeuroses pass anterior to the rectus muscle. Superior to the arcuate line, the internal oblique tendon splits to surround the rectus abdominis, so that only the external oblique and part of internal oblique contribute to the anterior layer of the sheath; the remaining part of the internal oblique and transversus abdominis form the posterior layer of the sheath. The primary muscles of the posterior abdominal wall are the **psoas major** and **minor**, **iliacus**, and **quadratus lumborum**. The psoas muscles and iliacus mainly flex the thigh at the hip joint, although they can flex the trunk if the lower extremity is fixed. The quadratus lumborum laterally flexes the trunk and stabilizes the twelfth rib.

MUSCLE	GENERAL ORIGIN	GENERAL INSERTION	INNERVATION	MAIN ACTIONS
External oblique	Lower ribs	Linea alba, pubic tubercle, iliac crest	Anterior rami of T7–T12 spinal nerves	Flexes and rotates trunk, compresses and supports abdominal contents
Internal oblique	Thoracolumbar fascia, iliac crest, inguinal ligament	Lower ribs, linea alba, pubic bone	Anterior rami of T7–T12, L1 spinal nerves	Flexes and rotates trunk, compresses and supports abdominal contents
Transversus abdominis	Thoracolumbar fascia, iliac crest, inguinal ligament	Linea alba, pubic bone	Anterior rami of T7–T12, L1 spinal nerves	Compresses and supports abdominal contents
Rectus abdominis	Pubic symphysis, pubic crest	Costal margin, xiphoid process	Anterior rami of T7–T12 spinal nerves	Flexes trunk, supports abdominal contents
Psoas major	Lumbar vertebrae	Lesser trochanter of femur	Anterior rami of L1–L3 spinal nerves	Flexes thigh at hip joint
Iliacus	Iliac fossa	Lesser trochanter of femur	Femoral nerve	Flexes thigh at hip joint
Quadratus lumborum	Iliac crest	12th rib	Anterior rami of T12–L4 spinal nerves	Laterally flexes trunk, stabilizes 12th rib

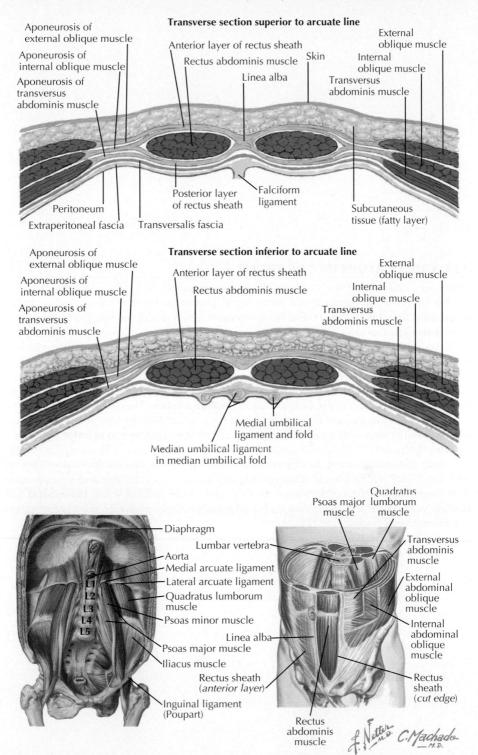

Transverse section superior to arcuate line

Aponeurosis of external oblique muscle
Aponeurosis of internal oblique muscle
Aponeurosis of transversus abdominis muscle

Anterior layer of rectus sheath
Rectus abdominis muscle
Linea alba
Skin

External oblique muscle
Internal oblique muscle
Transversus abdominis muscle

Peritoneum
Extraperitoneal fascia
Transversalis fascia
Posterior layer of rectus sheath
Falciform ligament
Subcutaneous tissue (fatty layer)

Transverse section inferior to arcuate line

Aponeurosis of external oblique muscle
Aponeurosis of internal oblique muscle
Aponeurosis of transversus abdominis muscle

Anterior layer of rectus sheath
Rectus abdominis muscle

External oblique muscle
Internal oblique muscle
Transversus abdominis muscle

Medial umbilical ligament and fold
Median umbilical ligament in median umbilical fold

Diaphragm
Lumbar vertebra
Aorta
Medial arcuate ligament
Lateral arcuate ligament
Quadratus lumborum muscle
Psoas minor muscle
Linea alba
Psoas major muscle
Iliacus muscle
Inguinal ligament (Poupart)

L1
L2
L3
L4
L5

Quadratus lumborum muscle
Psoas major muscle

Transversus abdominis muscle
External abdominal oblique muscle
Internal abdominal oblique muscle
Rectus sheath (cut edge)
Rectus abdominis muscle
Rectus sheath (anterior layer)

Figure 3.33 MUSCLES OF THE TRUNK

3.34 VASCULATURE OF THE TRUNK

The layered muscles and skin of the trunk receive arterial blood mainly via segmental arteries that travel around the body wall. In the upper part of the trunk these arteries are called **intercostal arteries** and they travel along the inferior surfaces of the ribs (5.11). **Posterior intercostal arteries** arise from the thoracic aorta and supply the posterior and lateral parts of the trunk. **Anterior intercostal arteries** originate from the internal thoracic arteries and deliver blood to the anterior part of the trunk. In the event of an occlusion in either the aorta or internal thoracic artery, the anterior and posterior intercostal arteries can develop anastomotic connections to facilitate uninterrupted blood flow. The segmental arteries that arise from the abdominal part of the aorta are called **lumbar arteries.** These supply muscles of the posterior abdominal wall and then travel around the trunk to feed the layered muscles. Blood supply from the segmental arteries is supplemented by the **superior** and **inferior epigastric arteries** that travel within the rectus sheath deep to the rectus muscles. These arteries supply the rectus abdominis, as well as adjacent skin and musculature. Venous drainage occurs via both superficial and deep veins. **Thoracoepigastric veins** drain the skin and subcutaneous tissue superiorly to the axillary veins and inferiorly to the femoral veins. **Intercostal** and **lumbar veins** travel with their companion arteries and drain mainly to the azygos system and inferior vena cava (4.12, 6.12).

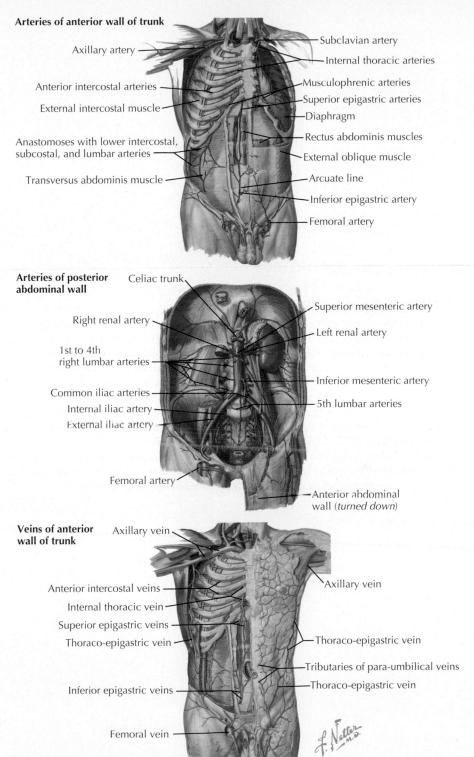

Arteries of anterior wall of trunk

Axillary artery

Anterior intercostal arteries

External intercostal muscle

Anastomoses with lower intercostal, subcostal, and lumbar arteries

Transversus abdominis muscle

Subclavian artery

Internal thoracic arteries

Musculophrenic arteries

Superior epigastric arteries

Diaphragm

Rectus abdominis muscles

External oblique muscle

Arcuate line

Inferior epigastric artery

Femoral artery

Arteries of posterior abdominal wall

Celiac trunk

Right renal artery

1st to 4th right lumbar arteries

Common iliac arteries

Internal iliac artery

External iliac artery

Femoral artery

Superior mesenteric artery

Left renal artery

Inferior mesenteric artery

5th lumbar arteries

Anterior abdominal wall (*turned down*)

Veins of anterior wall of trunk

Axillary vein

Anterior intercostal veins

Internal thoracic vein

Superior epigastric veins

Thoraco-epigastric vein

Inferior epigastric veins

Femoral vein

Axillary vein

Thoraco-epigastric vein

Tributaries of para-umbilical veins

Thoraco-epigastric vein

Figure 3.34 VESSELS OF THE TRUNK

3.35 NERVES OF THE TRUNK

The skin and musculature of the trunk receive innervation from the thoracic and lumbar spinal nerves. The anterolateral portion is innervated by the anterior rami of the T1–T11 spinal nerves (**intercostal nerves**), **subcostal nerves** (T12), and **iliohypogastric nerves** (L1). As the anterior rami travel around the body wall from posterior to anterior, they give off lateral cutaneous branches and then terminate as anterior cutaneous branches. Notice that the T7 dermatome is located approximately at the level of the xiphoid process, T10 is at the umbilicus, and the L1 dermatome is associated with the pubic bone. The muscles of the posterior abdominal wall receive innervation from branches of the **lumbar plexus**, which is formed by the anterior rami of L1–L4. These nerves intermingle within the substance of the psoas major muscle before giving rise to various branches that are destined for the trunk, pelvis, or lower extremity. The psoas muscles and quadratus lumborum receive direct muscular branches from the plexus, while the iliacus is innervated by the femoral nerve.

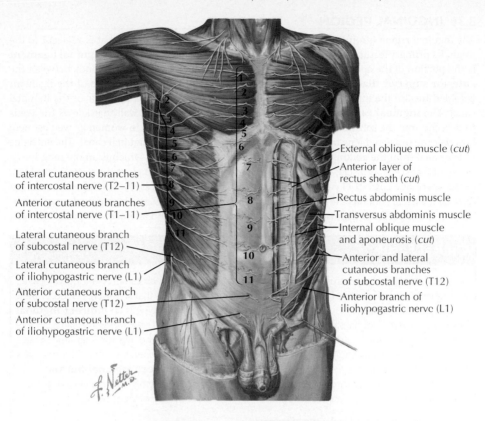

Lateral cutaneous branches
of intercostal nerve (T2–11)

Anterior cutaneous branches
of intercostal nerve (T1–11)

Lateral cutaneous branch
of subcostal nerve (T12)

Lateral cutaneous branch
of iliohypogastric nerve (L1)

Anterior cutaneous branch
of subcostal nerve (T12)

Anterior cutaneous branch
of iliohypogastric nerve (L1)

External oblique muscle (*cut*)

Anterior layer of
rectus sheath (*cut*)

Rectus abdominis muscle

Transversus abdominis muscle

Internal oblique muscle
and aponeurosis (*cut*)

Anterior and lateral
cutaneous branches
of subcostal nerve (T12)

Anterior branch of
iliohypogastric nerve (L1)

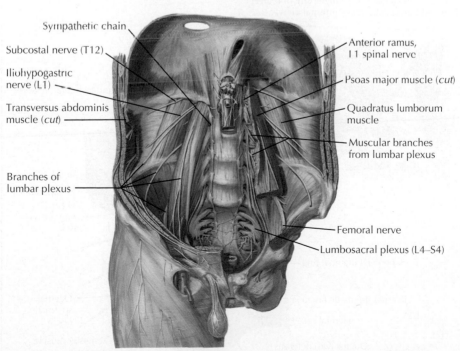

Sympathetic chain

Subcostal nerve (T12)

Iliohypogastric
nerve (L1)

Transversus abdominis
muscle (*cut*)

Branches of
lumbar plexus

Anterior ramus,
11 spinal nerve

Psoas major muscle (*cut*)

Quadratus lumborum
muscle

Muscular branches
from lumbar plexus

Femoral nerve

Lumbosacral plexus (L4–S4)

Figure 3.35 NERVES OF THE TRUNK

3.36 INGUINAL REGION

The inguinal region (groin) is the inferior portion of the abdominal wall that is adjacent to the thigh. Its primary features are the inguinal ligament and inguinal canal. The **inguinal ligament** is the portion of the aponeurosis of the external abdominal oblique that extends between the **anterior superior iliac spine** and **pubic tubercle** (3.32). The inferior edge of the ligament is folded toward the interior so that it creates a "trough" that forms the floor of the inguinal canal. The **inguinal canal** is a passageway through the abdominal wall that allows the testis to descend into the scrotum during development. The canal forms in women as well as men; however the ovary remains in the pelvis and does not traverse the inguinal canal. The entrance to the canal from the abdominal cavity is the **deep inguinal ring**, which is an opening into a sleeve of transversalis fascia, similar to the opening of a finger on a glove. In men the contents of the spermatic cord (9.11) are enclosed by this fascia as they traverse the inguinal canal; in women the canal contains the round ligament of the uterus (Fig. 9.4). The inguinal canal terminates at the **superficial inguinal ring** that is located superior and lateral to the pubic tubercle.

Clinical Focus

An inguinal hernia is a protrusion of intra-abdominal contents, such as fat or a loop of bowel, through the abdominal wall. There are two types of inguinal hernias that are distinguished by their relationship to the inferior epigastric vessels. The most common type is an **indirect inguinal hernia** where the hernial sac protrudes through the deep inguinal ring, taking the same course as the testis did during its descent. Indirect hernias are lateral to the inferior epigastric vessels and are surrounded by the same fascial layers that surround the spermatic cord. Hernial sacs that project medial to the inferior epigastric vessels are called **direct inguinal hernias**. This type of hernia protrudes through an area called the inguinal (Hesselbach's) triangle and is most often due to factors that weaken the abdominal wall, such as aging or obesity.

Inguinal (Hesselbach's) triangle: site of a direct inguinal hernia (posterior, internal view)

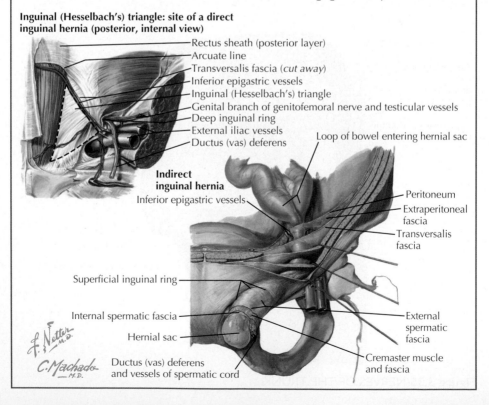

Rectus sheath (posterior layer)
Arcuate line
Transversalis fascia (*cut away*)
Inferior epigastric vessels
Inguinal (Hesselbach's) triangle
Genital branch of genitofemoral nerve and testicular vessels
Deep inguinal ring
External iliac vessels
Ductus (vas) deferens

Loop of bowel entering hernial sac

Indirect inguinal hernia
Inferior epigastric vessels

Peritoneum
Extraperitoneal fascia
Transversalis fascia

Superficial inguinal ring

Internal spermatic fascia

Hernial sac

External spermatic fascia

Cremaster muscle and fascia

Ductus (vas) deferens and vessels of spermatic cord

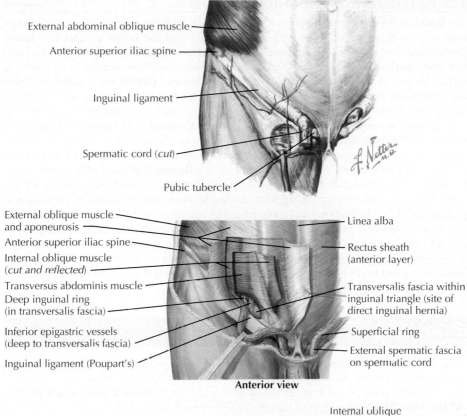

Anterior view

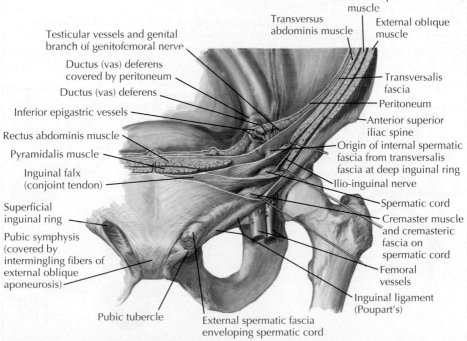

Figure 3.36 INGUINAL REGION

3.37 OSTEOLOGY OF THE THIGH AND HIP

The **femur** is the bone of the thigh that participates in both the hip and knee joints. Proximally the femur exhibits a **head** with a small divot called the **fovea**; **greater** and **lesser trochanters** that serve as sites of muscle attachment; and an **intertrochanteric crest** and **line** between the trochanters. The shaft is unremarkable apart from a ridge on its posterior surface known as the **linea aspera**. The distal end features **lateral** and **medial condyles** and an articular surface for the patella. The **hip joint** is a ball-and-socket synovial joint that allows flexion, extension, abduction, adduction, medial rotation, and lateral rotation (Fig. 1.4). The joint is comprised of an articulation between the **head of the femur** and the lunate surface of the **acetabulum**. The acetabular notch between the edges of the lunate surface is spanned by the **transverse acetabular ligament**. A ring of fibrocartilage, the **labrum**, deepens the acetabulum to help hold the femoral head. The **ligament of head of femur** connects the fovea to the acetabulum and conveys blood vessels to the femoral head. There are three major ligaments that support the hip joint, named by the bones they connect (**iliofemoral**, **pubofemoral**, and **ischiofemoral ligaments**). The ligaments spiral around the joint so that they become looser during flexion and tighter during extension; thus they are designed to prevent hyperextension of the femur. This is important during standing because the weight of the body is directed posterior to the hip joint, which promotes extension of the femur. The ligaments tighten to counteract this, helping to maintain upright posture without significant muscle fatigue.

Clinical Focus

Hip dislocations are typically due to trauma or a congenital condition. Motor vehicle accidents are a common source of trauma to the hip, for example, the femur can be pushed out of the hip socket if the knee collides with the dashboard. **Developmental dysplasia of the hip (DDH)** is a congenital condition where the acetabulum does not form properly, predisposing the femur to dislocation. It is common in babies that were in breech position during pregnancy, as this position may prevent normal hip development. **Hip fractures** are common in the elderly and frequently occur in the femoral neck or along the intertrochanteric line. Fractures of the femoral neck often disrupt arteries that supply the femoral head, putting the head at risk for necrosis.

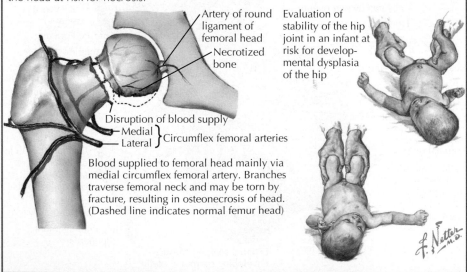

Artery of round ligament of femoral head

Necrotized bone

Evaluation of stability of the hip joint in an infant at risk for developmental dysplasia of the hip

Disruption of blood supply
Medial
Lateral } Circumflex femoral arteries

Blood supplied to femoral head mainly via medial circumflex femoral artery. Branches traverse femoral neck and may be torn by fracture, resulting in osteonecrosis of head. (Dashed line indicates normal femur head)

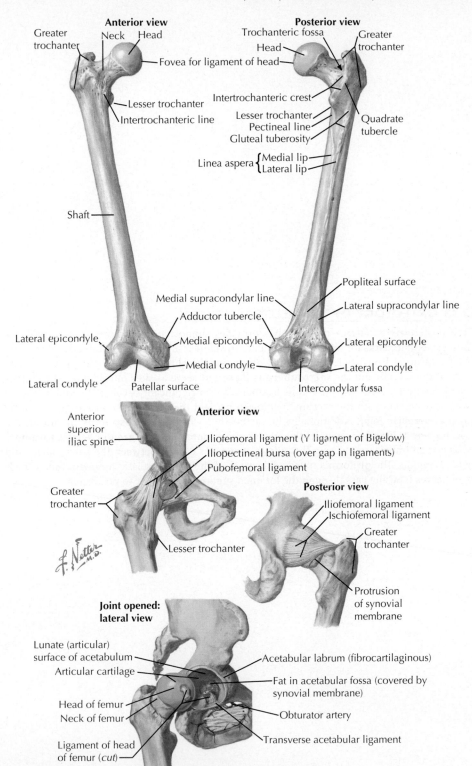

Anterior view

Greater trochanter

Neck

Head

Fovea for ligament of head

Lesser trochanter

Intertrochanteric line

Shaft

Lateral epicondyle

Lateral condyle

Medial supracondylar line

Adductor tubercle

Medial epicondyle

Medial condyle

Patellar surface

Posterior view

Trochanteric fossa

Head

Greater trochanter

Intertrochanteric crest

Lesser trochanter

Pectineal line

Gluteal tuberosity

Quadrate tubercle

Linea aspera { Medial lip / Lateral lip }

Popliteal surface

Lateral supracondylar line

Lateral epicondyle

Lateral condyle

Intercondylar fossa

Anterior view

Anterior superior iliac spine

Iliofemoral ligament (Y ligament of Bigelow)

Iliopectineal bursa (over gap in ligaments)

Pubofemoral ligament

Greater trochanter

Lesser trochanter

Posterior view

Iliofemoral ligament

Ischiofemoral ligament

Greater trochanter

Protrusion of synovial membrane

f. Netter
m.d.

Joint opened: lateral view

Lunate (articular) surface of acetabulum

Articular cartilage

Head of femur

Neck of femur

Ligament of head of femur (cut)

Acetabular labrum (fibrocartilaginous)

Fat in acetabular fossa (covered by synovial membrane)

Obturator artery

Transverse acetabular ligament

Figure 3.37 OSTEOLOGY OF THE THIGH AND HIP

3.38 OSTEOLOGY OF THE GLUTEAL REGION

The posterolateral surface of the pelvis provides support for the gluteal region and has numerous landmarks for muscle attachment. The gluteal surface of the ilium exhibits several ridges (**gluteal lines**) that separate the origins of the gluteal muscles. The posterior surface of the sacrum and the **sacrotuberous ligament** serve as sites of origin for the gluteus maximus muscle. The sacrotuberous ligament is also significant because it counteracts the weight of the body on the sacrum, helping to prevent the sacrum from rotating anteriorly in the sacroiliac joint. Additionally, in partnership with the **sacrospinous ligament**, the sacrotuberous ligament converts the greater sciatic notch into the **greater sciatic foramen**, which is an important opening that allows structures to pass between the pelvic cavity and gluteal region. The piriformis muscle fills most of the greater sciatic foramen; thus vessels and nerves typically pass through the foramen superior or inferior to piriformis.

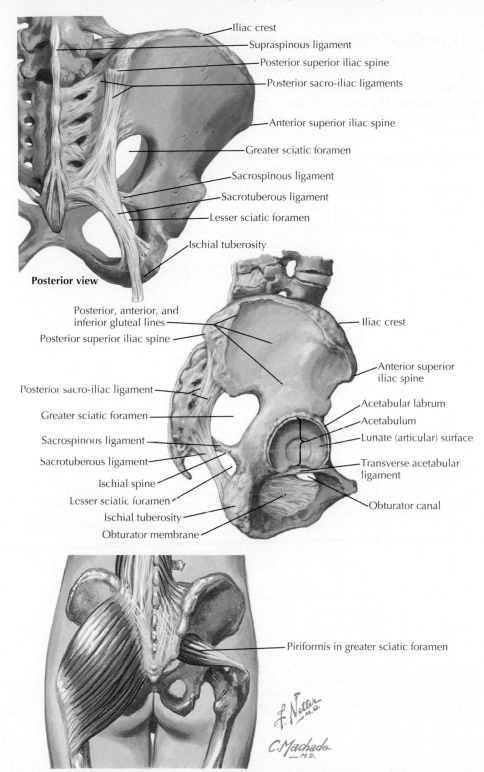

Iliac crest
Supraspinous ligament
Posterior superior iliac spine
Posterior sacro-iliac ligaments
Anterior superior iliac spine
Greater sciatic foramen
Sacrospinous ligament
Sacrotuberous ligament
Lesser sciatic foramen
Ischial tuberosity

Posterior view

Posterior, anterior, and inferior gluteal lines
Posterior superior iliac spine
Posterior sacro-iliac ligament
Greater sciatic foramen
Sacrospinous ligament
Sacrotuberous ligament
Ischial spine
Lesser sciatic foramen
Ischial tuberosity
Obturator membrane

Iliac crest
Anterior superior iliac spine
Acetabular labrum
Acetabulum
Lunate (articular) surface
Transverse acetabular ligament
Obturator canal

Piriformis in greater sciatic foramen

Figure 3.38 OSTEOLOGY OF THE GLUTEAL REGION

3.39 MUSCLES OF THE THIGH AND GLUTEAL REGION

The deep fascia of the thigh **(fascia lata)** surrounds the thigh like a stocking and has intermuscular septa that divide the thigh into three compartments. The **anterior compartment** contains muscles that primarily flex the hip joint and extend the knee joint; these muscles are mainly innervated by the femoral nerve. The **medial compartment** is comprised of muscles that adduct the thigh at the hip joint. The adductors are innervated by the obturator nerve, except for pectineus that is innervated by the femoral nerve.

Anterior Compartment of Thigh

MUSCLE	GENERAL ORIGIN	GENERAL INSERTION	INNERVATION	MAIN ACTIONS
Sartorius	Anterior superior iliac spine (ASIS)	Anteromedial aspect of proximal tibia	Femoral nerve	Flexes, abducts, and laterally rotates thigh at hip joint; flexes leg at knee joint
Iliopsoas	Lumbar vertebrae (psoas), iliac fossa (iliacus)	Lesser trochanter of femur	Anterior rami of L1–L3 spinal nerves (psoas), femoral nerve (iliacus)	Flexes thigh at hip joint
Quadriceps				
Rectus femoris	Anterior inferior iliac spine (AIIS)	Tibial tuberosity via the patellar ligament	Femoral nerve	Flexes thigh at hip joint, extends leg at knee joint
Vastus lateralis	Linea aspera			Extends leg at knee joint
Vastus medialis	Linea aspera			
Vastus intermedius	Anterior/lateral surfaces of femur			

Medial Compartment of Thigh

MUSCLE	GENERAL ORIGIN	GENERAL INSERTION	INNERVATION	MAIN ACTIONS
Pectineus	Superior ramus of pubis	Posteromedial part of proximal femur	Femoral nerve	Adducts and flexes thigh at hip joint
Adductor longus	Body of pubis	Linea aspera	Obturator nerve	Adducts thigh at hip joint
Adductor brevis	Body and inferior ramus of pubis	Linea aspera	Obturator nerve	Adducts thigh at hip joint
Adductor magnus	Ischiopubic ramus, ischial tuberosity	Linea aspera (adductor part), adductor tubercle (hamstring part)	Obturator nerve (adductor part), tibial division of sciatic nerve (hamstring part)	Adducts thigh at hip joint; hamstring part also extends the thigh
Gracilis	Body and inferior ramus of pubis	Anteromedial aspect of proximal tibia	Obturator nerve	Adducts thigh at hip joint, flexes leg at knee joint

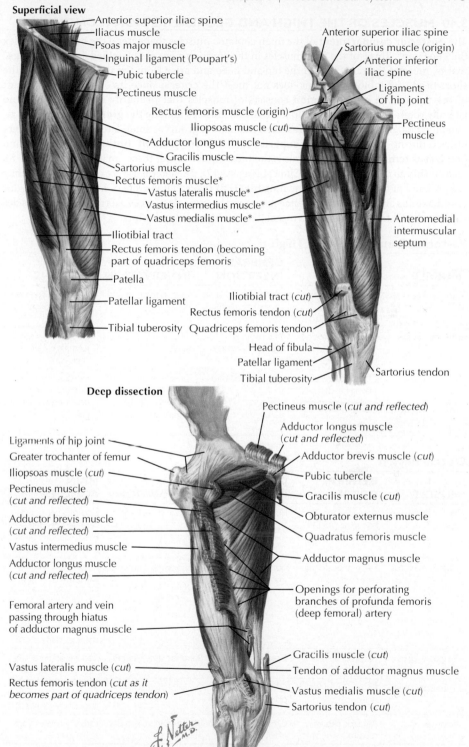

Figure 3.39 MUSCLES OF THE ANTERIOR AND MEDIAL THIGH.
*Muscles of quadriceps femoris.

3.40 MUSCLES OF THE THIGH AND GLUTEAL REGION *(CONTINUED)*

The **posterior compartment** of the thigh contains muscles that extend the hip joint and flex the knee joint. Three of the four muscles in the compartment are classified as "**hamstrings**," that is, muscles that act on both the hip and knee and arise from the ischial tuberosity. The short head of the biceps femoris does not meet the criteria since its origin is on the shaft of the femur. The **gluteal region** consists of muscles that primarily extend, abduct, and laterally rotate the femur at the hip joint. These muscles include the **gluteal muscles** (maximus, medius, minimus), **tensor fasciae latae**, and a group of small lateral rotators that are utilized during gait (**piriformis**, **superior** and **inferior gemelli**, **obturator internus**, and **quadratus femoris**). The piriformis is the most significant of these small muscles due to its relationship to the sciatic nerve (Clinical Focus 3.42). The lateral aspect of the thigh exhibits a thick band of fascia lata called the **iliotibial (IT) tract** that is a site of insertion for the gluteus maximus and tensor fasciae latae muscles. The opposing forces exerted by these muscles support the IT tract, which helps to stabilize the hip and knee joints.

Posterior Compartment of Thigh

MUSCLE	GENERAL ORIGIN	GENERAL INSERTION	INNERVATION	MAIN ACTIONS
Semimembranosus	Ischial tuberosity	Medial tibial condyle (posteromedial part)	Tibial division of sciatic nerve	Extends thigh at hip joint, flexes leg at knee joint
Semitendinosus	Ischial tuberosity	Anteromedial aspect of proximal tibia	Tibial division of sciatic nerve	Extends thigh at hip joint, flexes leg at knee joint
Biceps femoris	Ischial tuberosity (long head), linea aspera (short head)	Head of the fibula	Tibial division of sciatic nerve (long head), Common fibular division of sciatic nerve (short head)	Extends thigh at hip joint (long head), flexes leg at knee joint

Gluteal Region

MUSCLE	GENERAL ORIGIN	GENERAL INSERTION	INNERVATION	MAIN ACTIONS
Tensor fasciae latae	Anterior superior iliac spine (ASIS)	Iliotibial tract	Superior gluteal nerve	Stabilizes pelvis and helps to keep the knee extended by tensing the IT tract
Gluteus maximus	Sacrum, posterior surface of ilium, sacrotuberous ligament	Iliotibial tract, gluteal tuberosity	Inferior gluteal nerve	Extends and laterally rotates thigh at hip joint (extension occurs mainly when working against resistance, e.g., climbing stairs), stabilizes pelvis
Gluteus medius	Posterior surface of ilium	Greater trochanter of femur	Superior gluteal nerve	Abducts and medially rotates thigh at hip joint; prevents tilting of the pelvis when opposite leg is raised
Gluteus minimus	Posterior surface of ilium	Greater trochanter of femur	Superior gluteal nerve	
Piriformis	Anterior part of sacrum	Greater trochanter of femur	Branches from sacral plexus	Laterally rotates thigh at hip joint

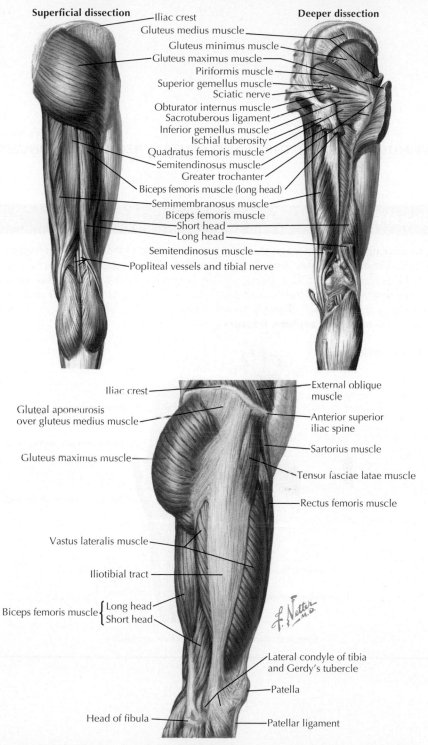

Superficial dissection

Iliac crest
Gluteus medius muscle
Gluteus minimus muscle
Gluteus maximus muscle
Piriformis muscle
Superior gemellus muscle
Sciatic nerve
Obturator internus muscle
Sacrotuberous ligament
Inferior gemellus muscle
Ischial tuberosity
Quadratus femoris muscle
Semitendinosus muscle
Greater trochanter
Biceps femoris muscle (long head)
Semimembranosus muscle
Biceps femoris muscle
Short head
Long head
Semitendinosus muscle
Popliteal vessels and tibial nerve

Deeper dissection

Iliac crest
External oblique muscle
Gluteal aponeurosis over gluteus medius muscle
Anterior superior iliac spine
Gluteus maximus muscle
Sartorius muscle
Tensor fasciae latae muscle
Rectus femoris muscle
Vastus lateralis muscle
Iliotibial tract
Biceps femoris muscle { Long head
Short head
Lateral condyle of tibia and Gerdy's tubercle
Patella
Head of fibula
Patellar ligament

Figure 3.40 MUSCLES OF THE POSTERIOR THIGH AND GLUTEAL REGION

3.40 MUSCLES OF THE THIGH AND GLUTEAL REGION (*CONTINUED*)

Clinical Focus

A hamstring strain is an injury where muscles or tendons of the hamstrings are stretched or torn. Hamstring strains are common in athletes that quickly accelerate because this requires strong extension at the hip joint. Kicking with an extended knee may also tear the hamstrings by stretching them beyond their normal extent. Severe injuries may produce a complete tear of the hamstrings from their origin on the ischial tuberosity, or cause a small piece of bone to detach with the tendon (**avulsion fracture**).

Hamstring strains

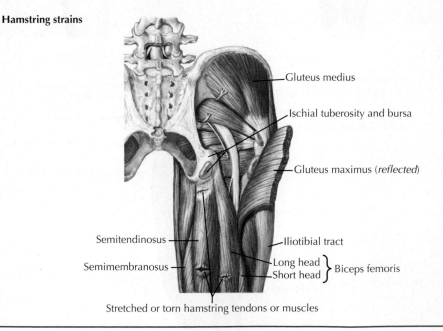

- Gluteus medius
- Ischial tuberosity and bursa
- Gluteus maximus (*reflected*)
- Semitendinosus
- Iliotibial tract
- Semimembranosus
- Long head
- Short head
- Biceps femoris

Stretched or torn hamstring tendons or muscles

Clinical Focus (Continued)

The gluteus medius and minimus stabilize the pelvis during walking (i.e., keep it level when one foot is lifted off the ground). The **Trendelenburg test** is one method of testing the strength of these muscles and the stability of the pelvis. A positive test is when the pelvis drops on the side that is lifted from the floor, indicating that the hip is unstable or that the gluteus medius and minimus on the side of the weight-bearing leg are not functioning properly to hold the pelvis and greater trochanter in close proximity. Injury to the superior gluteal nerve is one potential cause of a positive Trendelenburg test.

Iliotibial tract (band) syndrome is a condition common in athletes that frequently flex and extend the knee (e.g., runners, cyclists). This repetitive motion can cause inflammation of the bursa between the IT tract and the lateral epicondyle of the femur, which produces pain and allows friction between these structures.

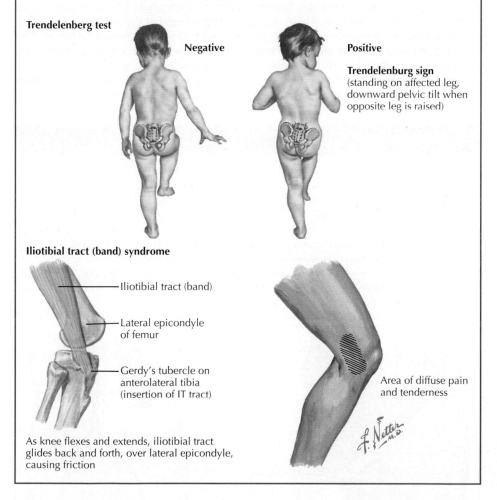

Trendelenberg test

Negative

Positive

Trendelenburg sign
(standing on affected leg, downward pelvic tilt when opposite leg is raised)

Iliotibial tract (band) syndrome

Iliotibial tract (band)

Lateral epicondyle of femur

Gerdy's tubercle on anterolateral tibia (insertion of IT tract)

Area of diffuse pain and tenderness

As knee flexes and extends, iliotibial tract glides back and forth, over lateral epicondyle, causing friction

3.41 VASCULATURE OF THE THIGH AND GLUTEAL REGION

The neurovascular structures in the proximal thigh are located in the **femoral triangle**, a region defined by the inguinal ligament, sartorius, and adductor longus. The femoral vessels are continuous with the external iliac vessels—the name "femoral" is applied when the vessels pass deep to the inguinal ligament. The femoral vessels and deep inguinal lymph nodes are surrounded by a fascial sheath known as the **femoral sheath**; the medial compartment of the sheath that contains lymph nodes and lymphatic vessels is called the **femoral canal**. The **femoral artery** and its **deep femoral branch** provide most of the arterial blood to the thigh. **Perforating branches** of the deep femoral artery supply the posterior compartment of the thigh, while **medial** and **lateral femoral circumflex branches** feed the hip joint. The medial circumflex artery is the primary source that supplies the head of the femur. The gluteal region receives blood supply from branches of the internal iliac artery, specifically the **superior** and **inferior gluteal arteries**. The superior gluteal artery enters the gluteal region superior to piriformis and travels between the gluteus medius and gluteus minimus. The inferior gluteal artery emerges from the pelvic cavity inferior to piriformis and subsequently divides into multiple branches that mainly supply gluteus maximus. Veins accompany the femoral and gluteal vessels and are tributaries of the inferior vena cava. Tributaries of the **great saphenous vein** drain the skin and superficial fascia of the thigh. An opening in the fascia lata, the **saphenous opening**, allows the great saphenous vein to drain into the femoral vein. The lymphatics of the lower extremity drain to the **superficial** and **deep inguinal lymph nodes** that are located in the groin near the saphenous opening.

Clinical Focus

A **femoral hernia** is a protrusion of fat or a loop of bowel through the femoral canal. Both femoral hernias and inguinal hernias occur in the groin; however they can be distinguished by the location of the hernial sac relative to the inguinal ligament. Inguinal hernias produce a bulge superior to the inguinal ligament, while femoral hernias produce a lump inferior to the inguinal ligament. The femoral artery is found at the midpoint of the inguinal ligament ("midinguinal point") and is identified in this location for **catheterization** or to take a **femoral pulse**. In clinical settings the portion of the femoral artery proximal to the deep femoral branch is often called the "common" femoral artery, while distal to the branch it is called the "superficial" femoral artery. Although inconsistent with standard nomenclature, this usage is helpful in more precisely describing the location of arterial disease.

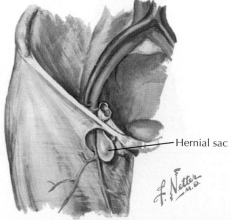

Hernial sac

Course of hernial sac through femoral ring, femoral canal, and saphenous hiatus

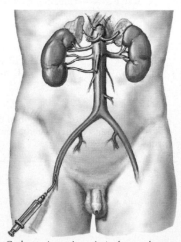

Catheter introduced via femoral artery

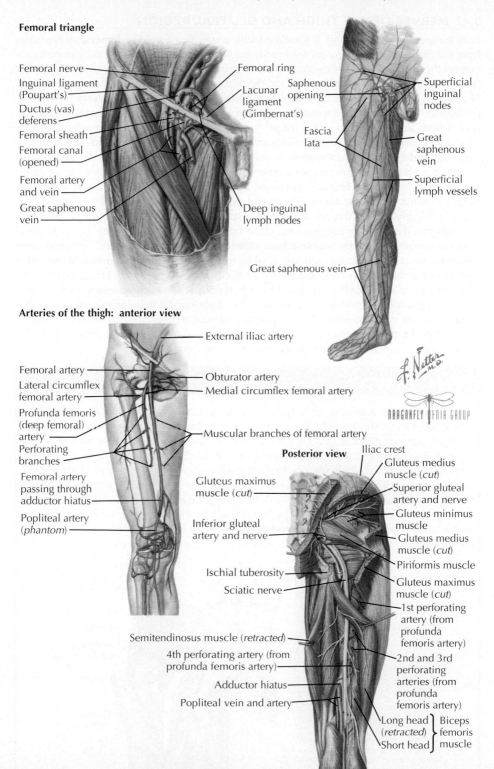

Femoral triangle

Femoral nerve

Inguinal ligament (Poupart's)

Ductus (vas) deferens

Femoral sheath

Femoral canal (opened)

Femoral artery and vein

Great saphenous vein

Femoral ring

Lacunar ligament (Gimbernat's)

Saphenous opening

Deep inguinal lymph nodes

Superficial inguinal nodes

Fascia lata

Great saphenous vein

Superficial lymph vessels

Great saphenous vein

Arteries of the thigh: anterior view

Femoral artery

Lateral circumflex femoral artery

Profunda femoris (deep femoral) artery

Perforating branches

Femoral artery passing through adductor hiatus

Popliteal artery (*phantom*)

External iliac artery

Obturator artery

Medial circumflex femoral artery

Muscular branches of femoral artery

Posterior view   Iliac crest

Gluteus maximus muscle (*cut*)

Inferior gluteal artery and nerve

Ischial tuberosity

Sciatic nerve

Semitendinosus muscle (*retracted*)

4th perforating artery (from profunda femoris artery)

Adductor hiatus

Popliteal vein and artery

Gluteus medius muscle (*cut*)

Superior gluteal artery and nerve

Gluteus minimus muscle

Gluteus medius muscle (*cut*)

Piriformis muscle

Gluteus maximus muscle (*cut*)

1st perforating artery (from profunda femoris artery)

2nd and 3rd perforating arteries (from profunda femoris artery)

Long head (*retracted*) / Short head } Biceps femoris muscle

Figure 3.41 VESSELS OF THE THIGH AND GLUTEAL REGION

3.42 NERVES OF THE THIGH AND GLUTEAL REGION

Each compartment of the thigh is associated with a specific nerve. The **femoral nerve** arises from the lumbar plexus and passes deep to the inguinal ligament to enter the anterior compartment of the thigh. Its branches innervate all the muscles in the anterior compartment, one muscle in the medial compartment (pectineus), and the skin of the anterior thigh and anteromedial leg. The skin on the lateral thigh is innervated by the **lateral femoral cutaneous nerve**. Apart from pectineus, the muscles in the medial compartment are innervated by the **obturator nerve**. This nerve travels along the lateral wall of the pelvic cavity and enters the thigh through the obturator canal. The obturator nerve divides into anterior and posterior branches that are named by their relationship to the adductor brevis muscle. In addition to supplying adductor muscles, the anterior branch also provides cutaneous innervation to skin on the medial thigh. The posterior compartment of the thigh receives innervation from the two divisions of the sciatic nerve—the **tibial** and **common fibular nerves**. The **sciatic nerve** is the largest branch of the sacral plexus. It leaves the pelvic cavity through the greater sciatic foramen inferior to piriformis, and then descends into the posterior compartment of the thigh. It typically divides into its two terminal branches just proximal to the popliteal fossa, although the branch point varies. The tibial nerve innervates the three hamstrings and part of adductor magnus, while the common fibular nerve innervates the short head of the biceps femoris. Neither nerve innervates skin of the posterior thigh; cutaneous innervation is provided by the **posterior femoral cutaneous nerve**. The gluteal region receives innervation primarily from the **superior** and **inferior gluteal nerves** that travel with their companion vessels. The gluteus maximus is innervated by the inferior gluteal nerve, while the gluteus medius and minimus are innervated by the superior gluteal nerve. The small lateral rotators receive muscular branches from the sacral plexus.

Clinical Focus

The lateral femoral cutaneous nerve typically travels deep to the inguinal ligament or pierces it near the ASIS. It may be compressed in this location (**meralgia paresthetica**), resulting in tingling, pain, or numbness over the lateral thigh. Individuals that wear tight pants or accessories in this region (e.g., a tool belt) are particularly at risk. **Sciatica** is a common ailment and is characterized by nerve pain that radiates from the lower back or buttock down the posterior part of the thigh. Sciatica is often caused by compression of one or more of the spinal nerves that contribute to the sciatic nerve (L4–S3), for example due to a herniated disc or vertebral bone spur. The sciatic nerve itself can be compressed by the piriformis muscle as it exits the greater sciatic foramen (**piriformis syndrome**). In some individuals a portion of the sciatic nerve passes through the piriformis muscle, putting it at greater risk for compression.

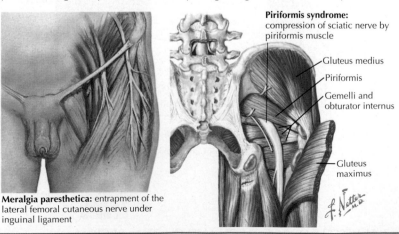

Piriformis syndrome: compression of sciatic nerve by piriformis muscle

Gluteus medius

Piriformis

Gemelli and obturator internus

Gluteus maximus

Meralgia paresthetica: entrapment of the lateral femoral cutaneous nerve under inguinal ligament

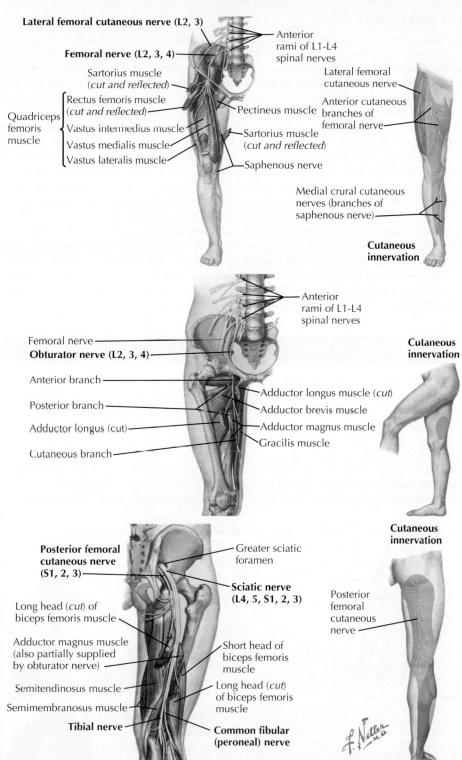

Figure 3.42 NERVES OF THE THIGH AND GLUTEAL REGION

3.43 KNEE JOINT

The **knee joint** is a large synovial hinge joint that includes tibiofemoral and patellofemoral articulations. Its primary movements are flexion and extension, although the laxity between the joint surfaces allows some degree of rotation. The tibiofemoral articulation is between the **condyles** of the femur and the **superior articular surface** of the tibia (see also 3.37 and 3.44). Two C-shaped rings of fibrocartilage, the **medial** and **lateral menisci**, are interspersed between the bones to improve compatibility between the articular surfaces. In the patellofemoral articulation, the posterior part of the patella interacts with the smooth **patellar surface** of the femur. The **patella** is a sesamoid bone because it is embedded in a tendon (3.39). Its primary role is to allow the quadriceps tendon to cross the knee joint without being "pinched" between the joint surfaces during extension of the knee. The knee joint is supported by numerous ligaments including the collateral ligaments and cruciate ligaments. The **tibial (medial)** and **fibular (lateral) collateral ligaments** provide stability on the sides of the knee to prevent medial and lateral displacement of the tibia with respect to the femur. The tibial collateral ligament and medial meniscus are connected, but a similar linkage is not present between the fibular collateral ligament and lateral meniscus. The **anterior cruciate ligament (ACL)** and **posterior cruciate ligament (PCL)** connect the femur to the anterior and posterior parts of the intercondylar area on the tibia; they are designed to prevent anteroposterior displacement between the femur and tibia. Numerous **bursae** surround the knee joint and prevent friction between multiple structures including skin, bones, tendons, and ligaments.

Clinical Focus

The knee is the most common joint affected by **osteoarthritis**, characterized by pain with movement and loss of flexibility (3.2). Injuries of the knee are also common, such as **fractures**, **sprains**, or **meniscal tears**. The collateral ligaments are typically stretched or torn by forces directed at the sides of the knee. A tear of the tibial collateral ligament may be accompanied by a tear of the medial meniscus since these two structures are fused. The ACL is frequently injured during athletic activities that involve sudden stops or twisting motions of the knee. Several physical exam maneuvers are used to identify a torn ACL, such as the **anterior drawer test**. Sprains involving the PCL are not common but may occur during motor vehicle accidents when the knee hits the dashboard and the tibia is forcefully pushed posteriorly.

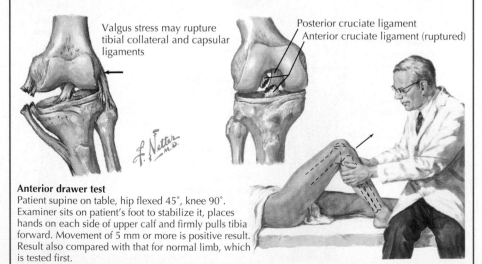

Valgus stress may rupture tibial collateral and capsular ligaments

Posterior cruciate ligament
Anterior cruciate ligament (ruptured)

Anterior drawer test
Patient supine on table, hip flexed 45°, knee 90°. Examiner sits on patient's foot to stabilize it, places hands on each side of upper calf and firmly pulls tibia forward. Movement of 5 mm or more is positive result. Result also compared with that for normal limb, which is tested first.

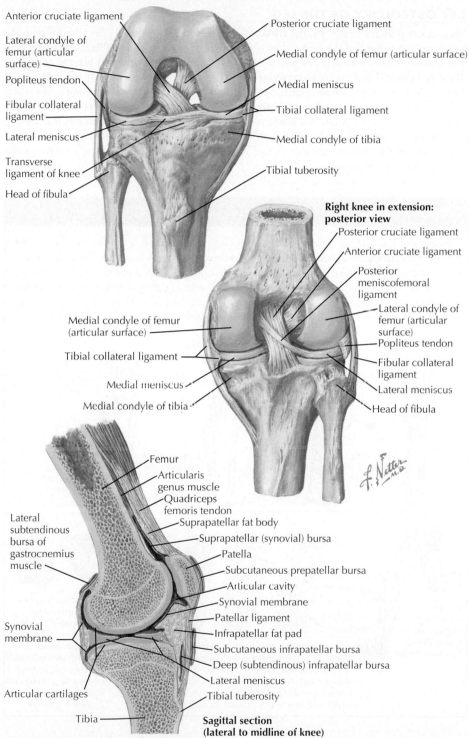

Right knee in flexion: anterior view

Anterior cruciate ligament

Lateral condyle of femur (articular surface)

Popliteus tendon

Fibular collateral ligament

Lateral meniscus

Transverse ligament of knee

Head of fibula

Posterior cruciate ligament

Medial condyle of femur (articular surface)

Medial meniscus

Tibial collateral ligament

Medial condyle of tibia

Tibial tuberosity

Right knee in extension: posterior view

Posterior cruciate ligament

Anterior cruciate ligament

Posterior meniscofemoral ligament

Lateral condyle of femur (articular surface)

Popliteus tendon

Fibular collateral ligament

Lateral meniscus

Head of fibula

Medial condyle of femur (articular surface)

Tibial collateral ligament

Medial meniscus

Medial condyle of tibia

Femur

Articularis genus muscle

Quadriceps femoris tendon

Suprapatellar fat body

Suprapatellar (synovial) bursa

Patella

Subcutaneous prepatellar bursa

Articular cavity

Synovial membrane

Patellar ligament

Infrapatellar fat pad

Subcutaneous infrapatellar bursa

Deep (subtendinous) infrapatellar bursa

Lateral meniscus

Tibial tuberosity

Lateral subtendinous bursa of gastrocnemius muscle

Synovial membrane

Articular cartilages

Tibia

Sagittal section (lateral to midline of knee)

Figure 3.43 KNEE JOINT

3.44 OSTEOLOGY OF THE LEG

There are two bones in the leg, the **tibia** (medial) and **fibula** (lateral). The tibia is the bone that bears the weight of the body; thus it has a wide proximal end ("tibial plateau") where it articulates with the femur. Prominent features include the **medial** and **lateral condyles**, **tibial tuberosity**, and the **intercondylar area**. The condyles have articular surfaces for the femur, while the latter two structures serve as sites of attachment for ligaments. The distal end of the tibia has an **inferior articular surface** and **medial malleolus**, both of which participate in the ankle joint. The fibula is joined to the tibia by an interosseous membrane. At its proximal end it has a **head** that articulates with the tibia; the distal end exhibits the **lateral malleolus** that contributes to the ankle joint. The shaft of the fibula serves as the origin for numerous muscles.

Clinical Focus

The tibia and fibula are commonly fractured during motor vehicle accidents, falls, and sports injuries. **Fractures** can be classified by their direction (transverse = across the shaft; spiral = wrapping around the shaft), the number of breaks (comminuted = three or more breaks), and the arrangement of the pieces (segmented = fracture with a floating segment of bone). **Stress fractures** are tiny cracks in bones that are due to repetitive stress. They are very common in the bones of the leg, especially in runners or other athletes.

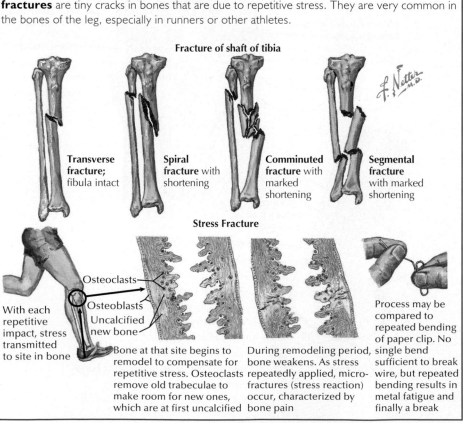

Fracture of shaft of tibia

Transverse fracture; fibula intact

Spiral fracture with shortening

Comminuted fracture with marked shortening

Segmental fracture with marked shortening

Stress Fracture

With each repetitive impact, stress transmitted to site in bone

Osteoclasts

Osteoblasts
Uncalcified new bone

Bone at that site begins to remodel to compensate for repetitive stress. Osteoclasts remove old trabeculae to make room for new ones, which are at first uncalcified

During remodeling period, bone weakens. As stress repeatedly applied, micro-fractures (stress reaction) occur, characterized by bone pain

Process may be compared to repeated bending of paper clip. No single bend sufficient to break wire, but repeated bending results in metal fatigue and finally a break

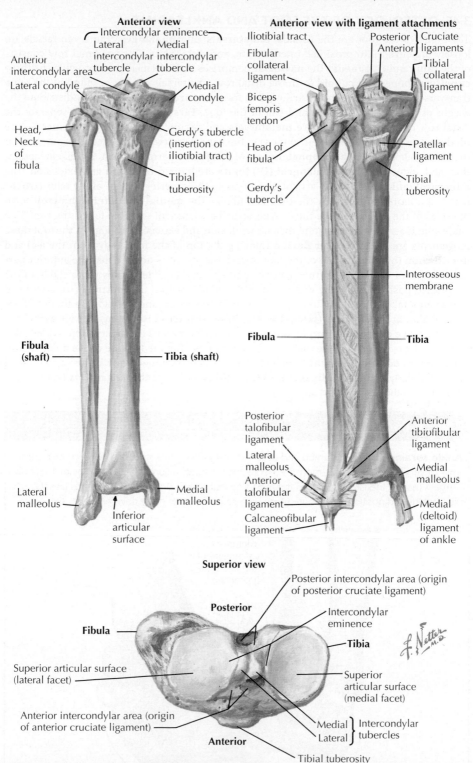

Figure 3.44 OSTEOLOGY OF THE LEG

3.45 OSTEOLOGY OF THE FOOT AND ANKLE JOINT

The bones of the foot are the **tarsals**, **metatarsals**, and **phalanges**. The seven tarsals are loosely organized into proximal, intermediate, and distal rows. The proximal row consists of the **talus** and **calcaneus**. The **navicular** comprises the intermediate row, while the three **cuneiform** bones and **cuboid** form the distal row. The tarsals are not oriented in the same transverse plane; rather they are arranged to form two **arches** that effectively distribute the weight of the body to the heel and ball of the foot. **Tarsometatarsal joints** separate the distal row of tarsals from the five **metatarsals** and permit slight gliding movements. The **phalanges** of the toes are similar to those in the hand, with two in the great toe and three in the other four toes. **Metatarsophalangeal (MTP) joints** permit flexion, extension, abduction, and adduction; **interphalangeal (IP) joints** are limited to flexion and extension. The **talocrural (ankle) joint** is an articulation between the superior surface of the talus (**trochlea**) and a mortise formed by the tibia and fibula. The **medial** and **lateral malleoli** form the sides of the mortise, while the inferior articular surface of the tibia forms the roof. The ankle joint is a synovial hinge joint that allows flexion and extension, though in the foot these movements are called **plantar flexion** (moving the top of the foot away from the leg) and **dorsiflexion** (moving the top of the foot toward the leg). It is notable that the anterior part of the trochlea is wider than the posterior part—thus the ankle joint is more stable in the dorsiflexed position when the wider part of the talus is within the mortise. Two additional movements take place in the region of the ankle (inversion and eversion), although these occur mainly at the **subtalar (talocalcaneal) joint**. **Inversion** is turning the sole of the foot medially, while **eversion** is turning the sole laterally. Numerous ligaments support the ankle joint and their names indicate their attachment points. The medial side of the ankle is supported by the **deltoid ligament**, which has four parts that connect the tibia to various tarsal bones. Similarly, the **lateral ligament of the ankle** consists of three ligaments that join the fibula to the talus and calcaneus.

Clinical Focus

Ankle sprains are very common and occur when ligaments are stretched beyond their normal limits. Inversion injuries occur more frequently than eversion injuries, and the anterior talofibular ligament (part of the lateral group) is the most frequently torn. Since the ankle joint is less stable in the plantarflexed position, injuries are more likely to occur when going downhill rather than uphill.

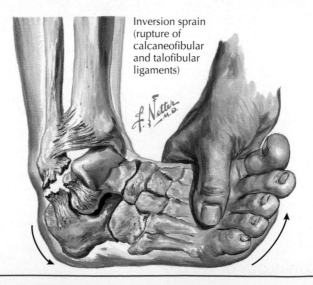

Inversion sprain
(rupture of
calcaneofibular
and talofibular
ligaments)

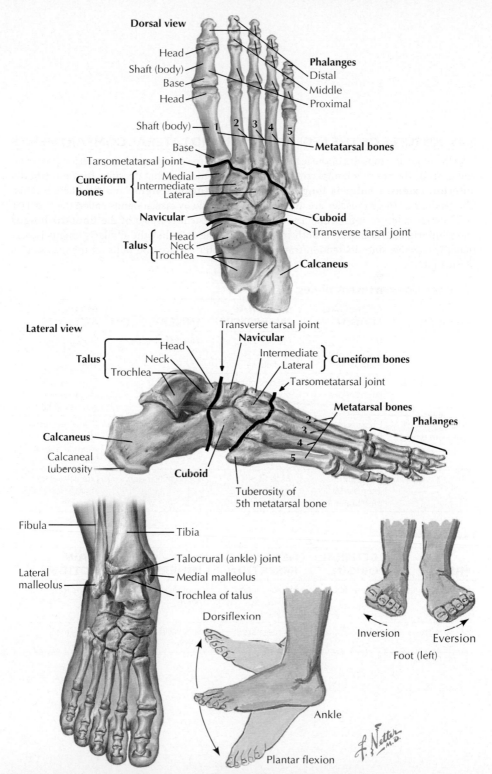

Figure 3.45 OSTEOLOGY OF THE FOOT AND ANKLE JOINT

3.46 MUSCLES OF THE LEG: ANTERIOR AND LATERAL COMPARTMENTS

Like the thigh, the muscles of the leg are arranged in three compartments (anterior, posterior, and lateral). The anterior compartment contains four muscles that dorsiflex the foot: **tibialis anterior**, **extensor hallucis longus**, **extensor digitorum longus**, and **fibularis tertius**. The tendons of these muscles are anchored at the ankle by fascial bands called the superior and inferior extensor retinacula. The lateral compartment consists of the **fibularis longus** and **fibularis brevis** muscles. Both muscles evert the foot, but the fibularis longus is particularly effective since its tendon traverses the plantar surface and pulls on the medial side of the foot.

Anterior Compartment of Leg

MUSCLE	GENERAL ORIGIN	GENERAL INSERTION	INNERVATION	MAIN ACTIONS
Tibialis anterior	Lateral side of tibia and interosseous membrane	Medial cuneiform, base of 1st metatarsal	Deep fibular nerve	Dorsiflexes foot at ankle joint, inverts foot
Extensor hallucis longus	Fibula and interosseous membrane	Base of distal phalanx of great toe	Deep fibular nerve	Dorsiflexes foot at ankle joint, extends great toe
Extensor digitorum longus	Fibula and interosseous membrane	Middle and distal phalanges of lateral four toes	Deep fibular nerve	Dorsiflexes foot at ankle joint, extends lateral four toes
Fibularis tertius	Fibula and interosseous membrane	Base of 5th metatarsal	Deep fibular nerve	Dorsiflexes foot at ankle joint, aids eversion

Lateral Compartment of Leg

MUSCLE	GENERAL ORIGIN	GENERAL INSERTION	INNERVATION	MAIN ACTIONS
Fibularis longus	Lateral fibula	Medial cuneiform, base of 1st metatarsal	Superficial fibular nerve	Everts foot
Fibularis brevis	Lateral fibula	5th metatarsal	Superficial fibular nerve	Everts foot

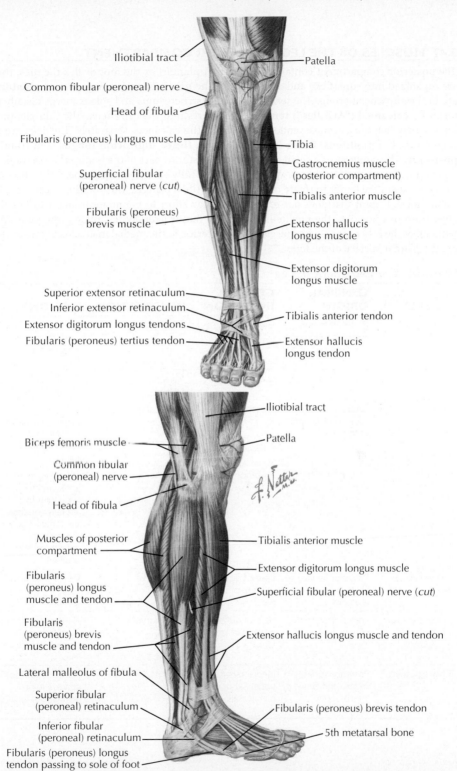

Iliotibial tract

Patella

Common fibular (peroneal) nerve

Head of fibula

Fibularis (peroneus) longus muscle

Tibia

Gastrocnemius muscle (posterior compartment)

Superficial fibular (peroneal) nerve (*cut*)

Tibialis anterior muscle

Fibularis (peroneus) brevis muscle

Extensor hallucis longus muscle

Extensor digitorum longus muscle

Superior extensor retinaculum

Inferior extensor retinaculum

Extensor digitorum longus tendons

Fibularis (peroneus) tertius tendon

Tibialis anterior tendon

Extensor hallucis longus tendon

Iliotibial tract

Biceps femoris muscle

Patella

Common fibular (peroneal) nerve

Head of fibula

Muscles of posterior compartment

Tibialis anterior muscle

Extensor digitorum longus muscle

Fibularis (peroneus) longus muscle and tendon

Superficial fibular (peroneal) nerve (*cut*)

Fibularis (peroneus) brevis muscle and tendon

Extensor hallucis longus muscle and tendon

Lateral malleolus of fibula

Superior fibular (peroneal) retinaculum

Inferior fibular (peroneal) retinaculum

Fibularis (peroneus) brevis tendon

5th metatarsal bone

Fibularis (peroneus) longus tendon passing to sole of foot

Figure 3.46 MUSCLES OF THE LEG: ANTERIOR AND LATERAL COMPARTMENTS

3.47 MUSCLES OF THE LEG: POSTERIOR COMPARTMENT

The posterior compartment contains muscles that plantarflex the foot or flex the toes; they are organized into superficial and deep groups. The **gastrocnemius**, **soleus**, and **plantaris** are in the superficial group. The tendons of the gastrocnemius and soleus merge distally to form the **calcaneal ("Achilles") tendon** that inserts into the calcaneus. The thin plantaris tendon may join the calcaneal tendon or insert on the calcaneus separately. The deep group is comprised of **popliteus**, **flexor hallucis longus**, **flexor digitorum longus**, and **tibialis posterior**. The popliteus is a small muscle in the posterior part of the popliteal fossa (hollow on the posterior part of the knee). When the knee is fully extended, the shape of the articular surfaces causes the femur to rotate medially on the tibial plateau. This rotation creates a very stable "locked" joint that does not require muscular effort to maintain. In order to flex the knee from this position, the popliteus rotates the femur laterally to "unlock" the joint. The tendons of the other three deep muscles pass posterior to the medial malleolus before entering the plantar surface of the foot.

Posterior Compartment of Leg

MUSCLE	GENERAL ORIGIN	GENERAL INSERTION	INNERVATION	MAIN ACTIONS
Gastrocnemius	Posterior femur, superior to femoral condyles	Calcaneus	Tibial nerve	Plantarflexes foot at ankle joint, flexes leg at knee joint
Soleus	Fibula, soleal line of tibia	Calcaneus	Tibial nerve	Plantarflexes foot at ankle joint
Plantaris	Lateral supracondylar area of femur	Calcaneus	Tibial nerve	Weakly plantarflexes foot at ankle joint, flexes leg at knee joint
Popliteus	Lateral femoral condyle	Posterior surface of tibia	Tibial nerve	Flexes leg at knee joint, "unlocks" knee joint by laterally rotating the femur when the leg is in a weight-bearing position
Flexor hallucis longus	Posterior surface of fibula, interosseous membrane	Base of distal phalanx of the great toe	Tibial nerve	Flexes great toe
Flexor digitorum longus	Posterior surface of tibia	Base of distal phalanx of lateral four toes	Tibial nerve	Plantarflexes foot at ankle joint, flexes lateral four toes
Tibialis posterior	Posterior surfaces of tibia and fibula, interosseous membrane	Medial tarsal bones, 2nd—4th metatarsals	Tibial nerve	Plantarflexes foot at ankle joint, inverts foot

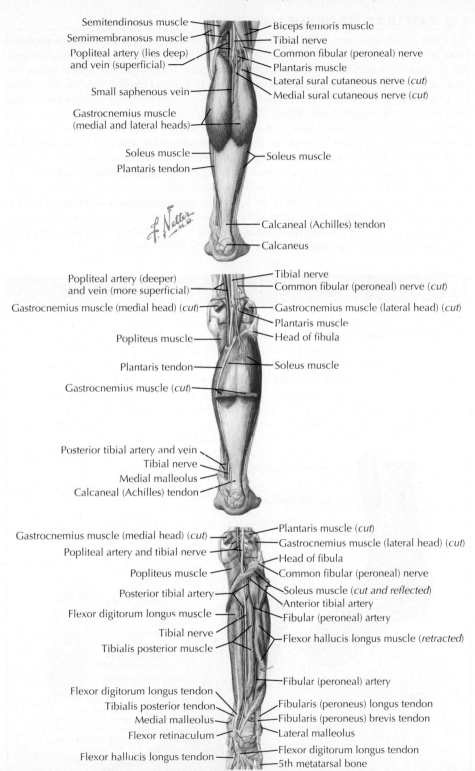

Semitendinosus muscle

Semimembranosus muscle

Popliteal artery (lies deep) and vein (superficial)

Small saphenous vein

Gastrocnemius muscle (medial and lateral heads)

Soleus muscle

Plantaris tendon

Biceps femoris muscle

Tibial nerve

Common fibular (peroneal) nerve

Plantaris muscle

Lateral sural cutaneous nerve (*cut*)

Medial sural cutaneous nerve (*cut*)

Soleus muscle

Calcaneal (Achilles) tendon

Calcaneus

Popliteal artery (deeper) and vein (more superficial)

Gastrocnemius muscle (medial head) (*cut*)

Popliteus muscle

Plantaris tendon

Gastrocnemius muscle (*cut*)

Tibial nerve

Common fibular (peroneal) nerve (*cut*)

Gastrocnemius muscle (lateral head) (*cut*)

Plantaris muscle

Head of fibula

Soleus muscle

Posterior tibial artery and vein

Tibial nerve

Medial malleolus

Calcaneal (Achilles) tendon

Gastrocnemius muscle (medial head) (*cut*)

Popliteal artery and tibial nerve

Popliteus muscle

Posterior tibial artery

Flexor digitorum longus muscle

Tibial nerve

Tibialis posterior muscle

Plantaris muscle (*cut*)

Gastrocnemius muscle (lateral head) (*cut*)

Head of fibula

Common fibular (peroneal) nerve

Soleus muscle (*cut and reflected*)

Anterior tibial artery

Fibular (peroneal) artery

Flexor hallucis longus muscle (*retracted*)

Fibular (peroneal) artery

Flexor digitorum longus tendon

Tibialis posterior tendon

Medial malleolus

Flexor retinaculum

Flexor hallucis longus tendon

Fibularis (peroneus) longus tendon

Fibularis (peroneus) brevis tendon

Lateral malleolus

Flexor digitorum longus tendon

5th metatarsal bone

Figure 3.47 MUSCLES OF THE LEG: POSTERIOR COMPARTMENT

3.48 VASCULATURE OF THE LEG

The major vessels and nerves that supply the leg pass through the diamond-shaped **popliteal fossa** on the posterior aspect of the knee before joining one of the three crural compartments. The femoral artery transitions to the **popliteal artery** after traversing the adductor hiatus. The popliteal artery gives off multiple **genicular branches** that provide collateral circulation around the knee joint before dividing into anterior and posterior tibial branches. The **anterior tibial artery** enters the anterior compartment of the leg through a gap in the proximal part of the interosseous membrane. It supplies muscles in the anterior and lateral compartments and then crosses the ankle joint where it changes names to the **dorsalis pedis artery**. The **posterior tibial artery** descends in the posterior leg between the superficial and deep compartments, supplying both. It also supplies the lateral compartment of the leg mainly via its **fibular branch**. The posterior tibial artery travels posterior to the medial malleolus before entering the plantar surface of the foot. The primary superficial veins of the leg are the **great** and **small saphenous veins** that ascend on the medial and posterior sides of the leg, respectively. These veins have connections with the deep veins via perforating veins that allow blood to move from superficial to deep. Deep veins travel with their companion arteries and drain to the inferior vena cava.

Clinical Focus

The posterior tibial artery has a superficial location posterior to the medial malleolus; thus the **posterior tibial pulse** can be obtained in this region. Effective venous drainage of the lower extremity relies on competent venous valves that help to move blood against gravity. Contraction of the muscles in the leg also helps with this effort. Veins can become damaged with aging, producing **chronic venous insufficiency**, that is, an inability to effectively move blood toward the heart. As blood backs up in the venous system, valves become incompetent because their cusps cannot completely close in a dilated vessel. The dilated, distorted veins are called **varicose veins** and they can be seen under the skin. In addition to aging, risk factors for varicose veins include obesity, pregnancy, and a sedentary lifestyle.

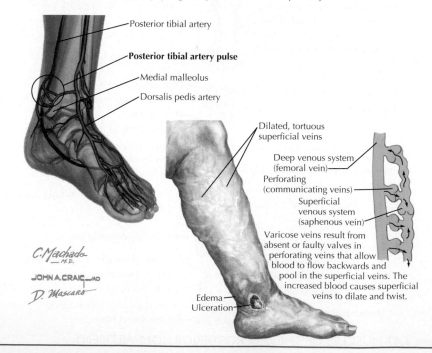

Posterior tibial artery

Posterior tibial artery pulse

Medial malleolus

Dorsalis pedis artery

C. Machado
—M.D.

JOHN A. CRAIG—MD

D. Mascaro

Dilated, tortuous superficial veins

Deep venous system (femoral vein)

Perforating (communicating veins)

Superficial venous system (saphenous vein)

Varicose veins result from absent or faulty valves in perforating veins that allow blood to flow backwards and pool in the superficial veins. The increased blood causes superficial veins to dilate and twist.

Edema
Ulceration

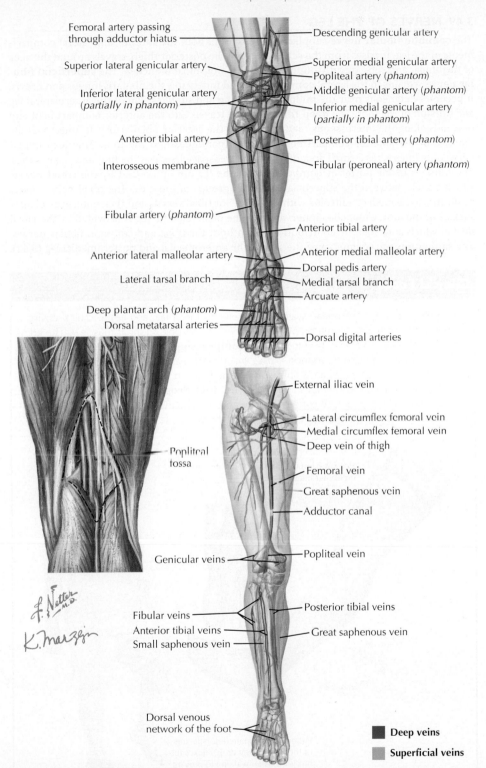

Femoral artery passing through adductor hiatus

Descending genicular artery

Superior lateral genicular artery

Superior medial genicular artery

Popliteal artery (*phantom*)

Inferior lateral genicular artery (*partially in phantom*)

Middle genicular artery (*phantom*)

Inferior medial genicular artery (*partially in phantom*)

Anterior tibial artery

Posterior tibial artery (*phantom*)

Interosseous membrane

Fibular (peroneal) artery (*phantom*)

Fibular artery (*phantom*)

Anterior tibial artery

Anterior lateral malleolar artery

Anterior medial malleolar artery

Dorsal pedis artery

Lateral tarsal branch

Medial tarsal branch

Arcuate artery

Deep plantar arch (*phantom*)

Dorsal metatarsal arteries

Dorsal digital arteries

Popliteal fossa

External iliac vein

Lateral circumflex femoral vein

Medial circumflex femoral vein

Deep vein of thigh

Femoral vein

Great saphenous vein

Adductor canal

Genicular veins

Popliteal vein

Posterior tibial veins

Fibular veins

Anterior tibial veins

Great saphenous vein

Small saphenous vein

Dorsal venous network of the foot

Deep veins

Superficial veins

Figure 3.48 VASCULATURE OF THE LEG

3.49 NERVES OF THE LEG

The **common fibular nerve** supplies the muscles of both the anterior and lateral compartments of the leg. It arises from the sciatic nerve in the posterior thigh, travels around the neck of the fibula, and subsequently bifurcates into two terminal branches. The **superficial fibular nerve** remains in the lateral compartment and innervates the fibularis longus and brevis. It becomes cutaneous near the midpoint of the leg and supplies skin of the anterolateral leg and dorsum of the foot. The **deep fibular nerve** travels into the anterior compartment and descends along the interosseous membrane with the anterior tibial artery. It innervates the muscles of the anterior compartment and then continues into the foot. The deep fibular nerve only innervates a small area of skin—the webspace between the first and second toes. The muscles in the posterior compartment of the leg are innervated by the **tibial nerve**, which travels between the superficial and deep groups of muscles. The tibial nerve passes posterior to the medial malleolus with the posterior tibial vessels and then enters the plantar surface of the foot. Cutaneous innervation of the posterolateral leg is provided by the **sural nerve**, which is formed by contributions from both the tibial and common fibular nerves. The **saphenous nerve** innervates the skin of the anteromedial and posteromedial leg (3.42).

Clinical Focus

Traditionally the term "peroneal" was used to refer to the fibula, and in the clinical environment it is still used (e.g., "common peroneal nerve" or "peroneus longus muscle"). The common fibular nerve is particularly vulnerable to **compression or injury** where it crosses the proximal part of the fibula. Common causes include dislocation of the knee, a tight splint or cast, and fractures of the proximal fibula. When the function of the common fibular nerve is compromised, patients exhibit a clinical sign called "**foot drop**." This is characterized by the inability to dorsiflex the foot, so patients flex their hip joint on the affected side when they walk in order to prevent their toes from dragging along the ground.

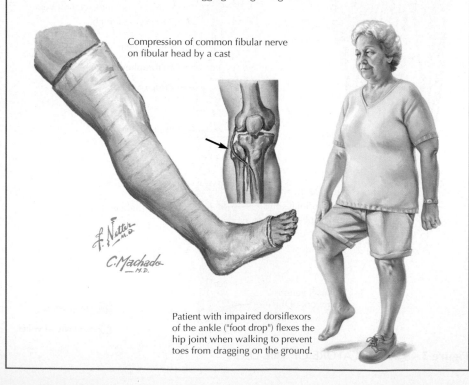

Compression of common fibular nerve on fibular head by a cast

Patient with impaired dorsiflexors of the ankle ("foot drop") flexes the hip joint when walking to prevent toes from dragging on the ground.

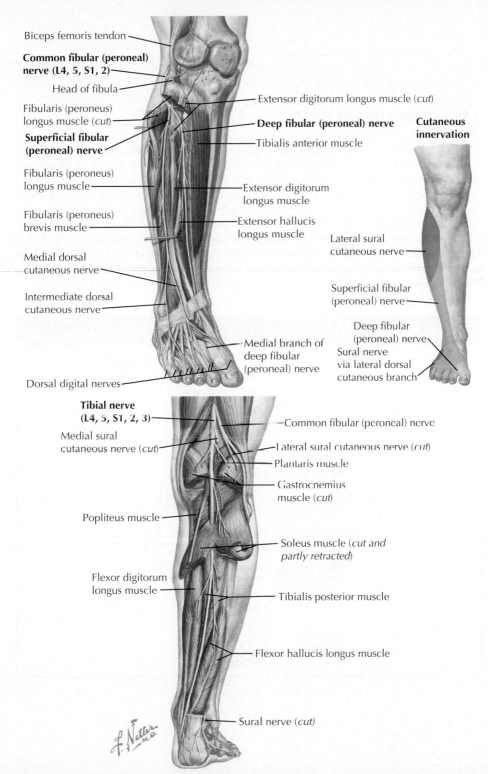

Biceps femoris tendon

Common fibular (peroneal) nerve (L4, 5, S1, 2)

Head of fibula

Fibularis (peroneus) longus muscle (*cut*)

Superficial fibular (peroneal) nerve

Fibularis (peroneus) longus muscle

Fibularis (peroneus) brevis muscle

Medial dorsal cutaneous nerve

Intermediate dorsal cutaneous nerve

Dorsal digital nerves

Extensor digitorum longus muscle (*cut*)

Deep fibular (peroneal) nerve

Tibialis anterior muscle

Extensor digitorum longus muscle

Extensor hallucis longus muscle

Medial branch of deep fibular (peroneal) nerve

Cutaneous innervation

Lateral sural cutaneous nerve

Superficial fibular (peroneal) nerve

Deep fibular (peroneal) nerve

Sural nerve via lateral dorsal cutaneous branch

Tibial nerve (L4, 5, S1, 2, 3)

Medial sural cutaneous nerve (*cut*)

Popliteus muscle

Flexor digitorum longus muscle

Common fibular (peroneal) nerve

Lateral sural cutaneous nerve (*cut*)

Plantaris muscle

Gastrocnemius muscle (*cut*)

Soleus muscle (*cut and partly retracted*)

Tibialis posterior muscle

Flexor hallucis longus muscle

Sural nerve (*cut*)

Figure 3.49 NERVES OF THE LEG

3.50 DORSUM OF THE FOOT

The dorsum of the foot contains the distal tendons of the anterior leg muscles, as well as two muscles that extend the toes—**extensor digitorum brevis** and **extensor hallucis brevis**. Both arise from the superolateral part of the calcaneus. The extensor digitorum brevis tendons merge with the extensor digitorum longus tendons and insert via a similar arrangement as in the hand, that is, tendons have a central band that terminates on the middle phalanx and two lateral bands that attach to the distal phalanx. The extensor hallucis brevis tendon inserts independently on the proximal phalanx of the great toe. Both muscles are innervated by the **deep fibular nerve** that terminates by dividing into two cutaneous dorsal digital branches. The blood supply to the dorsum of the foot is provided by the **dorsalis pedis artery**. Superficial venous drainage begins as a network of small veins that unite to form the **dorsal venous arch** (3.48). This arch is the source of the great and small saphenous veins.

Clinical Focus

The **dorsalis pedis pulse** is one of the commonly evaluated pulses during physical exam. It can be located on the dorsum of the foot just lateral to the extensor hallucis longus tendon (see also 4.12).

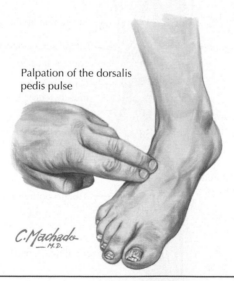

Palpation of the dorsalis pedis pulse

C. Machado
_M.D.

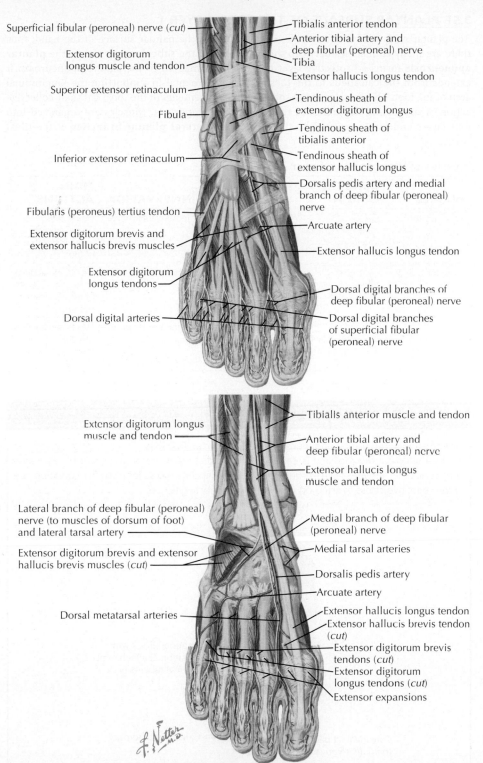

Superficial fibular (peroneal) nerve (*cut*)

Extensor digitorum longus muscle and tendon

Superior extensor retinaculum

Fibula

Inferior extensor retinaculum

Fibularis (peroneus) tertius tendon

Extensor digitorum brevis and extensor hallucis brevis muscles

Extensor digitorum longus tendons

Dorsal digital arteries

Tibialis anterior tendon

Anterior tibial artery and deep fibular (peroneal) nerve

Tibia

Extensor hallucis longus tendon

Tendinous sheath of extensor digitorum longus

Tendinous sheath of tibialis anterior

Tendinous sheath of extensor hallucis longus

Dorsalis pedis artery and medial branch of deep fibular (peroneal) nerve

Arcuate artery

Extensor hallucis longus tendon

Dorsal digital branches of deep fibular (peroneal) nerve

Dorsal digital branches of superficial fibular (peroneal) nerve

Extensor digitorum longus muscle and tendon

Lateral branch of deep fibular (peroneal) nerve (to muscles of dorsum of foot) and lateral tarsal artery

Extensor digitorum brevis and extensor hallucis brevis muscles (*cut*)

Dorsal metatarsal arteries

Tibialis anterior muscle and tendon

Anterior tibial artery and deep fibular (peroneal) nerve

Extensor hallucis longus muscle and tendon

Medial branch of deep fibular (peroneal) nerve

Medial tarsal arteries

Dorsalis pedis artery

Arcuate artery

Extensor hallucis longus tendon

Extensor hallucis brevis tendon (*cut*)

Extensor digitorum brevis tendons (*cut*)

Extensor digitorum longus tendons (*cut*)

Extensor expansions

Figure 3.50 DORSUM OF THE FOOT

3.51 PLANTAR SURFACE OF THE FOOT: LAYER I

The plantar surface of the foot (sole) is equivalent to the palmar surface of the hand; thus there are many similarities between the two. Deep to the subcutaneous tissue, the **plantar aponeurosis** forms a protective layer that can be compared to the palmar aponeurosis. It extends from the calcaneus to the toes and is instrumental in supporting the longitudinal arch of the foot. The muscles of the sole generate movements of the toes, but their collective action of supporting the arches of the foot is most important. Muscles are organized into four layers and are innervated by the **medial** and **lateral plantar branches** of the tibial nerve.

Muscles of Plantar Foot, Layer I

MUSCLE	GENERAL ORIGIN	GENERAL INSERTION	INNERVATION	MAIN ACTIONS
Flexor digitorum brevis	Calcaneal tuberosity, plantar aponeurosis	Middle phalanx of toes 2–5	Medial plantar nerve	Flexes toes 2–5, supports longitudinal arch of foot
Abductor hallucis	Calcaneal tuberosity, plantar aponeurosis	Proximal phalanx of great toe	Medial plantar nerve	Flexes and abducts great toe, supports longitudinal arch of foot
Abductor digiti minimi	Calcaneal tuberosity, plantar aponeurosis	Proximal phalanx of 5th toe	Lateral plantar nerve	Flexes and abducts 5th toe, supports longitudinal arch of foot

Clinical Focus

Inflammation of the plantar aponeurosis is called **plantar fasciitis**. This condition causes pain on the bottom of the foot and is common in individuals that are on their feet for extended periods of time. Athletes such as runners and ballet dancers also suffer from this condition due to the repetitive stress exerted on the heel and supportive tissues.

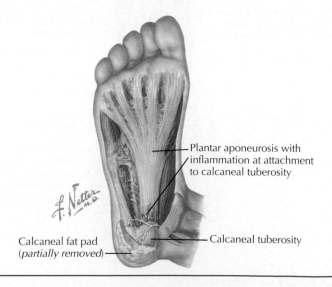

Plantar aponeurosis with inflammation at attachment to calcaneal tuberosity

Calcaneal fat pad (partially removed)

Calcaneal tuberosity

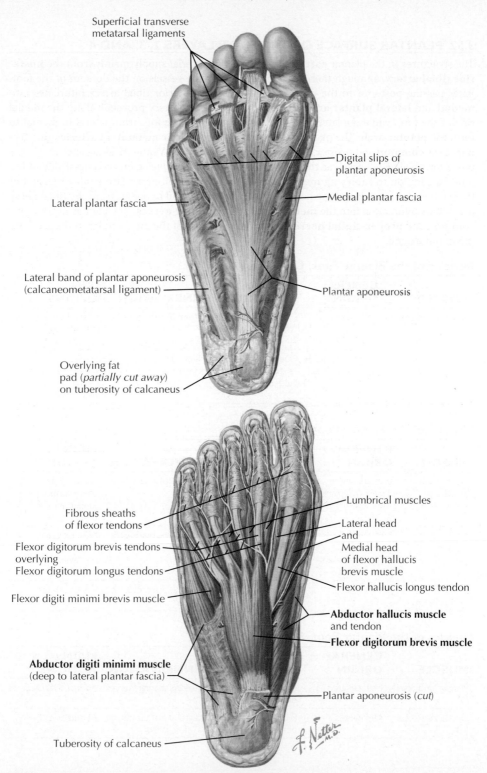

Superficial transverse
metatarsal ligaments

Digital slips of
plantar aponeurosis

Lateral plantar fascia

Medial plantar fascia

Lateral band of plantar aponeurosis
(calcaneometatarsal ligament)

Plantar aponeurosis

Overlying fat
pad (*partially cut away*)
on tuberosity of calcaneus

Lumbrical muscles

Fibrous sheaths
of flexor tendons

Lateral head
and
Medial head
of flexor hallucis
brevis muscle

Flexor digitorum brevis tendons
overlying
Flexor digitorum longus tendons

Flexor hallucis longus tendon

Flexor digiti minimi brevis muscle

Abductor hallucis muscle
and tendon

Flexor digitorum brevis muscle

Abductor digiti minimi muscle
(deep to lateral plantar fascia)

Plantar aponeurosis (*cut*)

Tuberosity of calcaneus

Figure 3.51 PLANTAR SURFACE OF THE FOOT: LAYER I

3.52 PLANTAR SURFACE OF THE FOOT: LAYERS 2, 3, AND 4

The structures in the plantar part of the foot receive arterial supply mainly from the **posterior tibial artery**, although there are connections to the vessels on the dorsum of the foot. After passing posterior to the medial malleolus, the posterior tibial artery bifurcates into **medial** and **lateral plantar arteries**. The medial plantar artery proceeds along the medial side of the foot, while the lateral plantar artery traverses the foot from lateral to medial to form the **plantar arch**. The plantar arch gives rise to **plantar metatarsal arteries** that terminate as **common** and **proper digital arteries** for the toes. Venous drainage occurs via the posterior tibial vein, as well as through connections with the veins on the dorsal side of the foot. In addition to supplying muscles, branches of the tibial nerve also supply the skin of the plantar foot. The skin of the heel receives direct calcaneal branches from the tibial nerve prior to its bifurcation into the **medial** and **lateral plantar nerves**. The plantar nerves emit **common** and **proper digital nerves** that supply the skin of the toes, similar to the arrangement in the hand.

Muscles of the Plantar Foot, Layer 2

MUSCLE	GENERAL ORIGIN	GENERAL INSERTION	INNERVATION	MAIN ACTIONS
Quadratus plantae	Calcaneus	Tendon of flexor digitorum longus	Lateral plantar nerve	Adjusts the pull of the flexor digitorum longus tendon
Lumbricals (4)	Tendons of flexor digitorum longus	Dorsal digital expansions of toes 2–5	Medial and lateral plantar nerves	Flexes metatarsophalangeal joints, extends IP joints of toes 2–5

Muscles of the Plantar Foot, Layer 3

MUSCLE	GENERAL ORIGIN	GENERAL INSERTION	INNERVATION	MAIN ACTIONS
Flexor hallucis brevis	Cuboid, lateral cuneiform (plantar surfaces)	Proximal phalanx of great toe	Medial plantar nerve	Flexes great toe, supports longitudinal arch of foot
Adductor hallucis	Metatarsals 2–4, ligaments of metatarsophalangeal joints of toes 3–5	Proximal phalanx of great toe	Lateral plantar nerve	Adducts great toe, supports transverse arch of foot
Flexor digiti minimi brevis	5th metatarsal	Proximal phalanx of 5th toe	Lateral plantar nerve	Flexes 5th toe

Muscles of the Plantar Foot, Layer 4

MUSCLE	GENERAL ORIGIN	GENERAL INSERTION	INNERVATION	MAIN ACTIONS
Plantar interossei (3)	Metatarsals 3–5	Proximal phalanges of toes 3–5	Lateral plantar nerve	Adduct toes 3–5
Dorsal interossei (4)	Metatarsals 1–5	Proximal phalanges of toes 2–4	Lateral plantar nerve	Abduct toes 2–4

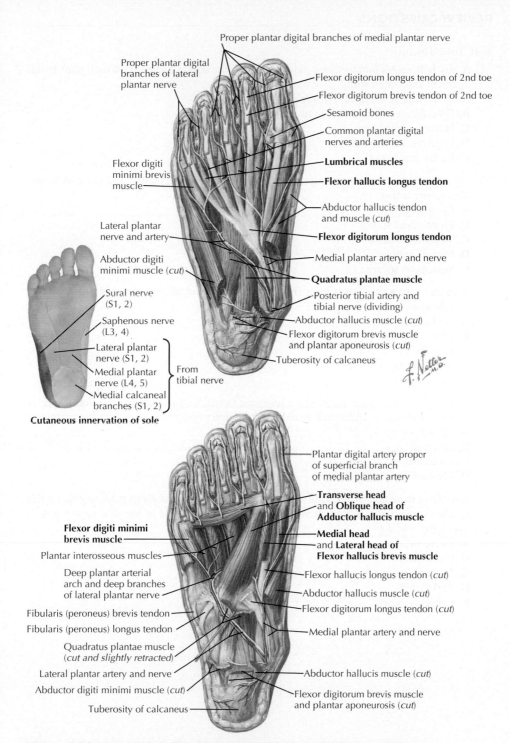

Proper plantar digital branches of medial plantar nerve

Proper plantar digital branches of lateral plantar nerve

Flexor digitorum longus tendon of 2nd toe

Flexor digitorum brevis tendon of 2nd toe

Sesamoid bones

Common plantar digital nerves and arteries

Lumbrical muscles

Flexor hallucis longus tendon

Flexor digiti minimi brevis muscle

Abductor hallucis tendon and muscle (*cut*)

Flexor digitorum longus tendon

Lateral plantar nerve and artery

Medial plantar artery and nerve

Abductor digiti minimi muscle (*cut*)

Quadratus plantae muscle

Sural nerve (S1, 2)

Posterior tibial artery and tibial nerve (dividing)

Saphenous nerve (L3, 4)

Abductor hallucis muscle (*cut*)

Lateral plantar nerve (S1, 2)

Flexor digitorum brevis muscle and plantar aponeurosis (*cut*)

Medial plantar nerve (L4, 5)

Tuberosity of calcaneus

Medial calcaneal branches (S1, 2)

From tibial nerve

Cutaneous innervation of sole

Plantar digital artery proper of superficial branch of medial plantar artery

Transverse head and **Oblique head of Adductor hallucis muscle**

Flexor digiti minimi brevis muscle

Medial head and **Lateral head of Flexor hallucis brevis muscle**

Plantar interosseous muscles

Flexor hallucis longus tendon (*cut*)

Deep plantar arterial arch and deep branches of lateral plantar nerve

Abductor hallucis muscle (*cut*)

Flexor digitorum longus tendon (*cut*)

Fibularis (peroneus) brevis tendon

Fibularis (peroneus) longus tendon

Medial plantar artery and nerve

Quadratus plantae muscle (*cut and slightly retracted*)

Lateral plantar artery and nerve

Abductor hallucis muscle (*cut*)

Abductor digiti minimi muscle (*cut*)

Flexor digitorum brevis muscle and plantar aponeurosis (*cut*)

Tuberosity of calcaneus

Figure 3.52 PLANTAR SURFACE OF THE FOOT: LAYERS 2, 3, AND 4

REVIEW QUESTIONS

Test Your Recall

1. A boy falls on his outstretched hand and tears the anular ligament. Which joint is this ligament associated with?
   A. Distal interphalangeal (DIP) joint
   B. Glenohumeral (shoulder) joint
   C. Humeroulnar joint
   D. Proximal radioulnar joint
   E. Radiocarpal joint

2. An infant has premature closure of the suture between the frontal and parietal bones. This suture is the:
   A. Coronal suture
   B. Frontonasal suture
   C. Lambdoid suture
   D. Sagittal suture
   E. Squamous suture

3. A soccer player executes a long shot into the goal and injures her hamstring. Which muscle was injured?
   A. Adductor longus
   B. Biceps femoris, short head
   C. Gracilis
   D. Semitendinosus
   E. Vastus lateralis

4. A cross-country runner steps into a hole and twists his ankle so that the bottom of his foot turns medially. This motion could best be described as:
   A. Dorsiflexion
   B. Eversion
   C. Inversion
   D. Plantarflexion

5. A medical student is prone to bruxism (teeth grinding) in her sleep prior to exams. You would expect that this student would experience tenderness in her oral region due to overactivity of the:
   A. Buccinator
   B. Genioglossus
   C. Lateral pterygoid
   D. Mylohyoid
   E. Orbicularis oris

Apply Your Knowledge

6. A piece of atherosclerotic plaque in the wall of the abdominal aorta breaks off and is carried downstream in the blood. It lodges in the deep femoral artery and forms a clot. In this patient you would be most concerned about loss of blood flow to the:
   A. Gluteal region
   B. Head of the femur
   C. Leg
   D. Popliteal fossa
   E. Quadriceps femoris

7. A patient has a bone spur that is compressing structures in the suprascapular notch. Which of the following would you expect to see in this individual?
   A. Loss of the ability to extend the arm
   B. Loss of the ability to adduct the arm
   C. Reduced blood supply to the infraspinous fossa
   D. Weakness in lateral (external) rotation of the arm
   E. Weakness in retraction of the scapula

8. An automotive mechanic comes into the ED with a piece of metal in his anterior abdominal wall superior to the umbilicus. The metal pierced the rectus sheath and lodged in the rectus abdominis muscle. Which of the following best describes the layers of the rectus sheath that were pierced?
   A. Aponeurosis of external oblique
   B. Aponeuroses of external oblique and half of internal oblique
   C. Aponeuroses of half of internal oblique and transversus abdominus
   D. Aponeuroses of external oblique, internal oblique and transversus abdominis

9. A carpenter severs her ulnar nerve at the wrist while feeding a board into a table saw. Which of the following would you most likely observe in this patient?
   A. Loss of abduction of the middle finger
   B. Loss of abduction of the thumb
   C. Loss of adduction of the wrist
   D. Loss of extension of the little finger
   E. Loss of flexion of the little finger

10. While undergoing a procedure to remove atherosclerotic plaque from the common carotid artery, a patient's ansa cervicalis is accidentally transected on the right side. Which of the following would you expect to see in the patient as a result of this error?
   A. Difficulty with swallowing and/or eating
   B. Inability to move the right vocal cord
   C. Inability to turn the chin to the left
   D. Loss of sensation on the anterior neck
   E. Weakness in elevation of the right shoulder

See Appendix for answers.

CHAPTER 4

CARDIOVASCULAR SYSTEM

4.1 THE CARDIOVASCULAR SYSTEM

The cardiovascular system is essentially the transportation system of the body, designed to convey materials to and from the cells. The **heart** functions as a pump to move blood through a system of tubes—the arteries and veins. **Arteries** conduct blood away from the heart and they become progressively smaller as they approach their targets; the smallest arteries are called **arterioles**. Small **venules** and **veins** convey blood towards the heart. A network of capillaries connects the arterioles and venules. **Capillaries** are the smallest vessels in the circulatory system, designed to facilitate the exchange of O_2, CO_2, nutrients, and wastes between the blood and body tissues. In general, capillaries are found between arterioles and venules; however, there are several locations in the body where a network of capillaries is found between two sets of venules. This arrangement is called a **portal system** and it is designed to fulfill a specific need for its associated organ. For example, the hepatic portal system allows nutrient-rich blood collected from the digestive tract to pass through the sinusoidal capillaries of the liver so nutrients can be extracted. The vasculature of the body as a whole is arranged in two distinct circuits. The short pulmonary circuit (**pulmonary circulation**) conveys blood between the heart and lungs for the purpose of continually supplying the blood with oxygen and removing wastes such as carbon dioxide. The **systemic circulation** is a longer circuit that is tasked with distributing oxygenated blood to all parts of the body, and then returning deoxygenated blood to the heart.

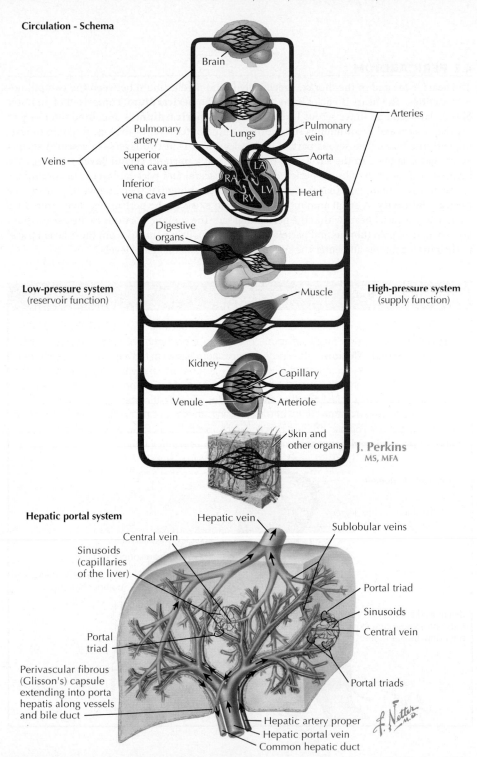

Circulation - Schema

Brain

Arteries

Pulmonary artery

Pulmonary vein

Lungs

Superior vena cava

Aorta

Veins

Inferior vena cava

RA   LA
RV   LV

Heart

Digestive organs

Low-pressure system
(reservoir function)

Muscle

High-pressure system
(supply function)

Kidney

Capillary

Venule

Arteriole

Skin and other organs

J. Perkins
MS, MFA

Hepatic portal system

Hepatic vein

Central vein

Sublobular veins

Sinusoids (capillaries of the liver)

Portal triad

Sinusoids

Central vein

Portal triad

Perivascular fibrous (Glisson's) capsule extending into porta hepatis along vessels and bile duct

Portal triads

Hepatic artery proper

Hepatic portal vein

Common hepatic duct

Figure 4.1 THE CARDIOVASCULAR SYSTEM

4.2 PERICARDIUM

The heart is located in the thorax, specifically in the mediastinum between the two pulmonary cavities. The heart is enclosed in a sac called the **pericardium**, comprised of an outer fibrous layer and an inner serous layer. The **fibrous pericardium** is anchored inferiorly to the diaphragm and is continuous superiorly with the outer layer of the vessels communicating with the heart. The serous part of the pericardium is in two layers—a **visceral serous layer** that is applied to the surface of the heart, and a **parietal serous layer** that lines the internal surface of the fibrous pericardium. The visceral and parietal layers are continuous at the superior boundary (base) of the heart, and the potential space between them is the **pericardial cavity**. A small amount of serous fluid exists in the pericardial cavity to reduce friction as the heart beats within the pericardial sac. The somatic portions of the pericardium are sensitive to pain (fibrous and parietal serous layers). Pain neurons from these layers travel in the phrenic nerves and enter the spinal cord at the C3–C5 spinal levels.

Clinical Focus

Inflammation of the pericardium, for example due to a bacterial or viral infection, is called **pericarditis**. Pericarditis may lead to an increase in the amount of fluid in the pericardial cavity (**pericardial effusion**). The fibrous pericardium has a limited capacity to stretch, thus pericardial effusions may compress the heart if they accumulate suddenly—for example, in the case of rapid bleeding into the pericardial cavity due to trauma. Compression of the heart due to pericardial effusion is called **cardiac tamponade**; it is a life-threatening condition because it compromises venous return and ventricular filling, thus reducing cardiac output. Pressure from pericardial effusion can be quickly relieved by removing the fluid with a needle—a procedure called **pericardiocentesis**, or more simply, a *pericardial tap*.

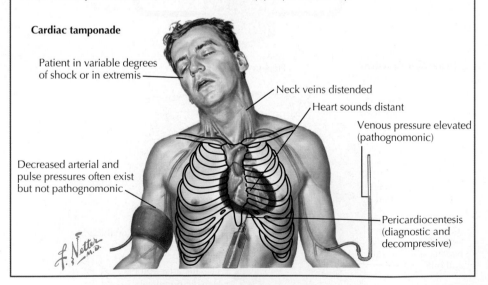

Cardiac tamponade

Patient in variable degrees of shock or in extremis

Neck veins distended

Heart sounds distant

Venous pressure elevated (pathognomonic)

Decreased arterial and pulse pressures often exist but not pathognomonic

Pericardiocentesis (diagnostic and decompressive)

Pericardial sac: anterior view

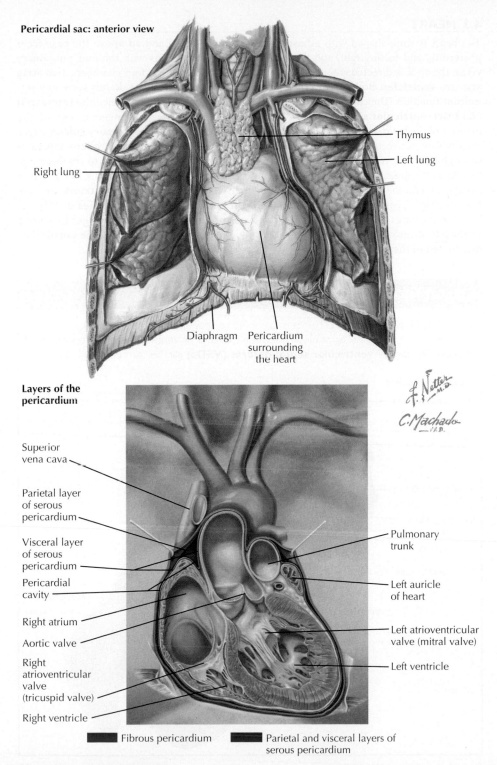

Thymus

Left lung

Right lung

Diaphragm   Pericardium surrounding the heart

Layers of the pericardium

Superior vena cava

Parietal layer of serous pericardium

Visceral layer of serous pericardium

Pericardial cavity

Right atrium

Aortic valve

Right atrioventricular valve (tricuspid valve)

Right ventricle

Pulmonary trunk

Left auricle of heart

Left atrioventricular valve (mitral valve)

Left ventricle

Fibrous pericardium   Parietal and visceral layers of serous pericardium

Figure 4.2 PERICARDIUM

4.3 HEART

The heart is cone-shaped with a **base** (flat part of the cone) and an **apex**. The base faces posteriorly and to the right, and is anchored by its connections with the four pulmonary veins; the apex is directed anteriorly and to the left. The heart has four chambers, two **atria** and two **ventricles**. Both atria have appendages called **auricles** that do not serve any significant function. The chambers are separated internally by partitions called the **interatrial** and **interventricular septa**. Evidence of the separations between chambers is seen on the exterior of the heart as grooves *(sulci)* between the musculature. The **coronary sulcus** marks the division between the atria and ventricles, while the **interventricular sulcus** separates the right and left ventricles. The large arteries and veins that are attached to the heart are known as the great vessels. The **superior** and **inferior venae cavae** (SVC and IVC) convey deoxygenated blood from the body into the right atrium. The **pulmonary trunk** emerges from the right ventricle and gives rise to the **right** and **left pulmonary arteries** that shuttle blood to the lungs to become oxygenated; four **pulmonary veins** carry the oxygenated blood to the left atrium of the heart. Oxygenated blood leaves the heart through the **aorta** to be distributed to the body.

Clinical Focus

If the septa between the heart chambers do not form properly during development, openings can remain that allow mixing of blood between the atria or ventricles. These **atrial septal defects (ASDs)** or **ventricular septal defects (VSDs)** can be corrected surgically.

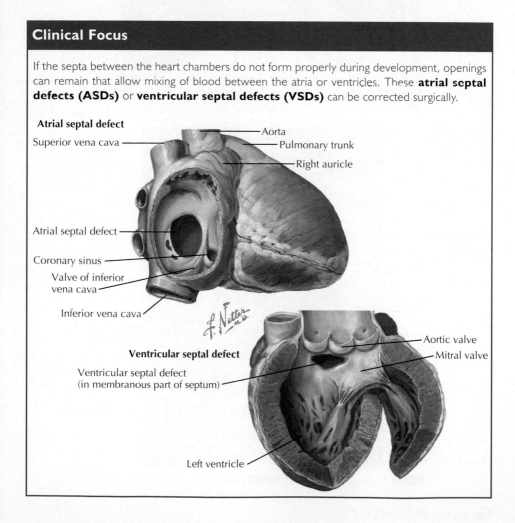

Atrial septal defect

Aorta
Superior vena cava
Pulmonary trunk
Right auricle

Atrial septal defect

Coronary sinus
Valve of inferior
vena cava

Inferior vena cava

Ventricular septal defect

Aortic valve
Mitral valve

Ventricular septal defect
(in membranous part of septum)

Left ventricle

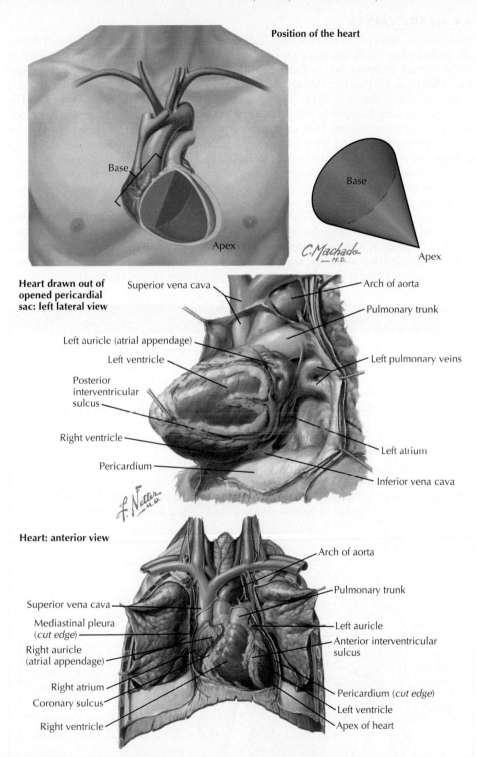

Position of the heart

Base

Base

Apex

Apex

C. Machado M.D.

Heart drawn out of opened pericardial sac: left lateral view

Superior vena cava

Arch of aorta

Pulmonary trunk

Left auricle (atrial appendage)

Left ventricle

Left pulmonary veins

Posterior interventricular sulcus

Right ventricle

Left atrium

Pericardium

Inferior vena cava

F. Netter M.D.

Heart: anterior view

Arch of aorta

Pulmonary trunk

Superior vena cava

Mediastinal pleura (*cut edge*)

Left auricle

Anterior interventricular sulcus

Right auricle (atrial appendage)

Right atrium

Pericardium (*cut edge*)

Coronary sulcus

Left ventricle

Right ventricle

Apex of heart

Figure 4.3 HEART

4.4 HEART VALVES

There are two types of valves in the heart—atrioventricular (AV) valves and semilunar valves. **AV valves** allow communication between the atria and ventricles; they are comprised of cusps that are anchored to ventricular **papillary muscles** via fibrous "strings" called **chordae tendineae**. On the right side of the heart, the AV valve is called the **tricuspid valve** due to the fact that it has three cusps. The left AV valve is most often called the **mitral valve**, although the term *bicuspid* is also used. **Semilunar valves** consist of three cuplike cusps with no chordae tendineae. They are located at the junction of the ventricles and the two outflow vessels of the heart (pulmonary trunk and aorta), thus they are logically named the **pulmonary** and **aortic valves**. During ventricular filling (diastole), blood flows with gravity from the atria to the ventricles and the AV valve cusps are passively opened; the semilunar valves are closed at this time. When the ventricles contract during systole, a mechanism is needed to prevent the AV valve cusps from flapping back into the atria, otherwise blood could pass from the ventricles to the atria. Contraction of the papillary muscles achieves this by putting tension on the chordae tendineae and holding the valve in a closed position. Thus blood is directed out of the ventricles through the pulmonary and aortic valves. The pressure of the blood passively pushes the semilunar valve cusps open; closure occurs when the ventricles relax and blood falls back toward the heart, filling the sinuses of the valves.

Clinical Focus

Auscultation of the heart with a stethoscope allows assessment of heart rate, heart rhythm, and valvular function. The sound produced by the heart is often described with the term *lub-dub*. The first portion of this two-syllable sound is produced by the closure of the AV valves; it is called the **first heart sound (S1)**. The **second heart sound (S2)** is generated by the closure of the semilunar valves. There are specific locations on the chest used to listen to each heart valve that do not correspond precisely with the location of the valve. This is because valve sounds are transmitted downstream of the valve by the flowing blood. Abnormalities of the heart valves produce stenosis or insufficiency. **Stenosis** is narrowing of the valve opening that reduces blood flow through the valve; one common cause is stiffening of the valve with age. **Valvular insufficiency**, or regurgitation, is lack of complete closure of a valve that allows leakage of blood "backwards" across the valve. Both of these conditions produce turbulence in blood flow that can be heard with a stethoscope as a **heart murmur**.

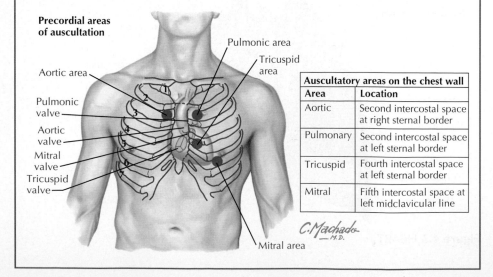

Precordial areas of auscultation

Aortic area

Pulmonic valve

Aortic valve

Mitral valve

Tricuspid valve

Pulmonic area

Tricuspid area

Auscultatory areas on the chest wall	
Area	**Location**
Aortic	Second intercostal space at right sternal border
Pulmonary	Second intercostal space at left sternal border
Tricuspid	Fourth intercostal space at left sternal border
Mitral	Fifth intercostal space at left midclavicular line

C. Machado
— M.D.

Mitral area

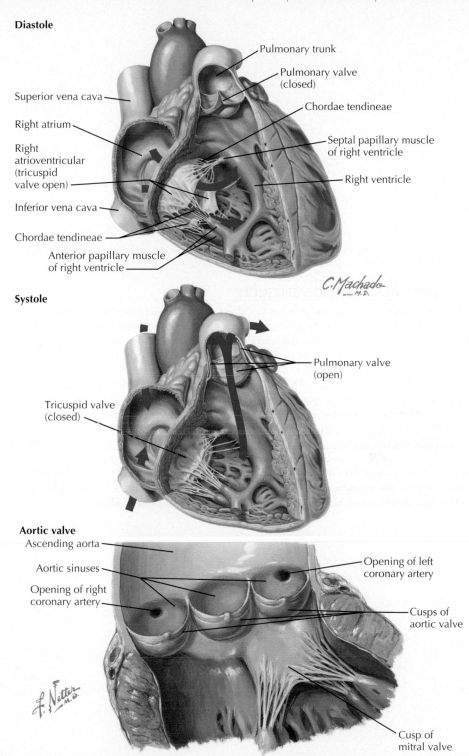

Diastole

Pulmonary trunk

Pulmonary valve (closed)

Superior vena cava

Chordae tendineae

Right atrium

Septal papillary muscle of right ventricle

Right atrioventricular (tricuspid valve open)

Right ventricle

Inferior vena cava

Chordae tendineae

Anterior papillary muscle of right ventricle

C. Machado
—M.D.

Systole

Pulmonary valve (open)

Tricuspid valve (closed)

Aortic valve

Ascending aorta

Opening of left coronary artery

Aortic sinuses

Opening of right coronary artery

Cusps of aortic valve

Cusp of mitral valve

F. Netter
M.D.

Figure 4.4 HEART VALVES

4.5 RIGHT ATRIUM AND VENTRICLE

The role of the right side of the heart is to collect deoxygenated blood and convey it to the lungs for gas exchange. Thus the interior of the **right atrium** exhibits openings of the great veins as well as the ostium of the **coronary sinus**—a venous structure that collects venous blood from the heart itself. These openings may have small flaps of tissue associated with them that have no role in the adult but functioned as valves in the fetus. Based on the way the right atrium develops, part of its wall consists of bands of muscle (**pectinate muscles**) while the remaining part is smooth; the ridge that indicates the transition between these two parts is the **crista terminalis**. The interatrial septum has an oval depression called the **fossa ovalis** that marks the location of the foramen ovale that was present in the fetus. The wall of the **right ventricle** is comprised of irregular ridges of muscle called **trabeculae carneae**. One particular band of muscle, the **moderator band**, is significant because it contains components of the conduction system of the heart. The vessel that conveys blood out of the right ventricle is the **pulmonary trunk**. The opening for this artery is located at the superior part of the right ventricle and blood flow is regulated by the **pulmonary valve**.

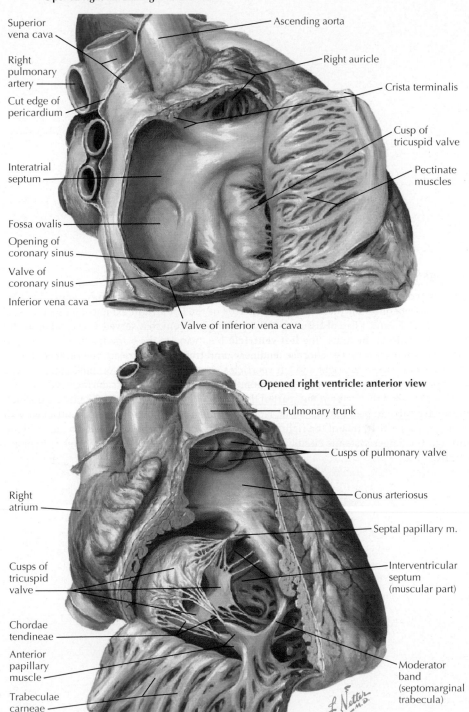

Opened right atrium: right lateral view

Superior vena cava

Right pulmonary artery

Cut edge of pericardium

Interatrial septum

Fossa ovalis

Opening of coronary sinus

Valve of coronary sinus

Inferior vena cava

Ascending aorta

Right auricle

Crista terminalis

Cusp of tricuspid valve

Pectinate muscles

Valve of inferior vena cava

Opened right ventricle: anterior view

Pulmonary trunk

Cusps of pulmonary valve

Conus arteriosus

Right atrium

Septal papillary m.

Cusps of tricuspid valve

Interventricular septum (muscular part)

Chordae tendineae

Anterior papillary muscle

Moderator band (septomarginal trabecula)

Trabeculae carneae

Figure 4.5 RIGHT ATRIUM AND VENTRICLE

4.6 LEFT ATRIUM AND VENTRICLE

Oxygenated blood from the lungs enters the **left atrium** via four **pulmonary veins**. In addition to the openings for these veins, the interior of the left atrium exhibits an opening into the left auricle, and a flap of tissue on the interatrial septum that served as the **valve of the foramen ovale** in the fetus. The **left ventricle** has many of the same features as the right ventricle: papillary muscles, chordae tendineae, and trabeculae carneae. The **interventricular septum** between the right and left ventricles is comprised mainly of muscle; however, a small portion near the aortic valve is not populated by myocardial cells during development, and thus is called the *membranous* part of the septum. Blood leaves the left ventricle through the **aortic valve** to pass into the aorta. Note that the myocardium of the left ventricular wall is much thicker than that of the right ventricle, since the left ventricle needs to pump blood through the longer systemic circuit of the circulation, in contrast to the shorter pulmonary circuit.

Flap opened in posterolateral wall of left ventricle

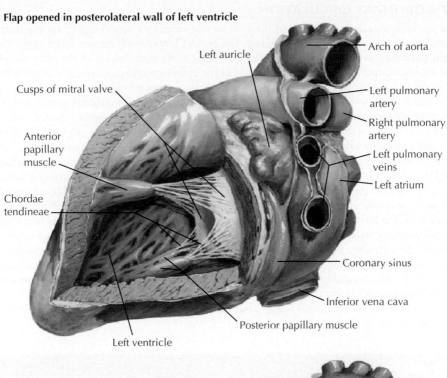

Left auricle

Arch of aorta

Cusps of mitral valve

Left pulmonary artery

Right pulmonary artery

Anterior papillary muscle

Left pulmonary veins

Left atrium

Chordae tendineae

Coronary sinus

Inferior vena cava

Posterior papillary muscle

Left ventricle

Section through left atrium and ventricle with mitral valve cut away

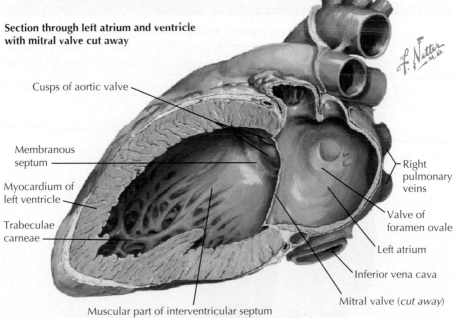

Cusps of aortic valve

Membranous septum

Right pulmonary veins

Myocardium of left ventricle

Valve of foramen ovale

Trabeculae carneae

Left atrium

Inferior vena cava

Mitral valve (*cut away*)

Muscular part of interventricular septum

Figure 4.6 LEFT ATRIUM AND VENTRICLE

4.7 CORONARY CIRCULATION

The coronary circulation consists of the arteries and veins that supply and drain the heart. Variations in these vessels exist, although the typical pattern will be described here. The **right coronary artery** emerges from the ascending aorta near the tip of the right auricle and travels around the right side of the heart in the coronary sulcus. It typically supplies the SA node via the **sinoatrial (SA) nodal artery,** and then gives off numerous branches to the right atrium and ventricle. Two primary branches are the **(acute) marginal artery** and the **posterior descending artery (PDA).** The right coronary artery also supplies the AV node in most individuals via several small **AV nodal branches** that arise near the origin of the PDA. The **left coronary artery** originates from the ascending aorta posterior to the pulmonary trunk. It subsequently bifurcates into two branches, the **left anterior descending artery (LAD)** and the **circumflex artery.** The LAD travels in the anterior interventricular sulcus and gives off branches to both ventricles. The circumflex branch travels in the coronary sulcus on the left side of the heart and supplies both the left atrium and left ventricle. Venous blood from the heart tissue is collected by the cardiac veins. Most cardiac veins terminate in the **coronary sinus,** a sac-like structure on the inferior surface of the heart that empties into the right atrium. Three primary veins are the **great cardiac vein** that travels with the LAD, the **middle cardiac vein** that travels with the PDA, and the **small cardiac vein** that travels with the marginal branch of the right coronary artery. Note that small **anterior cardiac veins** transmit blood from the right ventricle directly into the right atrium. The heart musculature also has very small veins ("least cardiac veins") that convey blood directly into the chambers of the heart.

Clinical Focus

Atherosclerosis of coronary arteries (**coronary artery disease** or **CAD**) reduces the blood supply to the heart muscle due to narrowing or occlusion of major arteries. Depending on the severity of the condition, the resultant ischemia can cause chest pain (angina) and/or myocardial infarction.

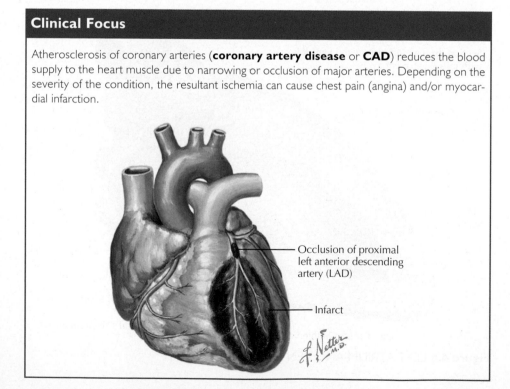

Occlusion of proximal left anterior descending artery (LAD)

Infarct

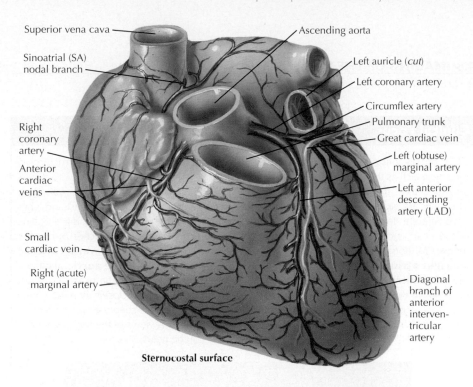

Superior vena cava

Sinoatrial (SA) nodal branch

Right coronary artery

Anterior cardiac veins

Small cardiac vein

Right (acute) marginal artery

Ascending aorta

Left auricle (*cut*)

Left coronary artery

Circumflex artery

Pulmonary trunk

Great cardiac vein

Left (obtuse) marginal artery

Left anterior descending artery (LAD)

Diagonal branch of anterior interventricular artery

Sternocostal surface

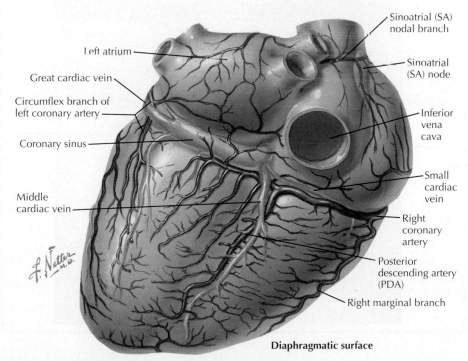

Left atrium

Great cardiac vein

Circumflex branch of left coronary artery

Coronary sinus

Middle cardiac vein

Sinoatrial (SA) nodal branch

Sinoatrial (SA) node

Inferior vena cava

Small cardiac vein

Right coronary artery

Posterior descending artery (PDA)

Right marginal branch

Diaphragmatic surface

Figure 4.7 CORONARY CIRCULATION

4.8 IMAGING OF THE HEART

Chest radiographs are commonly obtained to evaluate the heart, as well as other structures in the chest such as the lungs. The heart is mainly comprised of muscle, thus on x-ray it appears gray (structures that appear gray have what is called *soft tissue* or *water density* in radiology). The lungs are filled with air, thus they appear black *(air density)*. Because the heart and lungs have different densities, the boundaries between them can be seen on x-ray, and the outline of the heart is called the **cardiac silhouette**. On a posteroanterior (PA) chest x-ray, the mediastinal border adjacent to the right lung is comprised of the **superior vena cava** and the **right atrium**. On the left side, the border is comprised mainly of the **aortic arch** and the **left ventricle**. The right ventricle is the most anterior chamber of the heart and is just posterior to the sternum. The left atrium is posterior in location and is closely associated with the esophagus and vertebral column. These two chambers are not seen well on a PA chest x-ray; they can, however, be distinguished on a lateral view. Axial views of the heart produced with CT or MRI allow visualization of all four chambers of the heart.

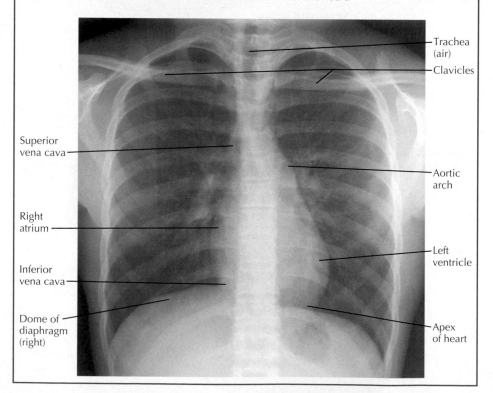

Clinical Focus (Continued)

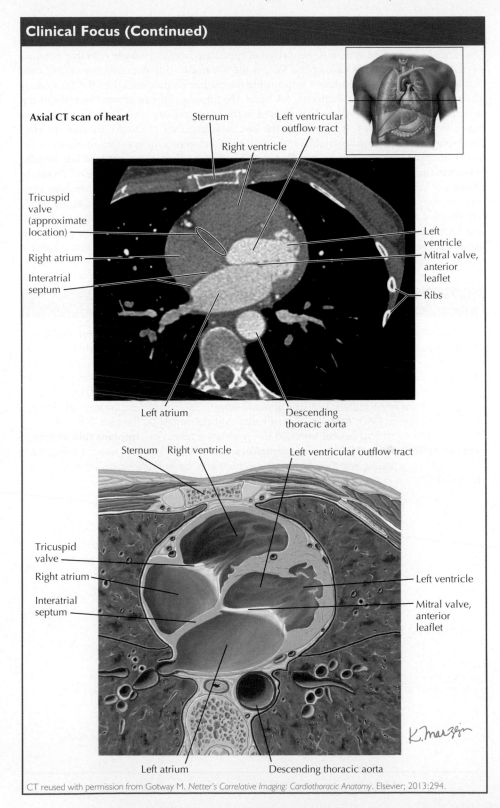

Axial CT scan of heart

Sternum

Left ventricular outflow tract

Right ventricle

Tricuspid valve (approximate location)

Right atrium

Interatrial septum

Left ventricle

Mitral valve, anterior leaflet

Ribs

Left atrium

Descending thoracic aorta

Sternum   Right ventricle

Left ventricular outflow tract

Tricuspid valve

Right atrium

Interatrial septum

Left ventricle

Mitral valve, anterior leaflet

Left atrium

Descending thoracic aorta

K. marzan

CT reused with permission from Gotway M. *Netter's Correlative Imaging: Cardiothoracic Anatomy.* Elsevier; 2013:294.

4.9 CONDUCTION SYSTEM

The cardiac conduction system is comprised of specialized cardiac muscle cells that conduct electrical impulses. At the base of the SVC is the **SA node**. This structure consists of cells that initiate the electrical impulses responsible for cardiac contraction, thus the SA node is often called the *pacemaker*. From the SA node, the impulses spread across the walls of the atria to the **AV node**. The AV node is located in the interatrial septum adjacent to the opening of the coronary sinus. It distributes the electrical impulses to the **AV bundle (of His)** that bridges the atrial and ventricular musculature and traverses the membranous part of the interventricular septum. The AV bundle subsequently branches into **right and left bundle branches** that conduct the impulses along the interventricular septum and give off **Purkinje fibers** that extend into the walls of the ventricles. In addition to stimulating ventricular contraction, the impulses conveyed by the Purkinje fibers also initiate contraction of the papillary muscles to promote closure of the AV valves in sync with contraction of the ventricles. The **septomarginal trabecula**, commonly known as the *moderator band*, is a prominent band of muscle in the right ventricle that conveys Purkinje fibers to the anterior papillary muscle of the tricuspid valve.

Clinical Focus

The electrical activity of the heart can be measured with an **electrocardiogram** (**ECG** or **EKG**), and abnormalities manifest as irregular heart rhythms (**arrhythmias**). Arrhythmias are classified by the chamber in which they originate, and the speed of the abnormal heart rate. **Tachycardia** refers to a resting heart rate that is too fast (greater than 100 beats/min in a typical patient), while **bradycardia** is a slow resting heart rate that is less than 60 beats/min. Arrhythmias are often caused by a lack of blood flow to the conduction tissue of the heart, for example due to CAD. A variety of treatments exist depending on the type of arrhythmia. In some patients artificial devices are used to regulate the heart rate. **Implantable cardioverter defibrillators (ICDs)** and **pacemakers** detect when the heart rate is tachycardic, bradycardic, or irregular, and then deliver an electrical impulse or defibrillation shock via leads (wires) implanted in the heart to restore a normal heartbeat.

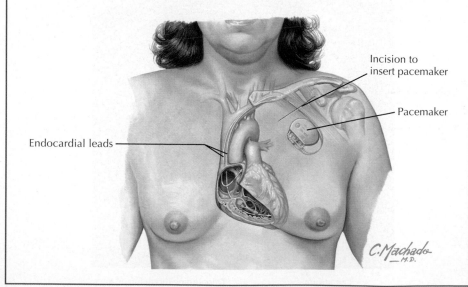

Incision to insert pacemaker

Pacemaker

Endocardial leads

C. Machado
_M.D.

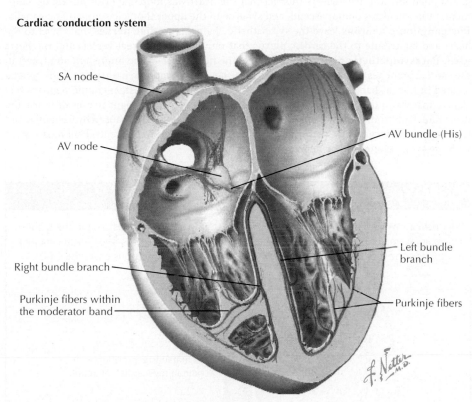

Cardiac conduction system

SA node

AV node

AV bundle (His)

Right bundle branch

Left bundle branch

Purkinje fibers within the moderator band

Purkinje fibers

Figure 4.9 CONDUCTION SYSTEM

4.10 INNERVATION OF THE HEART

The heart rate and force of contraction can be modified by autonomic input. **Sympathetic cardiac nerves** cause an increase in the heart rate and the strength of contraction via terminations on nodal tissue, conduction tissue, and heart muscle. The **preganglionic sympathetic neurons** have cell bodies in the lateral horns of the upper thoracic levels of the spinal cord (approximately T1–T4), and their axons enter the sympathetic chains. Once in the chains, many neurons ascend to the cervical region to synapse in cervical sympathetic ganglia, a phenomenon that reflects the fact that the heart was more superior during development. Other neurons do not ascend, and synapse in the upper thoracic sympathetic ganglia. **Postganglionic neurons** leave the sympathetic chains as **cardiac nerves** that travel to the heart and contribute to the cardiac plexus that ramifies on the great vessels and the heart itself. **Parasympathetic neurons** that supply the heart arise in the brainstem and travel in the cardiac branches of the **vagus nerves**. These neurons synapse in parasympathetic ganglia located in the cardiac plexus or on the wall of the heart; short postganglionic neurons terminate mainly on the SA and AV nodes. Cardiac branches of the vagus nerves decrease the heart rate. Pain from the heart is typically due to tissue damage (e.g., caused by ischemia) and is conveyed by **visceral afferent neurons** that primarily travel to the central nervous system with the sympathetic cardiac nerves.

Clinical Focus

Pain from a myocardial infarction ("heart attack") is often felt in the chest and in the left arm. This is an example of **referred pain**, a concept where visceral pain is referred to cutaneous territories corresponding to the spinal levels where the afferent neurons enter the CNS.

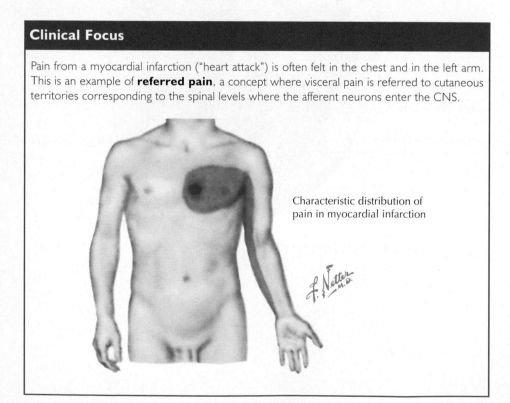

Characteristic distribution of pain in myocardial infarction

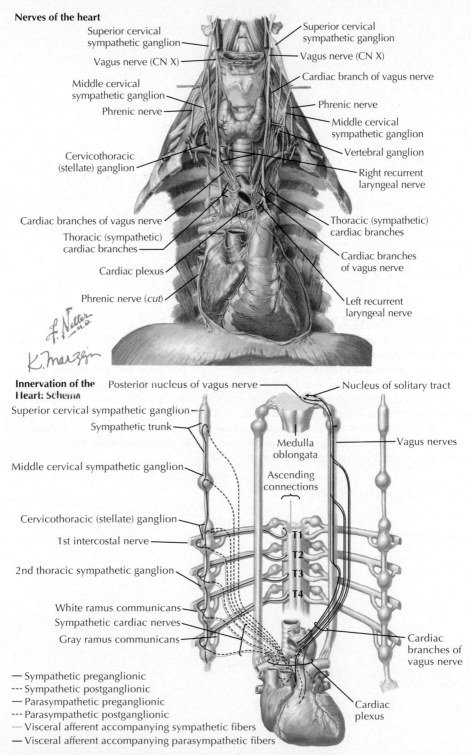

Nerves of the heart

Superior cervical sympathetic ganglion

Vagus nerve (CN X)

Middle cervical sympathetic ganglion

Phrenic nerve

Cervicothoracic (stellate) ganglion

Cardiac branches of vagus nerve

Thoracic (sympathetic) cardiac branches

Cardiac plexus

Phrenic nerve (*cut*)

Superior cervical sympathetic ganglion

Vagus nerve (CN X)

Cardiac branch of vagus nerve

Phrenic nerve

Middle cervical sympathetic ganglion

Vertebral ganglion

Right recurrent laryngeal nerve

Thoracic (sympathetic) cardiac branches

Cardiac branches of vagus nerve

Left recurrent laryngeal nerve

Innervation of the Heart: Schema

Posterior nucleus of vagus nerve

Nucleus of solitary tract

Superior cervical sympathetic ganglion

Sympathetic trunk

Middle cervical sympathetic ganglion

Cervicothoracic (stellate) ganglion

1st intercostal nerve

2nd thoracic sympathetic ganglion

White ramus communicans

Sympathetic cardiac nerves

Gray ramus communicans

Medulla oblongata

Ascending connections

Vagus nerves

T1
T2
T3
T4

Cardiac branches of vagus nerve

Cardiac plexus

— Sympathetic preganglionic
--- Sympathetic postganglionic
— Parasympathetic preganglionic
--- Parasympathetic postganglionic
— Visceral afferent accompanying sympathetic fibers
— Visceral afferent accompanying parasympathetic fibers

Figure 4.10 INNERVATION OF THE HEART

4.11 PULMONARY CIRCULATION

Deoxygenated blood from the body enters the right side of the heart through the **superior** and **inferior venae cavae**. After passing into the right ventricle, the blood leaves the heart through the **pulmonary trunk** that bifurcates into the **right** and **left pulmonary arteries** (colored blue in the figures to indicate the lack of oxygen in the blood). Each pulmonary artery enters the hilum of the lung and subsequently branches into smaller **lobar arteries**, **segmental arteries**, and eventually **arterioles** that feed the capillary beds of the alveoli. Gas exchange occurs across the alveolar wall, and then oxygenated blood enters **venules** and subsequently larger tributaries of the **pulmonary veins**. Four pulmonary veins, two from each lung, convey blood to the left atrium of the heart.

Pulmonary circulation

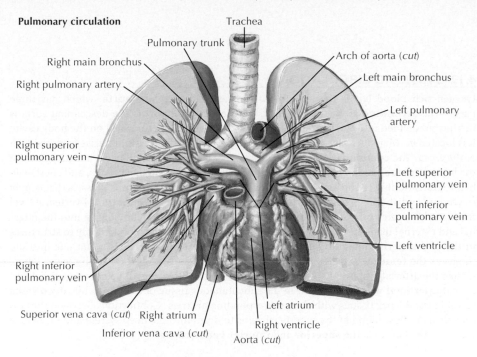

Trachea
Pulmonary trunk
Right main bronchus
Right pulmonary artery
Right superior pulmonary vein
Right inferior pulmonary vein
Superior vena cava (*cut*)   Right atrium
Inferior vena cava (*cut*)
Aorta (*cut*)
Right ventricle
Left atrium
Left ventricle
Left inferior pulmonary vein
Left superior pulmonary vein
Left pulmonary artery
Left main bronchus
Arch of aorta (*cut*)

Alveolar capillary beds

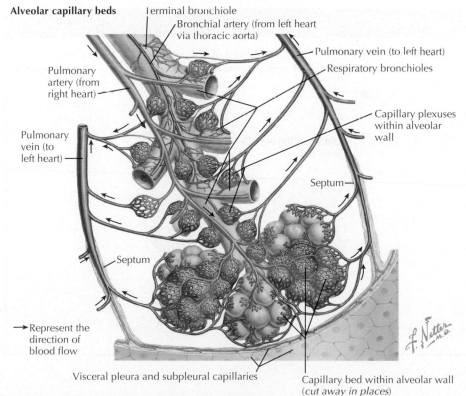

Terminal bronchiole
Bronchial artery (from left heart via thoracic aorta)
Pulmonary artery (from right heart)
Pulmonary vein (to left heart)
Septum
Septum
→ Represent the direction of blood flow
Visceral pleura and subpleural capillaries
Pulmonary vein (to left heart)
Respiratory bronchioles
Capillary plexuses within alveolar wall
Septum
Capillary bed within alveolar wall (*cut away in places*)

Figure 4.11 PULMONARY CIRCULATION

4.12 SYSTEMIC CIRCULATION

Oxygen-rich blood leaves the left side of the heart through the **aorta**, which has three parts—the **ascending aorta**, **aortic arch**, and **descending aorta**. The descending aorta is further subdivided into the **thoracic aorta** and **abdominal aorta**, based on the body cavity it is located in. Major arteries that supply the head, neck, and upper limbs arise from the arch of the aorta. The **common carotid arteries** supply both the head and neck, including part of the brain. The **subclavian arteries** provide branches to the brain, neck, back, and chest wall, before transitioning to the **axillary arteries** that supply the upper limbs. Vessels that supply the thorax and abdomen primarily arise from the descending aorta. At the L4 vertebral level the aorta bifurcates into the **common iliac arteries** that subsequently divide into the internal and external iliac arteries. The **internal iliac arteries** provide blood mainly to structures in the pelvis, perineum, and gluteal region. The **external iliac arteries** continue into the thighs as the **femoral arteries**, which are the primary source of blood to the lower limbs. Unlike the arterial system, the venous system consists of two sets of veins—superficial and deep. **Superficial veins** are located in the subcutaneous tissue of the skin, while **deep veins** travel in the deeper tissues with their corresponding arteries. Connections between the two sets of veins allow blood in the superficial veins to drain into the deep system and ultimately return to the heart via the **superior** and **inferior venae cavae**.

Clinical Focus

Assessment of arterial pulses is a fundamental part of a physical exam. Pulses commonly evaluated include the **carotid**, **brachial**, **radial**, **femoral**, **posterior tibial**, and **dorsalis pedis**.

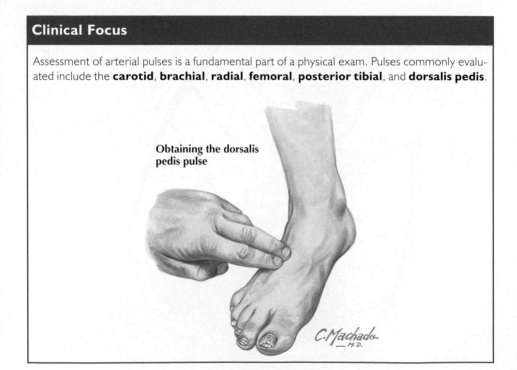

Obtaining the dorsalis pedis pulse

C. Machado
_M.D.

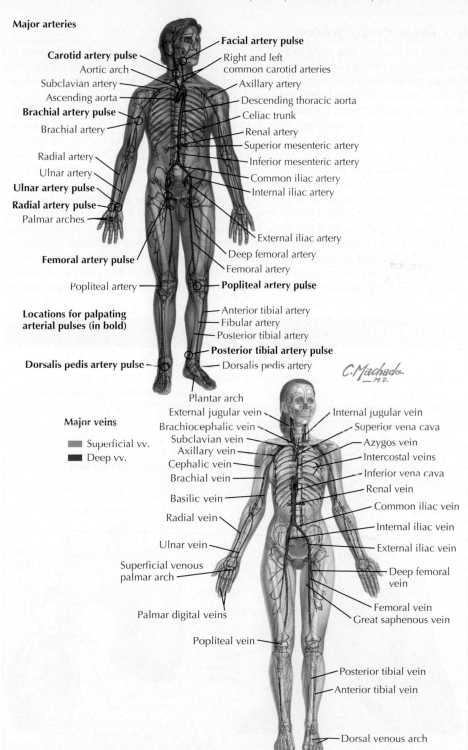

Major arteries

Facial artery pulse
Carotid artery pulse
Aortic arch
Right and left
common carotid arteries
Subclavian artery
Axillary artery
Ascending aorta
Descending thoracic aorta
Brachial artery pulse
Celiac trunk
Brachial artery
Renal artery
Superior mesenteric artery
Radial artery
Inferior mesenteric artery
Ulnar artery
Common iliac artery
Ulnar artery pulse
Internal iliac artery
Radial artery pulse
Palmar arches
External iliac artery
Deep femoral artery
Femoral artery pulse
Femoral artery
Popliteal artery
Popliteal artery pulse

**Locations for palpating
arterial pulses (in bold)**
Anterior tibial artery
Fibular artery
Posterior tibial artery
Posterior tibial artery pulse
Dorsalis pedis artery pulse
Dorsalis pedis artery

C. Machado
— M.D.

Plantar arch
External jugular vein
Internal jugular vein
Major veins
Brachiocephalic vein
Superior vena cava
Subclavian vein
Azygos vein
Superficial vv.
Axillary vein
Intercostal veins
Deep vv.
Cephalic vein
Inferior vena cava
Brachial vein
Renal vein
Basilic vein
Common iliac vein
Radial vein
Internal iliac vein
Ulnar vein
External iliac vein
Superficial venous
palmar arch
Deep femoral
vein
Palmar digital veins
Femoral vein
Great saphenous vein
Popliteal vein

Posterior tibial vein
Anterior tibial vein

Dorsal venous arch

Figure 4.12 SYSTEMIC CIRCULATION

4.13 FETAL CIRCULATION

In the fetus, nutrient-rich oxygenated blood is provided by the maternal placenta, thus the role of the circulation is primarily distribution. Blood from the placenta enters the fetus through the umbilical cord within the **umbilical vein**. Since this blood does not need to be filtered, a shunt called the **ductus venosus** allows it to bypass the liver and pass directly into the IVC and right atrium. The blood in the right atrium does not need to enter the pulmonary circulation for gas exchange, thus an opening in the interatrial septum, the **foramen ovale**, permits blood from the IVC to pass from the right atrium to the left atrium. Due to gravity, most of the blood that enters the right atrium through the SVC does not utilize the foramen ovale and passes through the tricuspid valve into the right ventricle. As this blood leaves the heart through the pulmonary trunk, it is directed away from the lungs by a shunt between the pulmonary trunk and aorta called the **ductus arteriosus**. Although the diameter of this shunt is small, blood preferentially flows through it in lieu of the pulmonary arteries because pulmonary resistance is high. After blood is distributed to the body via the aorta and its branches, it returns to the placenta within the paired **umbilical arteries**. At birth, when the infant no longer receives blood from the placenta, the three shunts close to create the postnatal pattern of pulmonary and systemic circulation. Remnants exist for each shunt; these are the **ligamentum venosum**, **fossa ovalis**, and the **ligamentum arteriosum**.

Clinical Focus

If the foramen ovale does not close after birth, an individual can have a **patent foramen ovale (PFO)**. This allows a small amount of mixing of oxygenated and deoxygenated blood between the atria, although it is typically a benign condition. **Patent ductus arteriosus (PDA)** is a congenital abnormality where the ductus arteriosus remains open. This is a more serious condition than a PFO, and management depends on factors such as the size of the PDA and the age of the patient. In some individuals, the lumen of the aorta can be affected by closure of the ductus arteriosus. It is thought that during the normal remodeling process, cells unintentionally migrate into the wall of the aorta producing a **coarctation** (narrowing) that hinders blood flow.

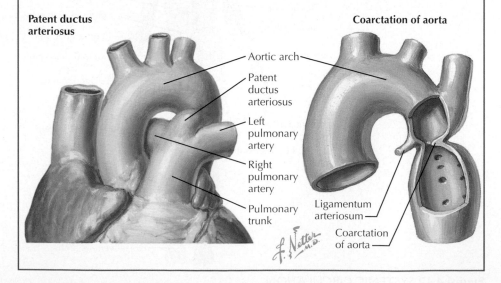

Patent ductus arteriosus

Coarctation of aorta

Aortic arch

Patent ductus arteriosus

Left pulmonary artery

Right pulmonary artery

Pulmonary trunk

Ligamentum arteriosum

Coarctation of aorta

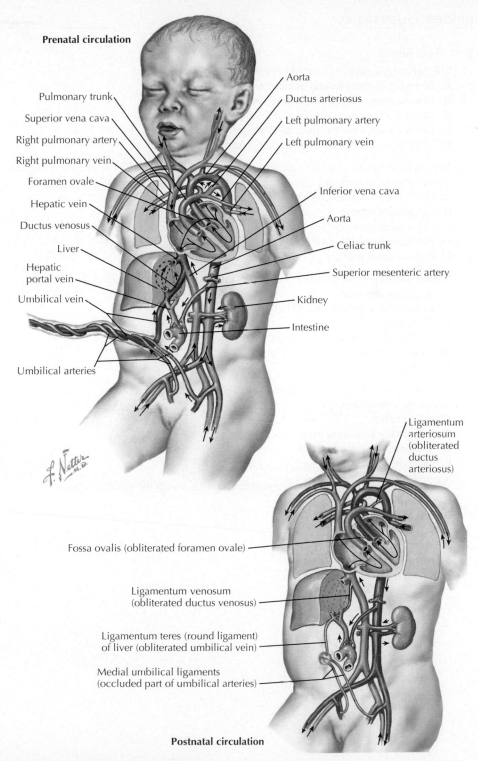

Prenatal circulation

Pulmonary trunk

Superior vena cava

Right pulmonary artery

Right pulmonary vein

Foramen ovale

Hepatic vein

Ductus venosus

Liver

Hepatic portal vein

Umbilical vein

Umbilical arteries

Aorta

Ductus arteriosus

Left pulmonary artery

Left pulmonary vein

Inferior vena cava

Aorta

Celiac trunk

Superior mesenteric artery

Kidney

Intestine

Ligamentum arteriosum (obliterated ductus arteriosus)

Fossa ovalis (obliterated foramen ovale)

Ligamentum venosum (obliterated ductus venosus)

Ligamentum teres (round ligament) of liver (obliterated umbilical vein)

Medial umbilical ligaments (occluded part of umbilical arteries)

Postnatal circulation

Figure 4.13 FETAL CIRCULATION

REVIEW QUESTIONS

Test Your Recall

1. The pericardial cavity is located between the:
   A. Fibrous pericardium and mediastinal pleura
   B. Fibrous pericardium and parietal serous pericardium
   C. Parietal serous pericardium and mediastinal pleura
   D. Parietal serous pericardium and visceral serous pericardium
   E. Visceral serous pericardium and myocardium

2. Your patient has an arterial occlusion affecting the sinoatrial (SA) node. Assuming the typical pattern of coronary circulation, which artery is most likely occluded?
   A. Left anterior descending artery (LAD)
   B. Circumflex artery
   C. Left coronary artery
   D. Posterior descending artery (PDA)
   E. Right coronary artery

3. Which portion of the cardiac conduction system directly conveys electrical impulses to the papillary muscles?
   A. Atrioventricular bundle (of His)
   B. AV node
   C. Left bundle branch
   D. Purkinje fibers
   E. SA node

4. After flowing through the tricuspid valve, blood flows through the:
   A. Aortic semilunar valve
   B. Mitral valve
   C. Pulmonary semilunar valve
   D. Right atrioventricular valve
   E. Valve of the foramen ovale

5. Which structure travels in the interventricular sulcus with the great cardiac vein?
   A. Circumflex artery
   B. Left anterior descending artery
   C. Left coronary artery
   D. Marginal artery
   E. Posterior descending artery
   F. Right coronary artery

Apply Your Knowledge

6. After being stationary on a long transcontinental flight, a patient develops a clot in a deep vein of their leg (deep vein thrombosis, or DVT). The clot breaks off and travels through the circulation; it then becomes lodged in the first capillary bed that it comes to. During its journey, how many valves of the heart did the clot pass through?
   A. 0
   B. 1
   C. 2
   D. 3
   E. 4

7. Your patient had rheumatic fever as a child that produced structural changes in one of the heart valves. A CT scan of the patient's heart shows that the wall of the right ventricle is hypertrophied, and one of the valves is stenotic (the valve opening is narrowed). Which of the four heart valves is most likely stenotic?
   A. Aortic semilunar valve
   B. Mitral valve
   C. Pulmonary semilunar valve
   D. Tricuspid valve

8. A patient enters the emergency department complaining of sharp pain in his chest and over his left shoulder. He reports that he recently had a respiratory infection with a fever, and he wondered if the two could be related. Which of the following is the most likely cause of the patient's pain?
   A. Heart block (abnormal heart rhythm)
   B. Heart failure
   C. Inflammation of the parietal pericardium (pericarditis)
   D. Inflammation of the heart muscle (myocarditis)
   E. Myocardial infarction ("heart attack")

9. An 8-year-old boy recently joined a soccer team and complains of pain and weakness in his legs. Physical exam reveals high blood pressure and a heart murmur. Simultaneous palpation of his brachial and femoral pulses indicates decreased femoral pulses. Imaging reveals mild hypertrophy of the left ventricle and a coarctation of the aorta (narrowing) just distal to the origin of the left subclavian artery. His physician shares that the coarctation is likely congenital and was caused by a problem with the normal changes that occur in circulation after birth. Which of the following processes most likely did not occur in a typical fashion?
   A. Closure of the ductus arteriosus
   B. Closure of the ductus venosus
   C. Closure of the foramen ovale
   D. Closure of the umbilical arteries
   E. Closure of the umbilical veins

10. A patient is brought to the emergency department after receiving a stab wound in his chest. The knife pierced the heart in the location indicated by the X on the chest x-ray. Which portion of the heart was punctured?

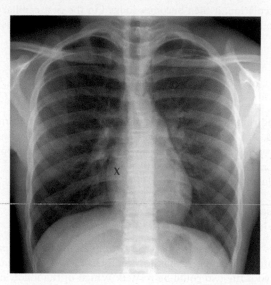

   A. Apex of the heart
   B. Left atrium
   C. Left ventricle
   D. Right atrium
   E. Right ventricle

See Appendix for answers.

CHAPTER 5

RESPIRATORY SYSTEM

5.1 THE RESPIRATORY SYSTEM

The major function of the respiratory system is to deliver oxygen to the body and remove carbon dioxide. The **conducting portion** of the system conveys air to and from the lungs, and is comprised of the **nasal cavities, pharynx, larynx, trachea,** and most of the **bronchial tree**. Structures of the conducting portion have the additional function of conditioning the inspired air, which includes removing debris and moistening and warming it. Gas exchange occurs in the **respiratory portion** of the respiratory system, which consists of **respiratory bronchioles, alveolar ducts,** and **alveoli** of the lungs. The walls of alveoli are specialized for exchange of oxygen and carbon dioxide between the air and the blood. It is the numerous sac-like alveoli that give the lungs a spongy appearance.

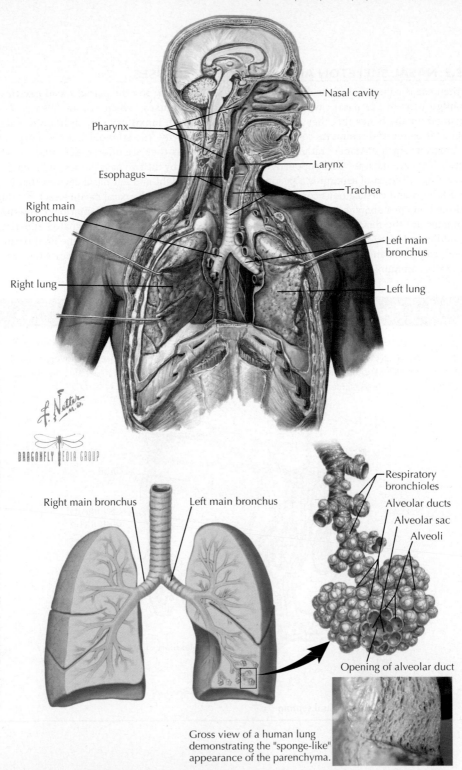

Nasal cavity

Pharynx

Esophagus

Larynx

Trachea

Right main
bronchus

Left main
bronchus

Right lung

Left lung

Right main bronchus   Left main bronchus

Respiratory
bronchioles

Alveolar ducts

Alveolar sac

Alveoli

Opening of alveolar duct

Gross view of a human lung
demonstrating the "sponge-like"
appearance of the parenchyma.

Figure 5.1 THE RESPIRATORY SYSTEM

5.2 NASAL SKELETON AND PARANASAL SINUSES

The nose is comprised of the **external nose**, **nasal septum**, and the paired **nasal cavities**. Outgrowths of the nasal cavity form the **paranasal sinuses**, which are air-filled spaces named for the bones that they invade: **frontal**, **ethmoid**, **maxillary**, and **sphenoid**. Each sinus is paired and retains its connection to the nasal cavity. The ethmoid sinuses consist of numerous small chambers rather than two cavities, thus they are often called *ethmoid air cells*. The external nose has a supportive skeleton formed by the two nasal bones and multiple cartilages. The nasal septum is a partition between the right and left nasal cavities that has both bony and cartilaginous components. The lateral walls of the nasal cavities each exhibit three bony protuberances called **turbinates** (conchae), and the grooves inferior to the turbinates are the **nasal meatuses**; both the turbinates and meatus are designated superior, middle, and inferior. The nasal cavities are separated from the oral cavity by the hard palate, and from the cranial cavity by the cribriform plate of the ethmoid bone. Posteriorly the nasal cavities communicate with the nasopharynx via openings called **choanae**.

Clinical Focus

In some individuals the nasal septum is not in the midline but is shifted toward one side of the body. This is called a **deviated septum**. Many people do not experience any adverse effects from a deviated septum, although if it is significantly displaced it may obstruct air flow through one nasal cavity and cause snoring.

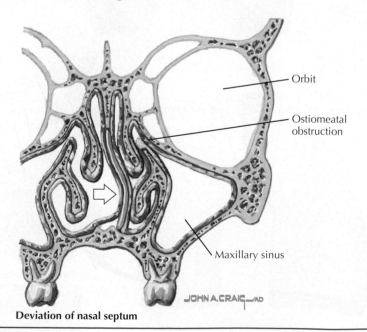

Orbit

Ostiomeatal obstruction

Maxillary sinus

JOHN A.CRAIG⎯MD

Deviation of nasal septum

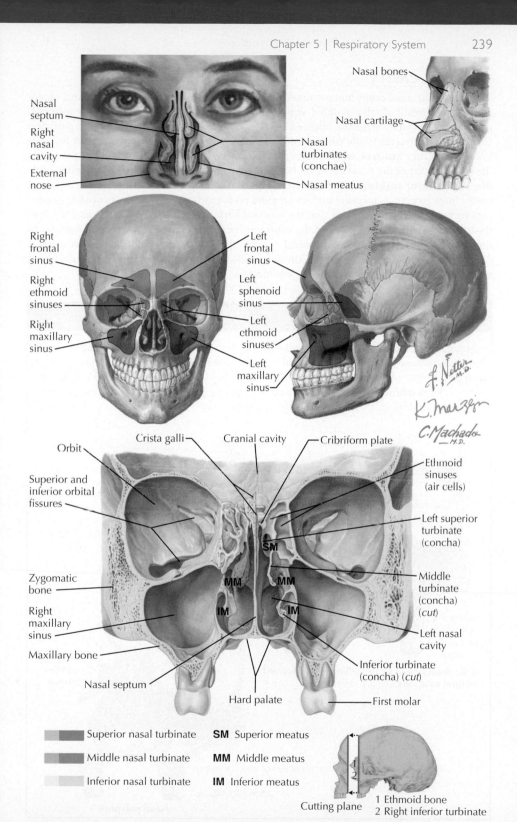

Nasal septum

Right nasal cavity

External nose

Nasal turbinates (conchae)

Nasal meatus

Nasal bones

Nasal cartilage

Right frontal sinus

Right ethmoid sinuses

Right maxillary sinus

Left frontal sinus

Left sphenoid sinus

Left ethmoid sinuses

Left maxillary sinus

Crista galli

Cranial cavity

Cribriform plate

Orbit

Superior and inferior orbital fissures

Zygomatic bone

Right maxillary sinus

Maxillary bone

Nasal septum

Ethmoid sinuses (air cells)

Left superior turbinate (concha)

Middle turbinate (concha) (cut)

Left nasal cavity

Inferior turbinate (concha) (cut)

Hard palate

First molar

SM

MM   MM

IM   IM

Superior nasal turbinate

Middle nasal turbinate

Inferior nasal turbinate

SM Superior meatus

MM Middle meatus

IM Inferior meatus

Cutting plane

1 Ethmoid bone
2 Right inferior turbinate

Figure 5.2 NASAL SKELETON AND PARANASAL SINUSES

5.3 NASAL CAVITY

The walls of the nasal cavity and paranasal sinuses are lined with a mucous membrane, except for the nasal vestibule that is lined with skin. Most regions have a **respiratory mucosa,** which moistens and warms the inspired air, and secretes mucus that traps foreign particles. Cilia sweep the mucus in the sinuses and nasal cavities toward the throat so it can be swallowed. **Olfactory mucosa,** which contains olfactory neurons that detect odors, is present in the superior part of the nasal cavity on both the septum and lateral wall. The **superior, middle,** and **inferior turbinates** and **meatuses** are the most prominent features of the lateral walls. These structures increase surface area and create turbulence, thereby providing greater contact between the inspired air and the mucosal surfaces. The paranasal sinuses drain into the meatuses, with the exception of the sphenoid sinus that drains into the space superior to the superior turbinate (sphenoethmoidal recess). Specifically, the superior meatus receives drainage from the posterior ethmoid sinuses, while the remaining sinuses (frontal, anterior, and middle ethmoid) drain into the middle meatus.

Clinical Focus

Inflammation of the nasal mucosa is called **rhinitis,** frequently caused by upper respiratory infections or allergies. Chronic inflammation may lead to the formation of benign growths called **polyps** that may obstruct airflow through the nose. Infections in the nasal cavities can spread to the sinuses (**rhinosinusitis**), and this often produces pain due to accumulation of mucus that cannot drain through swollen drainage openings.

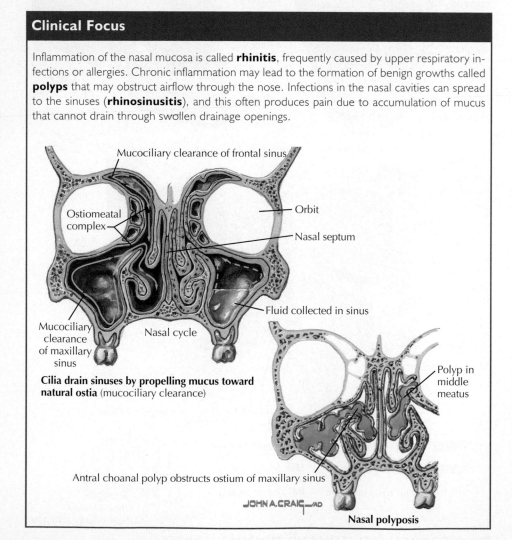

Mucociliary clearance of frontal sinus

Ostiomeatal complex

Orbit

Nasal septum

Fluid collected in sinus

Mucociliary clearance of maxillary sinus

Nasal cycle

Cilia drain sinuses by propelling mucus toward natural ostia (mucociliary clearance)

Polyp in middle meatus

Antral choanal polyp obstructs ostium of maxillary sinus

JOHN A.CRAIG—AD

Nasal polyposis

**Distribution of respiratory mucosa (*shaded pink*)
and olfactory mucosa (*shaded blue*)**

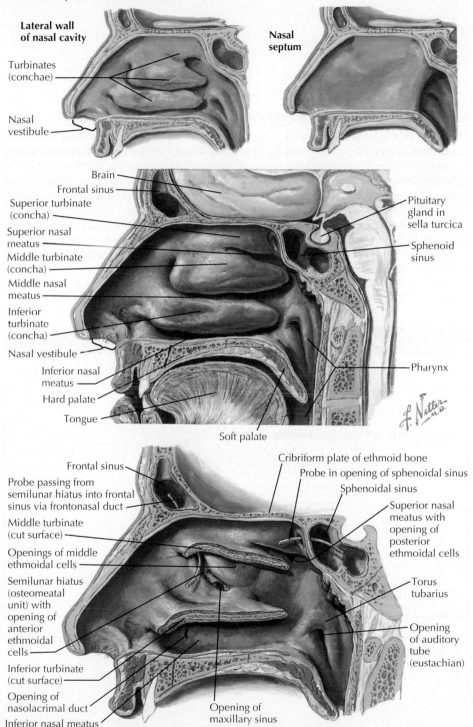

**Lateral wall
of nasal cavity**

Turbinates
(conchae)

Nasal
vestibule

**Nasal
septum**

Brain

Frontal sinus

Superior turbinate
(concha)

Superior nasal
meatus

Middle turbinate
(concha)

Middle nasal
meatus

Inferior
turbinate
(concha)

Nasal vestibule

Inferior nasal
meatus

Hard palate

Tongue

Soft palate

Pituitary
gland in
sella turcica

Sphenoid
sinus

Pharynx

Frontal sinus

Probe passing from
semilunar hiatus into frontal
sinus via frontonasal duct

Middle turbinate
(cut surface)

Openings of middle
ethmoidal cells

Semilunar hiatus
(osteomeatal
unit) with
opening of
anterior
ethmoidal
cells

Inferior turbinate
(cut surface)

Opening of
nasolacrimal duct

Inferior nasal meatus

Cribriform plate of ethmoid bone

Probe in opening of sphenoidal sinus

Sphenoidal sinus

Superior nasal
meatus with
opening of
posterior
ethmoidal cells

Torus
tubarius

Opening
of auditory
tube
(eustachian)

Opening of
maxillary sinus

Figure 5.3 NASAL CAVITY

5.4 VASCULATURE AND INNERVATION OF THE NASAL CAVITY

The blood supply of the nasal cavity is provided by the **ophthalmic branch of the internal carotid artery** (anterior ⅓) and the **maxillary branch of the external carotid artery** (posterior ⅔). Small branches from the facial artery contribute to the blood supply of the nasal septum and nasal vestibule. Veins of the nasal cavity primarily drain to the **pterygoid plexus of veins** that is located in the deep part of the face. Some venous blood also passes into the ophthalmic and facial veins. Sensory innervation of the nasal mucosa and paranasal sinuses is provided by the **trigeminal nerve** via its ophthalmic (CN V1) and maxillary (CN V2) branches. Sympathetic vasomotor fibers and parasympathetic secretomotor fibers also travel in CN V to supply vessels and mucosal glands, respectively. The **olfactory neurons** (CN I) that convey sensations of smell are located in the superior part of the nasal cavity and send axons through the cribriform plate to synapse in the olfactory bulbs within the cranial cavity (see Fig. 2.9).

Clinical Focus

Mucosal trauma or irritation often produces **epistaxis** (nosebleed). The majority of nosebleeds occur in Kiesselbach area, a region on the anterior nasal septum where multiple vessels anastomose.

Cauterization of Anterior Nasal Bleeding

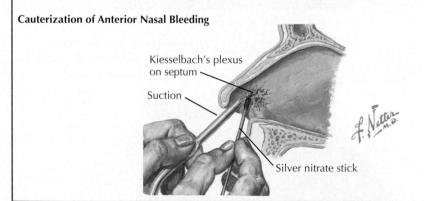

Kiesselbach's plexus on septum

Suction

Silver nitrate stick

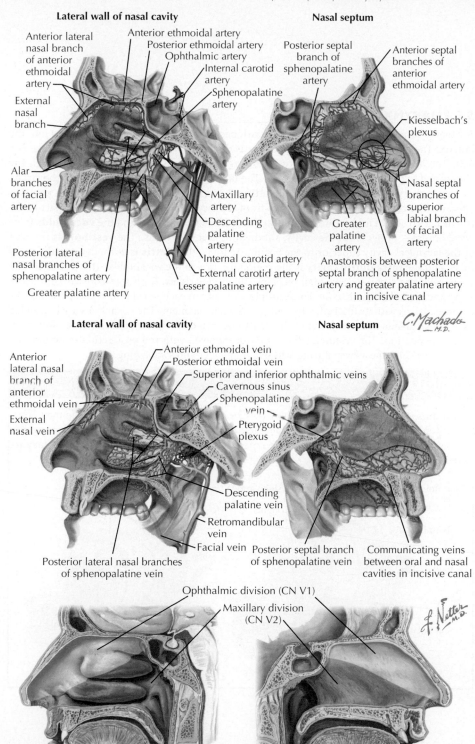

Lateral wall of nasal cavity

Anterior lateral nasal branch of anterior ethmoidal artery

External nasal branch

Alar branches of facial artery

Posterior lateral nasal branches of sphenopalatine artery

Greater palatine artery

Anterior ethmoidal artery
Posterior ethmoidal artery
Ophthalmic artery
Internal carotid artery
Sphenopalatine artery

Maxillary artery
Descending palatine artery
Internal carotid artery
External carotid artery
Lesser palatine artery

Nasal septum

Posterior septal branch of sphenopalatine artery

Anterior septal branches of anterior ethmoidal artery

Kiesselbach's plexus

Nasal septal branches of superior labial branch of facial artery

Greater palatine artery

Anastomosis between posterior septal branch of sphenopalatine artery and greater palatine artery in incisive canal

C. Machado M.D.

Lateral wall of nasal cavity

Anterior lateral nasal branch of anterior ethmoidal vein

External nasal vein

Anterior ethmoidal vein
Posterior ethmoidal vein
Superior and inferior ophthalmic veins
Cavernous sinus
Sphenopalatine vein
Pterygoid plexus

Descending palatine vein

Retromandibular vein

Facial vein

Posterior lateral nasal branches of sphenopalatine vein

Nasal septum

Posterior septal branch of sphenopalatine vein

Communicating veins between oral and nasal cavities in incisive canal

Ophthalmic division (CN V1)
Maxillary division (CN V2)

F. Netter M.D.

Figure 5.4 VASCULATURE AND INNERVATION OF THE NASAL CAVITY

5.5 PHARYNX AND LARYNX

Air that is inspired through the nose or mouth passes through the **pharynx** (throat) into the **larynx**. The detailed anatomy of the pharynx is discussed with the digestive system (see Fig. 6.3). The larynx has two basic functions: to regulate the passage of materials through the airway and to produce sound (phonation). The **laryngeal inlet** is the opening into the larynx from the pharynx, bounded by the epiglottis anteriorly and the aryepiglottic folds postero-laterally. The cavity of the larynx extends from the laryngeal inlet to the superior part of the trachea. Two sets of folds—the **vestibular folds** (false vocal cords) and the **vocal folds** (true vocal cords)— project into the cavity, subdividing it into regions. The **vestibule** is the part of the laryngeal cavity superior to the vestibular folds, the **glottis** is at the level of the vocal folds, and the **infraglottic cavity** is the region inferior to the vocal folds. The vestibular and vocal folds are separated by small recesses called **ventricles**. Each fold consists of mucosa surrounding a fibroelastic core. For example, the core of each vocal fold is comprised of the conus elasticus with its thickened free edge, the vocal ligament. The vocal folds are lubricated by mucous glands in the mucosa of the ventricles, which facilitates unrestricted movement during phonation. The vestibular folds are not involved with the production of sound, but function to close the airway during Valsalva maneuver and swallowing.

Clinical Focus

Anatomical variations (e.g., narrow pharynx, abnormally large tongue) may occlude the upper airway during sleep, a serious condition called **obstructive sleep apnea**. Infections in the respiratory tract or prolonged vocalization may cause inflammation of the vocal folds (**laryngitis**).

Anatomic representation of obstructive sleep apnea

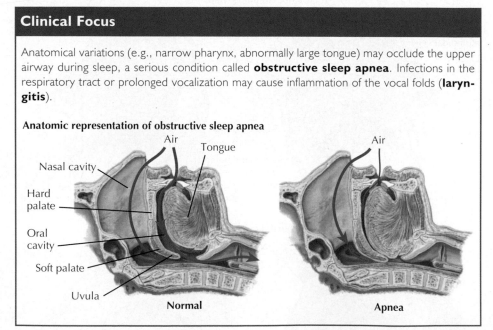

Nasal cavity

Hard palate

Oral cavity

Soft palate

Uvula

Air

Tongue

Air

Normal

Apnea

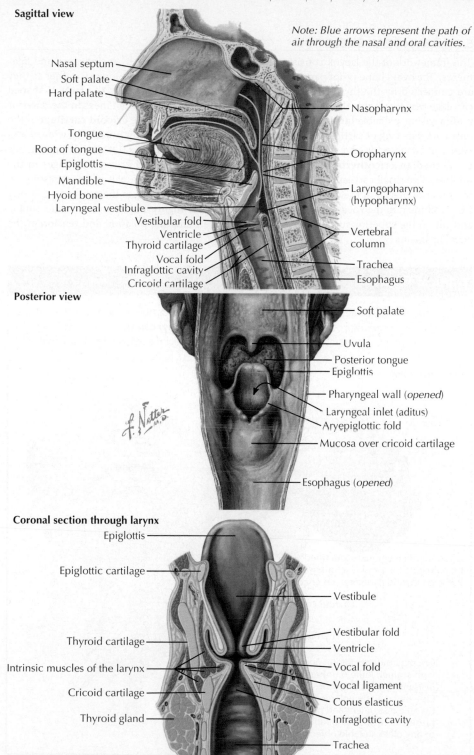

Sagittal view

Note: Blue arrows represent the path of air through the nasal and oral cavities.

Nasal septum
Soft palate
Hard palate

Nasopharynx

Tongue
Root of tongue
Epiglottis
Mandible
Hyoid bone
Laryngeal vestibule

Oropharynx

Laryngopharynx (hypopharynx)

Vestibular fold
Ventricle
Thyroid cartilage
Vocal fold
Infraglottic cavity
Cricoid cartilage

Vertebral column

Trachea
Esophagus

Posterior view

Soft palate

Uvula
Posterior tongue
Epiglottis

Pharyngeal wall (opened)
Laryngeal inlet (aditus)
Aryepiglottic fold
Mucosa over cricoid cartilage

Esophagus (opened)

Coronal section through larynx

Epiglottis

Epiglottic cartilage

Vestibule

Thyroid cartilage

Vestibular fold
Ventricle

Intrinsic muscles of the larynx

Vocal fold

Cricoid cartilage

Vocal ligament
Conus elasticus

Thyroid gland

Infraglottic cavity

Trachea

Figure 5.5 PHARYNX AND LARYNX

5.6 LARYNGEAL SKELETON

The framework of the larynx consists of multiple cartilages joined by membranes and ligaments. The hyoid bone is not part of the larynx, but the two structures move together as they are connected by the thyrohyoid membrane. The **thyroid cartilage** is the large V-shaped cartilage that surrounds the anterior part of the larynx. Its two laminae meet in the anterior midline as the palpable **laryngeal prominence** (Adam's apple). The **cricoid cartilage** is the only complete ring of cartilage that surrounds the airway. It is narrow anteriorly, wide posteriorly, and its inferior edge forms the inferior boundary of the larynx. Of clinical importance is the **median cricothyroid ligament** that joins the thyroid and cricoid cartilages in the midline. Two small cartilages, the **arytenoid cartilages**, resemble a pair of boots resting on the superior border of the cricoid cartilage. They have vocal processes that project anteriorly for attachment of the vocal ligaments. The arytenoids are highly mobile and can slide, rotate, and tilt on the superior surface of the cricoid, thus altering the position and tension of the vocal ligaments.

Clinical Focus

If the airway is obstructed superior to the level of the vocal cords, the median cricothyroid ligament can be incised to provide access to the airway (**cricothyrotomy**). This is typically only done in emergency situations, as there are other effective techniques that are less invasive.

Cricothyrotomy

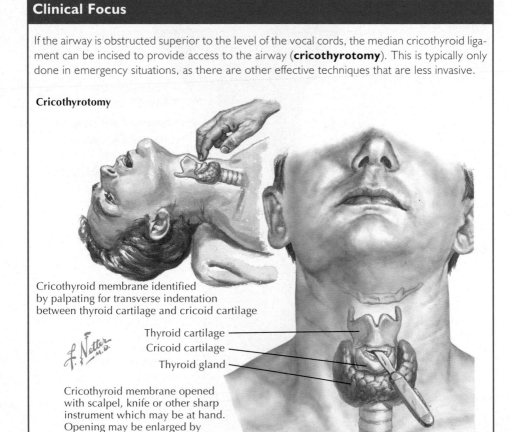

Cricothyroid membrane identified
by palpating for transverse indentation
between thyroid cartilage and cricoid cartilage

Thyroid cartilage
Cricoid cartilage
Thyroid gland

Cricothyroid membrane opened
with scalpel, knife or other sharp
instrument which may be at hand.
Opening may be enlarged by
twisting instrument and patency
preserved by inserting rubber tubing
or any other suitable object available

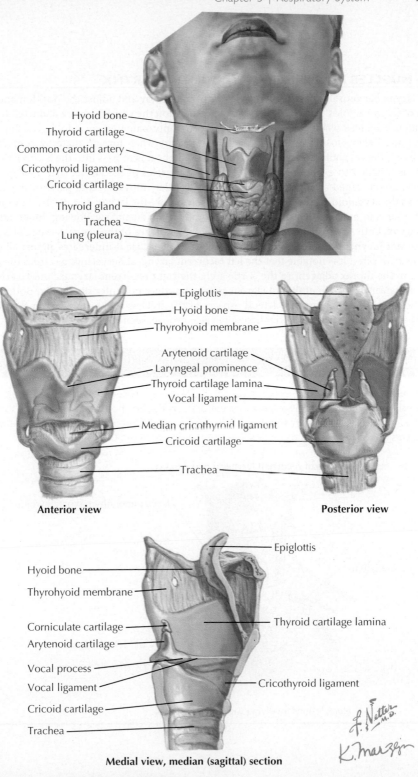

Hyoid bone
Thyroid cartilage
Common carotid artery
Cricothyroid ligament
Cricoid cartilage
Thyroid gland
Trachea
Lung (pleura)

Epiglottis
Hyoid bone
Thyrohyoid membrane
Arytenoid cartilage
Laryngeal prominence
Thyroid cartilage lamina
Vocal ligament
Median cricothyroid ligament
Cricoid cartilage
Trachea

Anterior view

Posterior view

Epiglottis
Hyoid bone
Thyrohyoid membrane
Corniculate cartilage
Arytenoid cartilage
Vocal process
Vocal ligament
Cricoid cartilage
Trachea
Thyroid cartilage lamina
Cricothyroid ligament

Medial view, median (sagittal) section

Figure 5.6 LARYNGEAL SKELETON

5.7 MUSCLES AND INNERVATION OF THE LARYNX

The larynx has muscles that regulate the size of the airway and adjust the position and tension of the vocal folds for phonation. During respiration the vocal folds are abducted (open). Sound is produced when air passes between closely approximated vocal folds, causing them to vibrate. Reflex closure of the laryngeal inlet occurs when foreign material contacts the mucosa of the vestibule (for example, if food or liquid begins to pass into the larynx); a cough reflex is initiated to expel the foreign object. The muscles of the larynx that mediate these actions are classified as **intrinsic muscles** because they move specific parts of the larynx, such as the arytenoid cartilages. **Extrinsic muscles** move the larynx *as a whole*, for example, the suprahyoid muscles that elevate the hyoid and larynx during swallowing. Innervation of the larynx, both sensory and motor, is provided by branches of the vagus nerve (CN X). The **recurrent laryngeal nerve** is particularly important because it innervates almost all of the intrinsic muscles. It is notable that the left recurrent laryngeal nerve emerges from the vagus nerve in the thorax adjacent to the aortic arch; the right recurrent laryngeal nerve arises in the neck near the origin of the subclavian artery, thus does not enter the thorax. Both nerves ascend to the larynx along the lateral aspects of the trachea and esophagus in the groove between these two structures (tracheoesophageal groove, see Fig. 7.3).

Clinical Focus

The recurrent laryngeal nerves are at risk for injury during procedures in the neck (e.g., thyroidectomy), from compression (e.g., by tumors), or due to thoracic pathology for the left nerve (e.g., aortic arch aneurysm). Unilateral injury to the recurrent laryngeal nerve often presents as hoarseness in a patient's voice due to vocal cord dysfunction.

Causes of recurrent laryngeal nerve injury

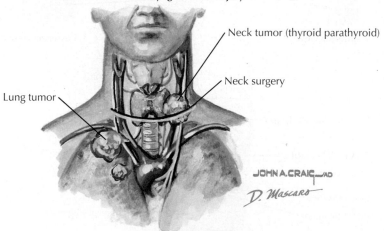

Neck tumor (thyroid parathyroid)

Neck surgery

Lung tumor

JOHN A.CRAIG—AD

D. Mascaro

Neck lesions involving vagus, RLN, or SLN

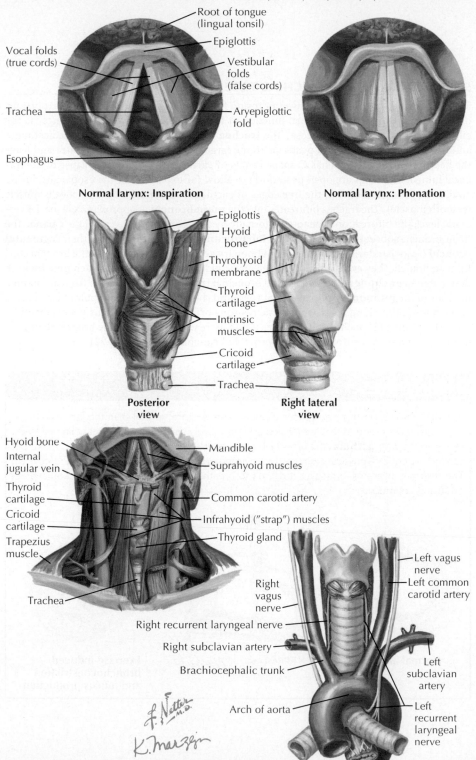

Figure 5.7 MUSCLES AND INNERVATION OF THE LARYNX

5.8 TRACHEA AND BRONCHIAL TREE

The trachea and bronchial tree convey air to and from the lungs. The more proximal portions of these airways have the additional function of moving debris away from the lungs via the ciliated epithelium in their mucosa. The **trachea** is located in the neck and mediastinum, anterior to the esophagus and posterior to the large arteries and veins that enter and leave the heart. The tracheal wall has C-shaped rings of cartilage that prevent collapse of the tracheal lumen. The rings are open posteriorly to allow for expansion of the esophagus during swallowing; the gap between the free edges of cartilage is spanned by the trachealis muscle (smooth muscle). The trachea bifurcates into the **main bronchi** at approximately the T4 vertebral level; the bifurcation is denoted internally by a ridge of cartilage called the **carina**. The main bronchi subsequently branch into **lobar bronchi** (one per lobe) and then **segmental bronchi** (associated with each bronchopulmonary segment of the lung). As the bronchi continue to branch, they eventually lose the cartilage plates in their walls, at which time they are designated **bronchioles**. The trachea and bronchial tree receive innervation from autonomic neurons of the **pulmonary plexuses** that surround the main bronchi and pulmonary vessels at the hilum of the lung. Parasympathetic neurons originating in the vagus nerves maintain the resting tone of bronchial smooth muscle and increase secretions of the bronchial mucous glands. Sympathetic neurotransmitters promote bronchodilation (see 2.22).

Clinical Focus

The right main bronchus has a wider diameter and is more vertical than the left main bronchus, thus foreign bodies that are inhaled are more likely to lodge in the right main bronchus. In individuals with **asthma**, the bronchial tree is overly sensitive to allergens (e.g., mold, pet dander), strenuous physical exercise, or environmental factors such as smoke and cold air. The resultant inflammation makes it difficult to breathe due to bronchial constriction and accumulation of mucus.

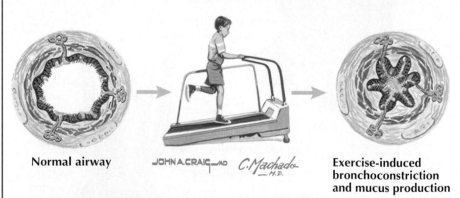

Normal airway   JOHN A.CRAIG—AD   C.Machado—M.D.   **Exercise-induced bronchoconstriction and mucus production**

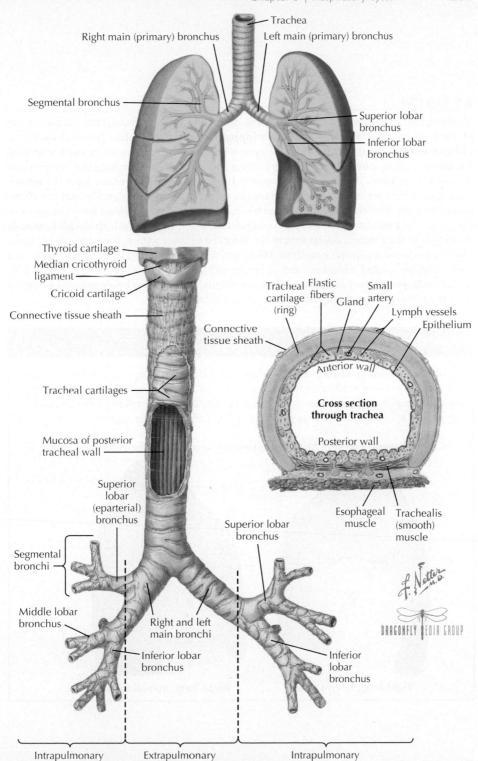

Figure 5.8 TRACHEA AND BRONCHIAL TREE

5.9 LUNGS

The **lungs** are the major organs of respiration, designed for gas exchange between the air and blood. Each lung is divided into a **superior (upper) lobe** and an **inferior (lower) lobe** by the **oblique fissure**. On the right side, the upper lobe is further subdivided by the **horizontal fissure**, producing a **middle lobe**. The pointed superior portion of the lung that extends into the neck is the **apex**. The prominent feature of the medial surface of each lung is the **hilum**, the region where vessels, nerves, and branches of the bronchial tree pass in and out of the lung. The right and left **pulmonary arteries** convey deoxygenated blood from the heart to the lungs; the **pulmonary veins** return oxygenated blood to the heart. **Bronchial arteries** (branches of the thoracic aorta) supply the lung tissue itself with oxygenated blood. Lymphatic vessels convey lymph away from the lungs, and this is filtered through various lymph nodes that are located along branches of the bronchial tree. Major groups of nodes include the **bronchopulmonary (hilar) nodes** at the hilum, **inferior tracheobronchial nodes** at the carina, and **paratracheal nodes** adjacent to the trachea.

Clinical Focus

Bronchopulmonary segments are functionally independent regions of the lung that are supplied by one segmental bronchus and a branch of the pulmonary artery. Knowledge of these segments is useful when surgical resection is warranted, for example in the treatment of lung cancer, as one segment can be removed without affecting other segments.

Colored areas represent bronchopulmonary segments of the right lung

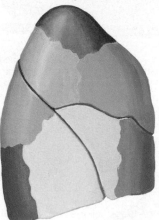
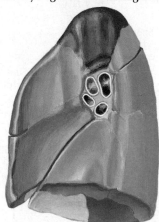

Right lung, lateral view   Right lung, medial view

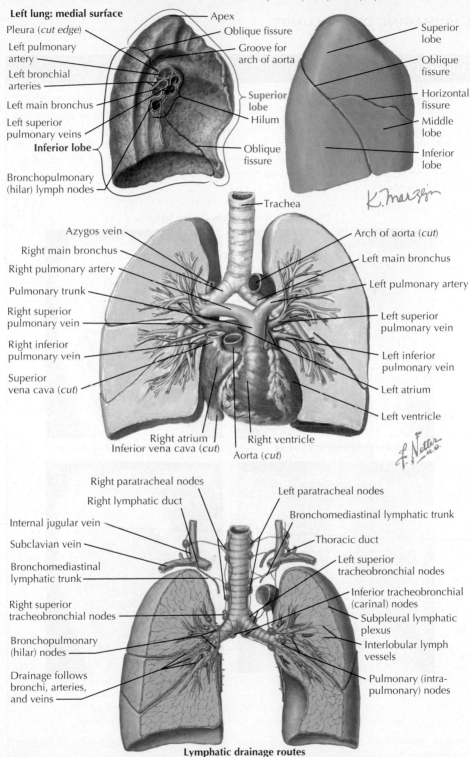

Left lung: medial surface

Apex

Pleura (*cut edge*)

Oblique fissure

Left pulmonary artery

Groove for arch of aorta

Left bronchial arteries

Superior lobe

Left main bronchus

Hilum

Left superior pulmonary veins

Inferior lobe

Oblique fissure

Bronchopulmonary (hilar) lymph nodes

Superior lobe

Oblique fissure

Horizontal fissure

Middle lobe

Inferior lobe

Trachea

Azygos vein

Arch of aorta (*cut*)

Right main bronchus

Right pulmonary artery

Left main bronchus

Pulmonary trunk

Left pulmonary artery

Right superior pulmonary vein

Left superior pulmonary vein

Right inferior pulmonary vein

Left inferior pulmonary vein

Superior vena cava (*cut*)

Left atrium

Left ventricle

Right atrium

Inferior vena cava (*cut*)

Right ventricle

Aorta (*cut*)

Right paratracheal nodes

Left paratracheal nodes

Right lymphatic duct

Bronchomediastinal lymphatic trunk

Internal jugular vein

Thoracic duct

Subclavian vein

Left superior tracheobronchial nodes

Bronchomediastinal lymphatic trunk

Inferior tracheobronchial (carinal) nodes

Right superior tracheobronchial nodes

Subpleural lymphatic plexus

Bronchopulmonary (hilar) nodes

Interlobular lymph vessels

Drainage follows bronchi, arteries, and veins

Pulmonary (intra-pulmonary) nodes

Lymphatic drainage routes

Figure 5.9 LUNGS

5.10 IMAGING OF THE LUNGS

Clinical Focus

Lung pathology is commonly evaluated with chest radiographs. Two views of the chest, posteroanterior (PA) and lateral, are required to fully evaluate the lobes of the lungs since they are superimposed on one another in two-dimensional images. The lungs appear black (radiolucent) on radiographs because they are filled with air that does not absorb (attenuate) x-rays. Computed tomography (CT) is used frequently to evaluate structures of the respiratory system and provides excellent soft-tissue contrast to distinguish structures that are not well seen in radiographs.

PA and lateral chest x-rays of the lungs

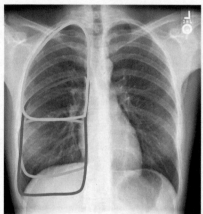

Lobes of the right lung in PA view

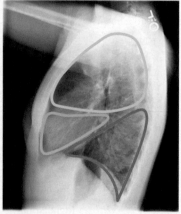

Lobes of the right lung in lateral view

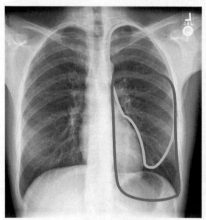

Lobes of the left lung in PA view

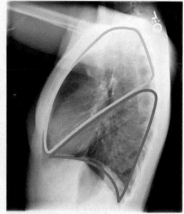

Lobes of the left lung in lateral view

===== = Upper lobe   ===== = Middle lobe   ==== = Lower lobe

Images reused with permission from Cochard LR, et al. *Netter's Introduction to Imaging.* Elsevier; 2011: 45.

Axial CT scan displayed in "soft tissue" window

Ascending aorta

Superior
vena cava

Main pulmonary
artery

Right
pulmonary
artery

Pulmonary vein

Left pulmonary
artery

Left mainstem
bronchus

Right
mainstem
bronchus

Descending
thoracic aorta

Esophagus

Axial CT scan displayed in "lung" window to highlight lung parenchyma

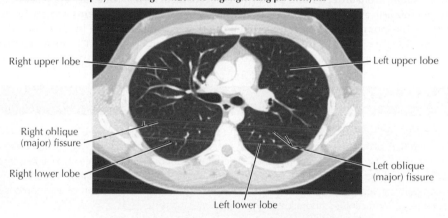

Right upper lobe

Left upper lobe

Right oblique
(major) fissure

Right lower lobe

Left oblique
(major) fissure

Left lower lobe

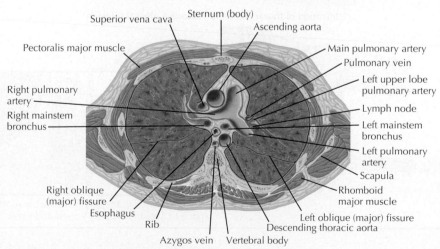

Superior vena cava

Sternum (body)

Ascending aorta

Pectoralis major muscle

Main pulmonary artery

Pulmonary vein

Right pulmonary
artery

Left upper lobe
pulmonary artery

Right mainstem
bronchus

Lymph node

Left mainstem
bronchus

Left pulmonary
artery

Scapula

Rhomboid
major muscle

Right oblique
(major) fissure

Esophagus

Rib

Azygos vein   Vertebral body

Left oblique (major) fissure

Descending thoracic aorta

Imaging reused with permission from Gotway M. *Netter's Correlative Imaging: Cardiothoracic Anatomy*. Elsevier; 2013: 47.

5.11 MUSCULOSKELETAL COMPONENTS OF THE THORAX

The lungs are located in the thorax, which consists of a musculoskeletal framework surrounding a roughly cylindrical cavity. The **thoracic wall** is comprised of skeletal elements (sternum, ribs, vertebrae) and soft-tissue elements (skin, fascia, muscle, pleura). The **sternum** forms the anterior part of the ribcage and has three components: the **manubrium**, **body**, and **xiphoid process**. The superior and inferior edges of the manubrium are associated with two important palpable landmarks: the **jugular notch** and **sternal angle**. Ribs articulate with the vertebrae posteriorly (costovertebral joints) and the sternum or costal margin anteriorly via costal cartilages (ribs 11 and 12 do not have anterior articulations). Small rotational and sliding movements at these joints allow elevation and depression of the ribs, which causes expansion and contraction of the thoracic cavity for respiration. The gaps between the ribs are spanned by three layers of muscle that are collectively called **intercostal muscles**. These muscles are accessory muscles of respiration as they help elevate and depress the ribs, especially during forced inspiration or expiration. The intercostal muscles receive arterial supply from **anterior and posterior intercostal arteries**, which are branches of the internal thoracic arteries and thoracic aorta, respectively; **intercostal veins** accompany the arteries. The intercostal vessels travel around the thoracic wall along the inferior borders of the ribs. They are joined by **intercostal nerves** (anterior rami of T1–T11), which innervate the intercostal muscles and the skin of the thoracic wall.

Clinical Focus

The costal cartilage of the second rib meets the sternum at the sternal angle, thus palpation of this landmark allows reliable identification of the second rib to begin counting ribs for clinical procedures (rib 1 is not typically palpable). The bifurcation of the trachea also typically occurs at the level of the sternal angle. Knowledge of the position of the intercostal nerves and their accompanying vessels is important for procedures that require penetration of an intercostal space (e.g., thoracentesis, thoracostomy).

Utilization of thoracentesis to remove a pleural effusion

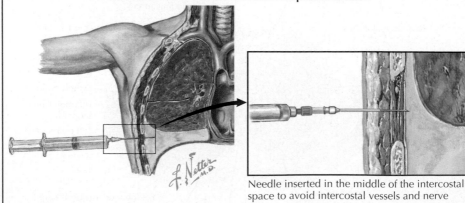

Needle inserted in the middle of the intercostal space to avoid intercostal vessels and nerve

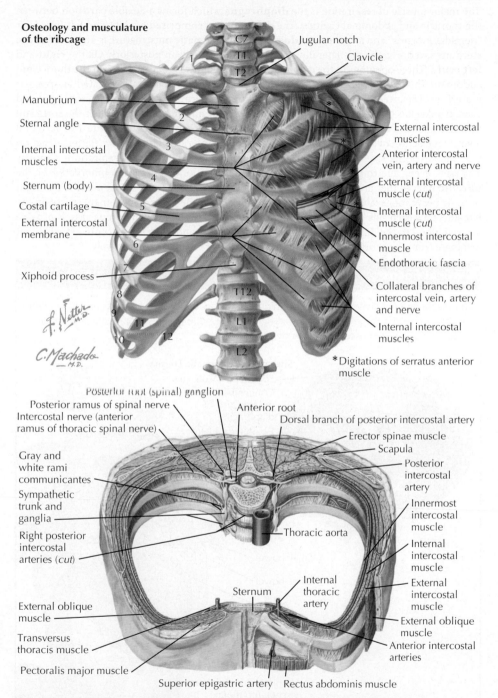

Osteology and musculature of the ribcage

Jugular notch

Clavicle

Manubrium

Sternal angle

Internal intercostal muscles

Sternum (body)

Costal cartilage

External intercostal membrane

Xiphoid process

C7
T1
T2

* External intercostal muscles

* Anterior intercostal vein, artery and nerve

External intercostal muscle (*cut*)

Internal intercostal muscle (*cut*)

Innermost intercostal muscle

Endothoracic fascia

Collateral branches of intercostal vein, artery and nerve

Internal intercostal muscles

*Digitations of serratus anterior muscle

Posterior root (spinal) ganglion
Posterior ramus of spinal nerve
Intercostal nerve (anterior ramus of thoracic spinal nerve)

Anterior root
Dorsal branch of posterior intercostal artery

Erector spinae muscle

Scapula

Gray and white rami communicantes

Sympathetic trunk and ganglia

Right posterior intercostal arteries (*cut*)

Posterior intercostal artery

Innermost intercostal muscle

Internal intercostal muscle

Thoracic aorta

External intercostal muscle

External oblique muscle

Transversus thoracis muscle

Pectoralis major muscle

Sternum

Internal thoracic artery

Superior epigastric artery   Rectus abdominis muscle

External oblique muscle

Anterior intercostal arteries

Figure 5.11 MUSCULOSKELETAL COMPONENTS OF THE THORAX

5.12 RESPIRATORY DIAPHRAGM

The major muscle of respiration is the **diaphragm**, which forms a flexible partition between the thoracic and abdominal cavities. The diaphragm is comprised of right and left muscular "hemidiaphragms" and a **central tendon**. The diaphragmatic musculature is anchored to the sternum anteriorly, the ribs laterally, and the vertebral column posteriorly via the **right** and **left crura**. Three openings in the diaphragm allow structures to pass between the thorax and abdomen. The **caval opening**, which conveys the inferior vena cava, is located at approximately the T8 vertebral level. The **esophageal hiatus** permits passage of the esophagus and vagal trunks; it is located at the T10 vertebral level. The **aortic hiatus** transmits the aorta and thoracic duct and is located posterior to the diaphragmatic musculature at the T12 vertebral level. Contraction of the diaphragm causes it to move inferiorly and become flatter, an action that increases the size of the thoracic cavity for inspiration. Normal expiration is mostly a passive event due to the elastic recoil of the lungs. The diaphragm is innervated by the **phrenic nerves** that are formed by contributions from the C3–C5 spinal nerves. The right phrenic nerve innervates the right hemidiaphragm, and the same arrangement exists on the left side; thus each side of the diaphragm functions independently. Numerous vessels provide arterial blood to the diaphragm, including the **superior** and **inferior phrenic arteries** that originate from the thoracic and abdominal portions of the aorta, respectively.

Clinical Focus

The diaphragm may have abnormal openings that allow abdominal contents to herniate into the thoracic cavity. Some openings are congenital (i.e., due to a developmental abnormality), while others can be caused by trauma or aging.

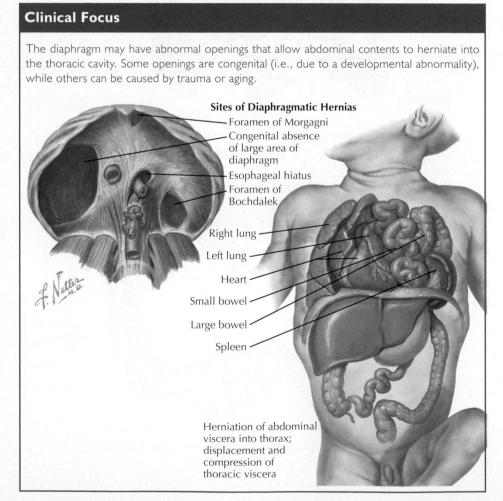

Sites of Diaphragmatic Hernias

- Foramen of Morgagni
- Congenital absence of large area of diaphragm
- Esophageal hiatus
- Foramen of Bochdalek

Right lung

Left lung

Heart

Small bowel

Large bowel

Spleen

Herniation of abdominal viscera into thorax; displacement and compression of thoracic viscera

Respiratory Diaphragm

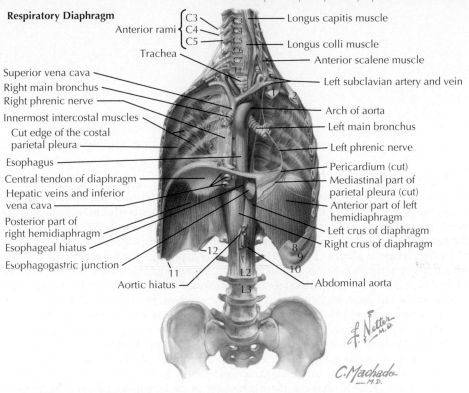

Anterior rami { C3, C4, C5

Longus capitis muscle
Trachea
Longus colli muscle
Anterior scalene muscle
Superior vena cava
Right main bronchus
Right phrenic nerve
Innermost intercostal muscles
Cut edge of the costal parietal pleura
Esophagus
Central tendon of diaphragm
Hepatic veins and inferior vena cava
Posterior part of right hemidiaphragm
Esophageal hiatus
Esophagogastric junction
Aortic hiatus
Left subclavian artery and vein
Arch of aorta
Left main bronchus
Left phrenic nerve
Pericardium (cut)
Mediastinal part of parietal pleura (cut)
Anterior part of left hemidiaphragm
Left crus of diaphragm
Right crus of diaphragm
Abdominal aorta

Diaphragm: Abdominal Surface

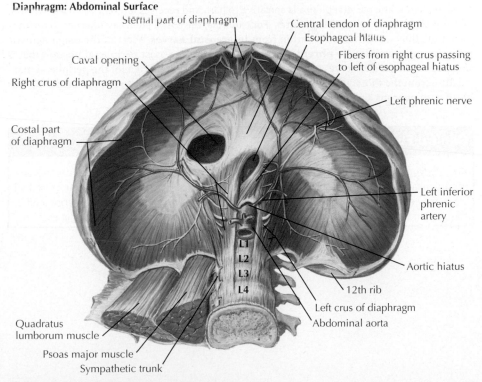

Sternal part of diaphragm
Central tendon of diaphragm
Esophageal hiatus
Fibers from right crus passing to left of esophageal hiatus
Caval opening
Right crus of diaphragm
Left phrenic nerve
Costal part of diaphragm
Left inferior phrenic artery
Aortic hiatus
12th rib
Left crus of diaphragm
Abdominal aorta
Quadratus lumborum muscle
Psoas major muscle
Sympathetic trunk

Figure 5.12 RESPIRATORY DIAPHRAGM

5.13 THORACIC CAVITY AND PLEURA

The thoracic cavity is subdivided into three compartments—bilateral **pulmonary cavities** for the lungs, and a centrally located compartment called the **mediastinum** that contains the heart and various other structures. Each pulmonary cavity is lined with a serous membrane, the **parietal pleura**, that is continuous at the hilum with a homologous layer on the surface of the lung (**visceral pleura**). Between the two layers of pleura is the **pleural cavity** (pleural space), which normally contains a small amount of serous fluid that allows the lung to move freely within the cavity. The parietal pleura is subdivided into parts, named by the structure with which a particular portion is in contact. For example, the parietal pleura in contact with the chest wall and ribs is the **costal pleura**, while that in contact with the diaphragm is **diaphragmatic pleura**. The **cervical pleura** extends over the apex of the lung and the **mediastinal pleura** borders the structures of the mediastinum. **Reflections** of the parietal pleura indicate locations where the pleura changes direction—for example, when it transitions from the costal pleura to the diaphragmatic pleura. In a few locations, most notably the **costodiaphragmatic recesses,** there is no intervening lung tissue between the layers of parietal pleura. The parietal pleura is sensitive to pain and receives afferent innervation from neurons that supply adjacent structures. For example, the costal pleura is adjacent to the thoracic wall, thus it receives innervation from **intercostal nerves**. Most of the diaphragmatic pleura is innervated by the **phrenic nerves,** apart from the most peripheral portion that is supplied by intercostal nerves (this is due to the developmental origin of the peripheral musculature from the thoracic wall). The mediastinal pleura is adjacent to the pericardium, thus its afferent neurons are conveyed in the phrenic nerves.

Clinical Focus

Knowledge of the position of the lungs and pleura with respect to the chest wall is important for auscultation of the lungs and to access the pleural cavity (e.g., to withdraw abnormal fluid via thoracentesis). A useful mnemonic is "6-8-10, 8-10-12" which refers to the inferior limit of the lung and pleura, respectively, at the midclavicular, midaxillary and midscapular lines.

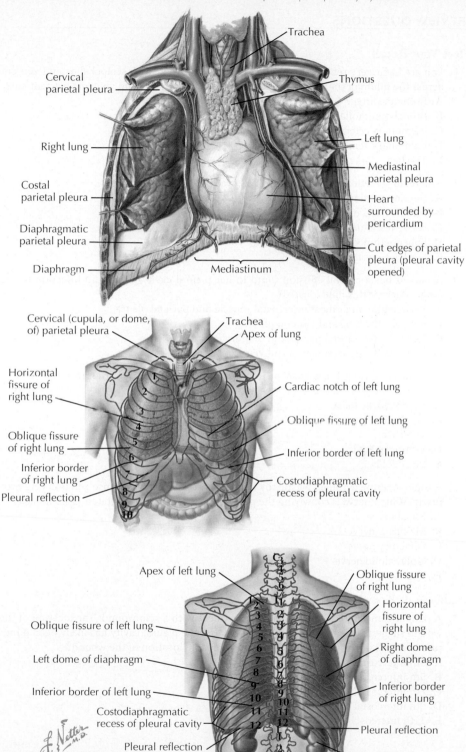

Trachea

Cervical parietal pleura

Thymus

Right lung

Left lung

Mediastinal parietal pleura

Costal parietal pleura

Heart surrounded by pericardium

Diaphragmatic parietal pleura

Diaphragm

Mediastinum

Cut edges of parietal pleura (pleural cavity opened)

Cervical (cupula, or dome, of) parietal pleura

Trachea
Apex of lung

Horizontal fissure of right lung

Cardiac notch of left lung

Oblique fissure of left lung

Oblique fissure of right lung

Inferior border of left lung

Inferior border of right lung

Pleural reflection

Costodiaphragmatic recess of pleural cavity

Apex of left lung

Oblique fissure of right lung

Oblique fissure of left lung

Horizontal fissure of right lung

Left dome of diaphragm

Right dome of diaphragm

Inferior border of left lung

Inferior border of right lung

Costodiaphragmatic recess of pleural cavity

Pleural reflection

Pleural reflection

Right kidney

Figure 5.13 THORACIC CAVITY AND PLEURA

REVIEW QUESTIONS

Test Your Recall

1. You are in surgery removing a mediastinal tumor, when your scalpel slips and you cut across the hilum of the lung. Which structure is not at risk from your inadvertent cut?
   A. Bronchial artery
   B. Bronchopulmonary (hilar) lymph nodes
   C. Pulmonary artery
   D. Pulmonary vein
   E. Trachea

2. Where do secretions in the frontal sinus drain into the nasal cavity?
   A. Inferior nasal meatus
   B. Middle nasal meatus
   C. Nasal vestibule
   D. Sphenoethmoidal recess
   E. Superior nasal meatus

3. A patient has a pleural effusion (fluid in her pleural cavity) due to an infection in her lung. Where is this fluid located?
   A. Between the innermost intercostal muscle and parietal pleura
   B. Between the lung and visceral pleura
   C. Between the parietal pleura and diaphragm
   D. Between the parietal pleura and visceral pleura

4. A physician is using a laryngoscope to investigate a foreign body in the larynx and inserts it as far as the glottis. This coincides with the level of the:
   A. Aryepiglottic folds
   B. Epiglottis
   C. Ventricle
   D. Vestibular folds
   E. Vocal folds

5. A toddler jammed a small plastic toy into the anterior part of his nose and is crying profusely. Which nerve is conveying the pain sensations from the irritated nasal mucosa?
   A. Facial nerve
   B. Maxillary nerve
   C. Olfactory nerve
   D. Ophthalmic nerve
   E. Vagus nerve

Apply Your Knowledge

6. A patient comes into the emergency department with a stab wound. The location of the wound suggests that the lung is not injured, but the pleural cavity has likely been punctured. Which of the following is the most probable location of the wound?
   A. 4th intercostal space at midclavicular line
   B. 5th intercostal space at midclavicular line
   C. 7th intercostal space at midclavicular line
   D. 9th intercostal space at midclavicular line
   E. 11th intercostal space at midclavicular line

7. A tumor adjacent to the left main bronchus is compressing the phrenic nerve. Which of the following would you expect to see on a chest x-ray of this patient during inspiration?
   A. Left hemidiaphragm would be abnormally high
   B. Left hemidiaphragm would be abnormally low
   C. Right hemidiaphragm would be abnormally high
   D. Right hemidiaphragm would be abnormally low
   E. Both halves of the diaphragm would be abnormally high
   F. Both halves of the diaphragm would be abnormally low

8. A patient visits an outpatient clinic complaining of chronic nasal congestion and sinus pain. The sinus pain is localized specifically to the forehead and cheek. Examination of the nasal cavity reveals a large polyp that is impeding normal drainage of mucus. Which of the following best describes the site of obstruction?
   A. Inferior meatus
   B. Middle meatus
   C. Sphenoethmoid recess
   D. Superior meatus

9. A patient has a small osteosarcoma (bone tumor) growing on her sternal angle. As it begins to spread laterally, you would most likely expect to find it infiltrating the:
   A. Body of the sternum
   B. Clavicle
   C. Manubrium
   D. Costal cartilage of rib 1
   E. Costal cartilage of rib 2
   F. Costal cartilage of rib 4

10. A woman visits her primary care physician with complaints of a hoarse voice that has gradually been getting worse over the past month. Laryngoscope examination reveals a paralyzed left vocal cord. Which of the following would most likely be the source of the patient's problem?
    A. Aortic arch aneurysm
    B. Bone tumor on the C3 vertebral body
    C. Cancerous tumor on the anterior aspect of the root of the left lung
    D. Enlarged tracheobronchial lymph nodes at the carina
    E. Small mass growing from the anterior part of the thyroid

CHAPTER 6

DIGESTIVE SYSTEM

6.1 THE DIGESTIVE SYSTEM

The gastrointestinal system is composed of organs that function in digestion—the process of breaking down ingested substances into forms the body can use for energy. Materials that cannot be used are eliminated as waste. Digestion begins in the **oral cavity**, where the teeth and tongue physically manipulate food and secretions from the **salivary glands** initiate enzymatic digestion. The **pharynx** (throat) and **esophagus** use muscular contractions to propel the food bolus to the stomach. Cells of the **stomach, pancreas, liver**, and **small intestine** all contribute to further chemical breakdown of the ingested material. The stomach also aids in mechanical digestion by churning the food, and the semisolid mass that is produced is called chyme. As the chyme passes through the intestines, nutrients and water are absorbed by intestinal cells, while waste products are compacted as feces and propelled toward the **rectum** to be defecated.

Organs of digestion are found in multiple locations in the body, although most are located in the abdominal cavity. The abdominal cavity is lined with a serous membrane called the **peritoneum**, and this membrane also forms an outer coating of most organs so they can move freely with respect to each other. The peritoneum on the body wall is called **parietal peritoneum**, while that on the abdominal organs is called **visceral peritoneum**.

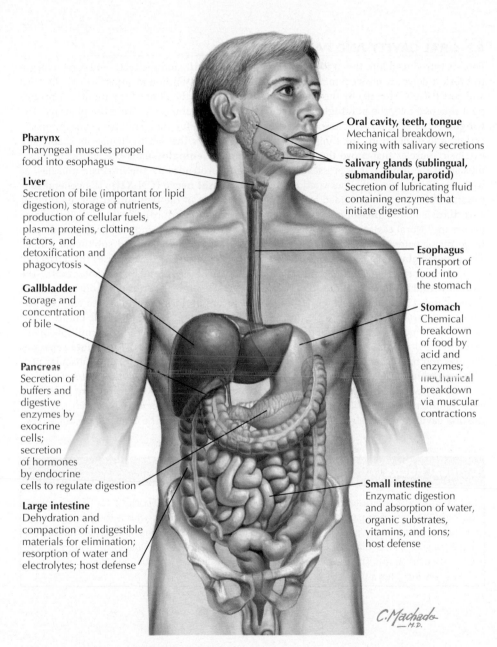

Pharynx
Pharyngeal muscles propel
food into esophagus

Liver
Secretion of bile (important for lipid
digestion), storage of nutrients,
production of cellular fuels,
plasma proteins, clotting
factors, and
detoxification and
phagocytosis

Gallbladder
Storage and
concentration
of bile

Pancreas
Secretion of
buffers and
digestive
enzymes by
exocrine
cells;
secretion
of hormones
by endocrine
cells to regulate digestion

Large intestine
Dehydration and
compaction of indigestible
materials for elimination;
resorption of water and
electrolytes; host defense

Oral cavity, teeth, tongue
Mechanical breakdown,
mixing with salivary secretions

**Salivary glands (sublingual,
submandibular, parotid)**
Secretion of lubricating fluid
containing enzymes that
initiate digestion

Esophagus
Transport of
food into
the stomach

Stomach
Chemical
breakdown
of food by
acid and
enzymes;
mechanical
breakdown
via muscular
contractions

Small intestine
Enzymatic digestion
and absorption of water,
organic substrates,
vitamins, and ions;
host defense

C.Machado
— M.D.

Figure 6.1 THE DIGESTIVE SYSTEM

6.2 ORAL CAVITY AND PALATE

Food is introduced into the oral cavity through the **mouth**, and the teeth and tongue begin to break it down by physical manipulation. The **oral cavity** is bound superiorly by the hard and soft palates, laterally by the cheeks, and inferiorly by the floor of the mouth. A prominent mucosal fold, the **palatoglossal arch**, separates the oral cavity from the pharynx. The **tongue** is the primary structure in the oral cavity, which functions in taste, speech, mastication, and deglutition. The tongue has intrinsic muscles that act to change its shape, and extrinsic muscles that move the tongue as a whole. **Genioglossus** is the largest extrinsic muscle of the tongue; it depresses the tongue and protrudes it. The intrinsic muscles, as well as genioglossus, are innervated by the **hypoglossal nerve (CN XII)**. The general sensation of the tongue is provided by the lingual branches of the **trigeminal nerve** (anterior two-thirds) and the **glossopharyngeal nerve** (posterior one-third). Chemical digestion also occurs in the oral cavity via saliva that is secreted by major and minor **salivary glands**. The three major paired salivary glands are the parotid, submandibular, and sublingual glands. The **parotid gland** is located on the face anterior to the ear; its duct crosses the surface of the masseter muscle and empties into the oral cavity near the second upper molar tooth. The **submandibular gland** straddles the mylohyoid muscle in the floor of the mouth; thus part of the gland is located in the neck. Its duct travels from posterior to anterior to empty at the sublingual caruncle adjacent to the frenulum of the tongue. The **sublingual gland** is just deep to the mucosa in the floor of the mouth, and it empties its secretions via multiple openings. The oral mucosa also contains numerous minor salivary glands. The **palate** separates the oral and nasal cavities and consists of a bony portion (**hard palate**) and muscular portion (**soft palate**). The inferior portion of the soft palate that is visible at the posterior part of the oral cavity is the **uvula**. The soft palate elevates during swallowing to prevent food from entering the nasal cavity. This action is mediated by the **vagus nerve (CN X)**. Structures of the oral cavity and palate receive blood supply from branches of the external carotid artery.

Clinical Focus

CN IX and CN X are tested clinically using the **gag reflex** (Clinical Focus 2.15). This involves touching the posterior part of the patient's tongue or oropharynx with a tongue depressor and noting whether the pharyngeal muscles contract (the oropharynx, like the posterior part of the tongue, is innervated by CN IX). The integrity of CN XII is evaluated with a similar test (Clinical Focus 2.18). The patient is asked to protrude his/her tongue, and deviation to one side usually indicates a problem with the hypoglossal nerve.

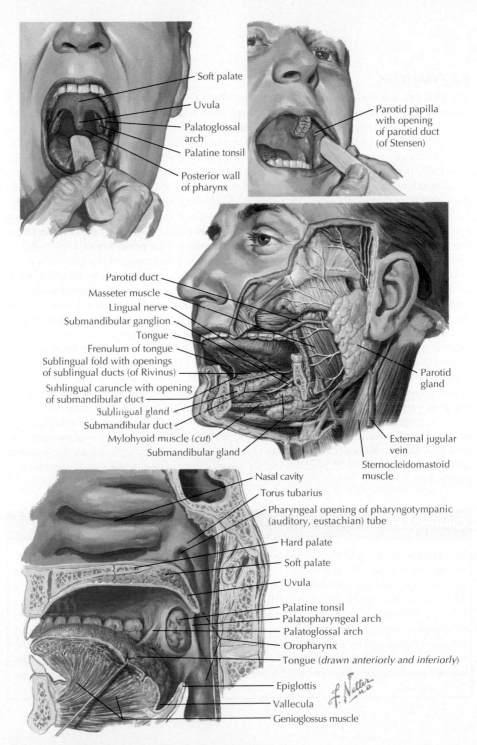

Soft palate

Uvula

Palatoglossal arch

Palatine tonsil

Posterior wall of pharynx

Parotid papilla with opening of parotid duct (of Stensen)

Parotid duct

Masseter muscle

Lingual nerve

Submandibular ganglion

Tongue

Frenulum of tongue

Sublingual fold with openings of sublingual ducts (of Rivinus)

Sublingual caruncle with opening of submandibular duct

Sublingual gland

Submandibular duct

Mylohyoid muscle (cut)

Submandibular gland

Parotid gland

External jugular vein

Sternocleidomastoid muscle

Nasal cavity

Torus tubarius

Pharyngeal opening of pharyngotympanic (auditory, eustachian) tube

Hard palate

Soft palate

Uvula

Palatine tonsil

Palatopharyngeal arch

Palatoglossal arch

Oropharynx

Tongue (drawn anteriorly and inferiorly)

Epiglottis

Vallecula

Genioglossus muscle

Figure 6.2 THE ORAL CAVITY AND PALATE

6.3 PHARYNX

The **pharynx** is a muscular channel that primarily functions in deglutition (swallowing); it also serves as a passageway for air during respiration and speech. The circular muscles that form the wall of the pharynx are called **constrictors** (superior, middle, inferior) because they constrict the lumen of the pharynx to propel the food bolus toward the esophagus. The constrictors are arranged in the shape of the letter C, with the open side of the C facing anteriorly. The most inferior part of the inferior constrictor that merges with the esophagus is called **cricopharyngeus**. Its lumen is the narrowest part of the entire gastrointestinal (GI) tract, and it functions as a sphincter between the pharynx and esophagus. The pharynx also has longitudinal bands of muscle (e.g., stylopharyngeus) that elevate the pharynx during swallowing. The interior of the pharynx is divided into three regions. The **nasopharynx** is the portion of the pharynx posterior to the nasal cavities. The **oropharynx** is posterior to the oral cavity, and the **laryngopharynx** (hypopharynx) is posterior to the larynx. The soft palate forms the boundary between the nasopharynx and oropharynx, while the epiglottis defines the border between the oropharynx and laryngopharynx. The **openings of the eustachian tubes** and surrounding cartilage (**torus tubarius**) are important landmarks in the nasopharynx. The pharyngeal tonsils (**adenoids**) are located in the posterosuperior part of the nasopharynx, while the **palatine tonsils** are found in the oropharynx posterior to the palatoglossal arches. The depression between the base of the tongue and anterior part of the epiglottis is the **vallecula**. The most prominent features of the laryngopharynx are the paired **piriform fossae** (recesses) on either side of the cricoid cartilage. Due to the length of the pharynx, the blood supply comes from numerous arteries that are mainly branches of the **external carotid artery**. The veins form a plexus on the posterior wall of the pharynx that drains to multiple veins in the neck including the superior and inferior thyroid veins, and the **internal jugular vein**. The innervation of the pharynx is primarily via the **glossopharyngeal (CN IX)** and **vagus (CN X) nerves** that intermingle to form a plexus on the posterior wall of the pharynx. CN IX provides mainly sensory innervation, while CN X provides primarily motor.

Clinical Focus

The **tonsils** are collections of lymphoid tissue that protect the body from pathogens entering through the nasal or oral cavities. Lymphocytes within the tonsils intercept antigens and can initiate an immune response. Tonsils that are activated by antigens swell and can become inflamed. Swollen adenoids can make it difficult to breathe through the nose and can also obstruct the opening of the eustachian tube, which can impair hearing. The **vallecula** is an important landmark for **intubation**, the process of inserting an endotracheal tube in patients who cannot maintain an airway. Part of the laryngoscope is inserted in the vallecula to pull the tongue forward and visualize the vocal cords before advancing the tube. The **piriform fossae** are also clinically important because ingested foreign bodies (e.g., fish bones) often lodge in this location.

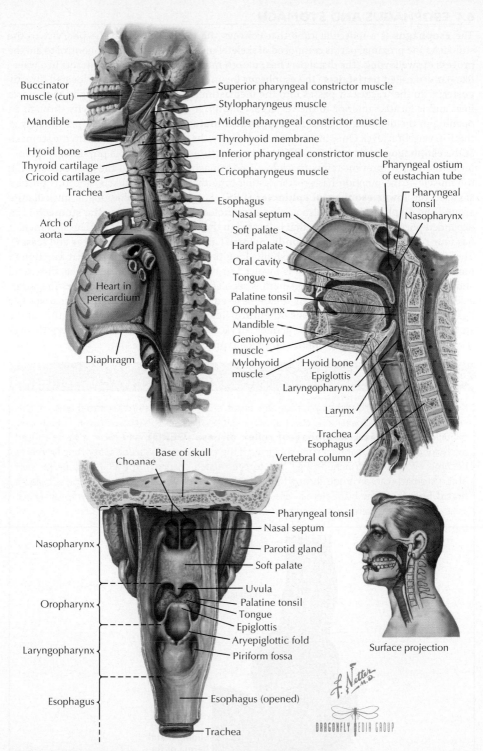

Figure 6.3 PHARYNX

Buccinator muscle (cut)
Mandible
Hyoid bone
Thyroid cartilage
Cricoid cartilage
Trachea
Arch of aorta
Heart in pericardium
Diaphragm

Superior pharyngeal constrictor muscle
Stylopharyngeus muscle
Middle pharyngeal constrictor muscle
Thyrohyoid membrane
Inferior pharyngeal constrictor muscle
Cricopharyngeus muscle
Esophagus
Nasal septum
Soft palate
Hard palate
Oral cavity
Tongue
Palatine tonsil
Oropharynx
Mandible
Geniohyoid muscle
Mylohyoid muscle
Hyoid bone
Epiglottis
Laryngopharynx
Larynx
Trachea
Esophagus
Vertebral column

Pharyngeal ostium of eustachian tube
Pharyngeal tonsil
Nasopharynx

Base of skull
Choanae

Nasopharynx
Oropharynx
Laryngopharynx
Esophagus

Pharyngeal tonsil
Nasal septum
Parotid gland
Soft palate
Uvula
Palatine tonsil
Tongue
Epiglottis
Aryepiglottic fold
Piriform fossa
Esophagus (opened)
Trachea

Surface projection

6.4 ESOPHAGUS AND STOMACH

The **esophagus** is a muscular tube that conveys the food bolus from the pharynx to the stomach. The proximal part is composed of skeletal muscle under voluntary control to aid the process of swallowing. The distal part has smooth muscle in its wall that contracts in a wave-like pattern called **peristalsis**. The esophagus begins in the neck where it is located directly posterior to the trachea. It passes into the mediastinum of the thorax through the thoracic inlet and is located anterior to the vertebral column. It exits the thoracic cavity through an opening in the diaphragm called the **esophageal hiatus**, which is located approximately at the T10 vertebral level. Once in the abdominal cavity, the esophagus merges with the stomach at the **esophagogastric junction (EGJ)**. Two structures contribute to a physiologic sphincter at the EGJ to prevent reflux (backflow) of stomach contents into the esophagus. First, the muscle at the junction has greater resting tone than adjacent muscle, and this portion is called the **lower esophageal sphincter (LES)**. Second, the diaphragmatic musculature around the esophageal hiatus also acts as a sphincter when it contracts. The **stomach** is an expanded portion of the gut tube that is located in the left upper quadrant of the abdomen. It has four regions (**cardia, fundus, body, pylorus**) and two curvatures (**greater** and **lesser**). The internal surface of the stomach exhibits longitudinal folds called **rugae** that function to increase surface area. The stomach is involved in both mechanical and chemical digestion, and passage of chyme into the duodenum is regulated by the **pyloric sphincter**. The stomach is anchored to other organs by double-layered folds of peritoneum. The hepatogastric ligament, which is part of the **lesser omentum**, links the liver to the lesser curvature of the stomach. The peritoneum along the greater curvature of the stomach extends inferiorly over the intestines as the **greater omentum**, which typically accumulates fat.

Clinical Focus

If the LES is weak or relaxes at inappropriate times, stomach acid can reflux into the esophagus causing heartburn—a pain in the chest due to irritation of the esophageal mucosa. This chronic condition is called **gastroesophageal reflex disease (GERD)**, and it can also be caused by dysfunction of the diaphragmatic sphincter. If the esophageal hiatus or supporting ligaments become excessively stretched (e.g., due to age-related changes), the EGJ or superior part of the stomach can protrude through the opening into the thorax. This condition is called a **hiatal hernia**. Some hiatal hernias are asymptomatic, but others can cause symptoms such as acid reflux, heartburn, and difficulty swallowing.

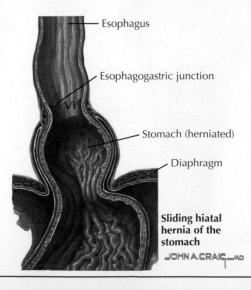

Esophagus

Esophagogastric junction

Stomach (herniated)

Diaphragm

**Sliding hiatal
hernia of the
stomach**

JOHN A.CRAIG—AD

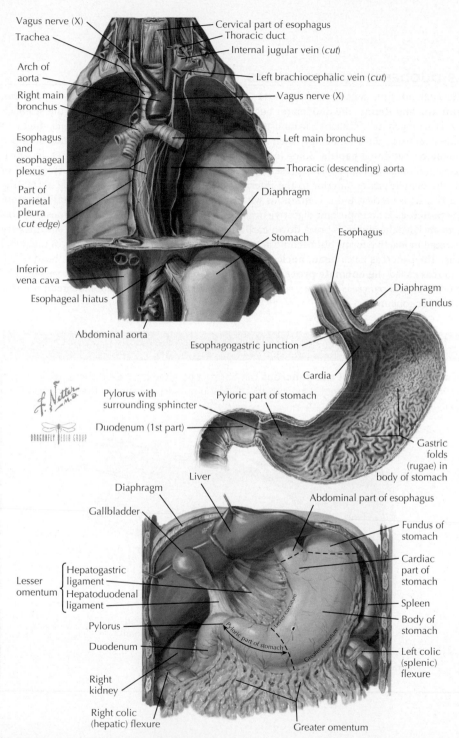

Figure 6.4 ESOPHAGUS AND STOMACH

6.5 DUODENUM AND PANCREAS

The small intestine consists of three parts—from proximal to distal they are the **duodenum**, **jejunum**, and **ileum**. The duodenum begins distal to the pyloric sphincter of the stomach and is arranged in a "C shape" around the head of the pancreas. The common bile duct and main pancreatic duct both empty their secretions into the second part of the duodenum via the **major duodenal papilla**. Some individuals have an accessory pancreatic duct, in which case a minor duodenal papilla is present to receive secretions. The third (transverse) part of the duodenum passes anterior to the inferior venae cavae (IVC) and abdominal aorta. The fourth part is vertical and is continuous with the jejunum at the **duodenojejunal junction**. The **pancreas** is an important digestive organ because it secretes multiple enzymes that collectively have the ability to break down carbohydrates, lipids, and proteins. The enzymes are secreted in inactive forms but become active when they interact with secretions of intestinal cells. The pancreas has a **head**, **neck**, **body**, and **tail**. A small projection of the head of the pancreas called the **uncinate process** extends deep to the superior mesenteric vessels. The duodenum and pancreas are both retroperitoneal organs because they are located posterior to the peritoneum.

Clinical Focus

Cancer of the head of the pancreas can obstruct both the pancreatic duct and the common bile duct. If bile cannot drain into the duodenum, it accumulates in the blood, causing jaundice.

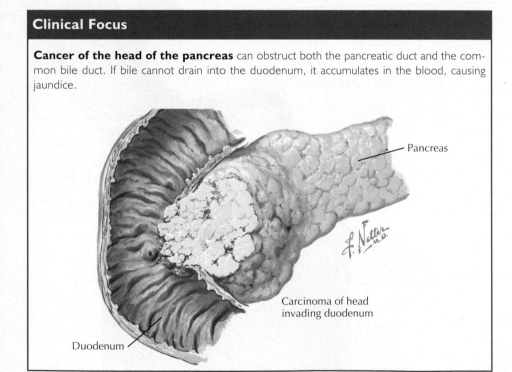

Pancreas

Carcinoma of head
invading duodenum

Duodenum

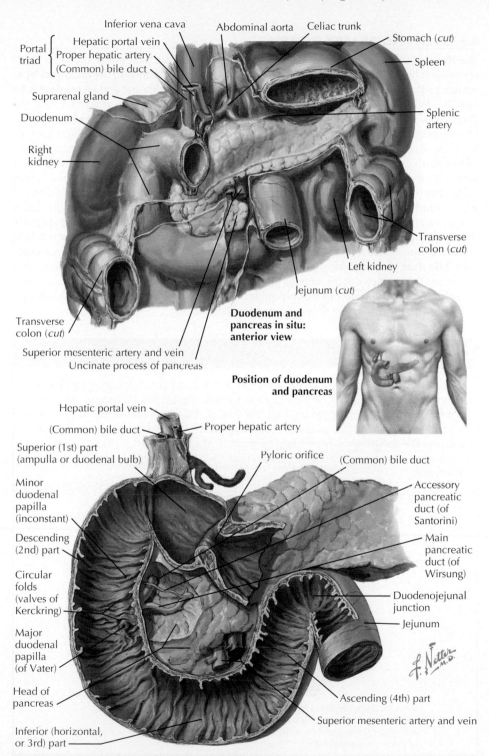

Inferior vena cava

Abdominal aorta   Celiac trunk

Stomach (*cut*)

Portal triad
- Hepatic portal vein
- Proper hepatic artery
- (Common) bile duct

Spleen

Suprarenal gland

Splenic artery

Duodenum

Right kidney

Transverse colon (*cut*)

Left kidney

Jejunum (*cut*)

Transverse colon (*cut*)

Duodenum and pancreas in situ: anterior view

Superior mesenteric artery and vein
Uncinate process of pancreas

Position of duodenum and pancreas

Hepatic portal vein

(Common) bile duct   Proper hepatic artery

Superior (1st) part (ampulla or duodenal bulb)

Pyloric orifice

(Common) bile duct

Minor duodenal papilla (inconstant)

Accessory pancreatic duct (of Santorini)

Descending (2nd) part

Main pancreatic duct (of Wirsung)

Circular folds (valves of Kerckring)

Duodenojejunal junction

Jejunum

Major duodenal papilla (of Vater)

Head of pancreas

Ascending (4th) part

Inferior (horizontal, or 3rd) part

Superior mesenteric artery and vein

Figure 6.5 DUODENUM AND PANCREAS

6.6 LIVER AND BILIARY SYSTEM

The **liver** is a solid organ located mainly in the upper right quadrant of the abdomen. Anatomically it has **right** and **left lobes** (separated by a fold of peritoneum, the **falciform ligament**), a square-shaped **quadrate lobe** adjacent to the gallbladder, and a small **caudate lobe** near the IVC. The liver has two surfaces—a **diaphragmatic surface** in contact with the diaphragm, and a **visceral surface** in contact with the abdominal viscera. The hilum of the liver is called the **porta hepatis**. The hepatic arteries, portal vein, and hepatic ducts enter or leave the liver in this location. The liver is mainly surrounded by visceral peritoneum, apart from a small area on the posterosuperior surface that is in contact with the diaphragm; this region is called the "**bare area**" of the liver. The **gallbladder** is a small pear-shaped hollow organ that is applied to the visceral surface of the liver. The liver has many functions, one of which contributes to the digestive process. Hepatic cells produce bile, which emulsifies lipids so they can be digested by enzymes. Bile leaves the liver through the **right** and **left hepatic ducts**, which merge to form the **common hepatic duct**. The **cystic duct** transports bile in and out of the gallbladder. The cystic duct and common hepatic duct merge to form the **common bile duct** that terminates at the **hepatopancreatic ampulla (of Vater)**. When fat is consumed the sphincter of the ampulla opens to release bile into the duodenal lumen. When the sphincter is closed, any bile that is produced backs up in the common bile duct and then flows through the cystic duct to be stored in the gallbladder.

Clinical Focus

Individuals that are overweight or eat a high-fat diet are at risk for developing **gallstones**. Gallstones are hard deposits of materials in bile, such as bilirubin and cholesterol. If a gallstone becomes lodged in one of the biliary ducts, the flow of bile can be obstructed. Buildup of bile can cause inflammation of the gallbladder (**cholecystitis**), which causes pain in the right upper quadrant. The gallbladder is located approximately at the intersection of the right midclavicular line and costal margin. Pain in this region upon palpation (**Murphy sign**) is indicative of cholecystitis.

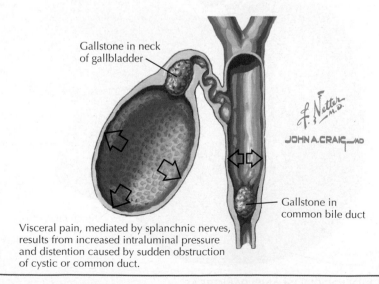

Gallstone in neck of gallbladder

JOHN A.CRAIG—MD

Gallstone in common bile duct

Visceral pain, mediated by splanchnic nerves, results from increased intraluminal pressure and distention caused by sudden obstruction of cystic or common duct.

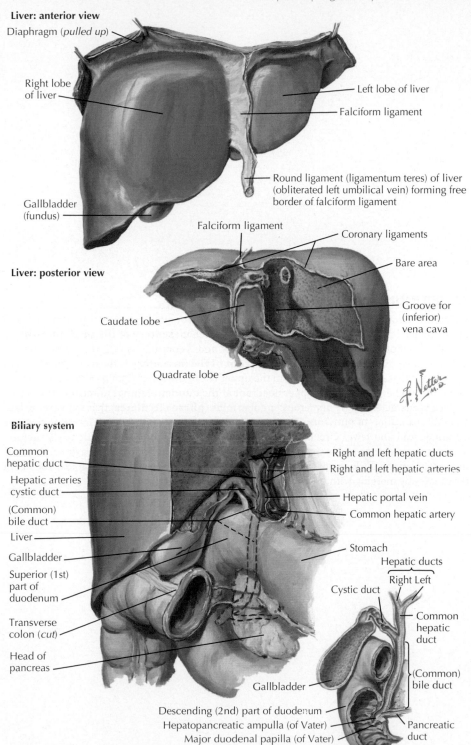

Liver: anterior view

Diaphragm (*pulled up*)

Right lobe of liver

Left lobe of liver

Falciform ligament

Round ligament (ligamentum teres) of liver (obliterated left umbilical vein) forming free border of falciform ligament

Gallbladder (fundus)

Falciform ligament

Coronary ligaments

Liver: posterior view

Bare area

Groove for (inferior) vena cava

Caudate lobe

Quadrate lobe

Biliary system

Common hepatic duct

Hepatic arteries cystic duct

(Common) bile duct

Liver

Gallbladder

Superior (1st) part of duodenum

Transverse colon (*cut*)

Head of pancreas

Right and left hepatic ducts

Right and left hepatic arteries

Hepatic portal vein

Common hepatic artery

Stomach

Hepatic ducts

Right Left

Cystic duct

Common hepatic duct

(Common) bile duct

Gallbladder

Descending (2nd) part of duodenum

Hepatopancreatic ampulla (of Vater)

Major duodenal papilla (of Vater)

Pancreatic duct

Figure 6.6 LIVER AND BILIARY SYSTEM

6.7 JEJUNUM AND ILEUM

Unlike the duodenum, the jejunum and ileum are surrounded by visceral peritoneum and are suspended from the body wall by a mesentery. The **mesentery of the small intestine** is a double layer of peritoneum that accumulates fat and is continuous with the parietal perito-neum on the posterior abdominal wall. The **root of the mesentery** is the name for its line of attachment that extends obliquely from the upper left to the lower right part of the abdomen. The **jejunum** begins in the left upper quadrant at the **duodenojejunal junction**. Its internal surface is characterized by numerous circular folds (**plicae circulares**) that increase surface area for absorption of nutrients. The **ileum** is the distal part of the small intestine that has a thinner wall and fewer circular folds than the jejunum. There is no particular structural feature that marks the end of the jejunum and beginning of the ileum, rather a gradual transi-tion occurs in the thickness of the intestinal wall and the number of circular folds. The ileum terminates by merging with the cecum at the **ileocecal junction**.

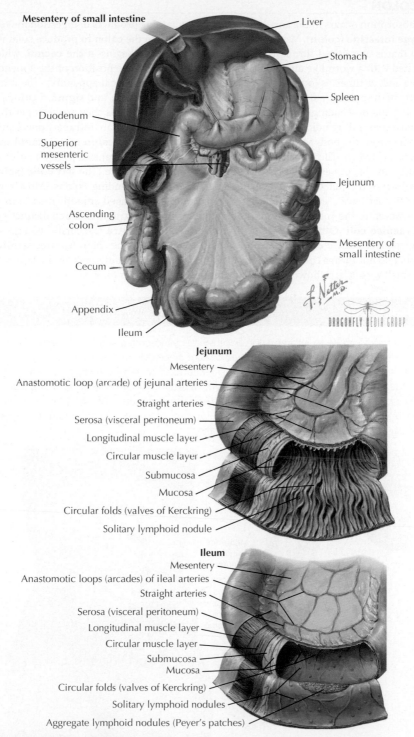

Mesentery of small intestine

Liver

Stomach

Spleen

Duodenum

Superior
mesenteric
vessels

Jejunum

Ascending
colon

Mesentery of
small intestine

Cecum

Appendix

Ileum

Jejunum

Mesentery

Anastomotic loop (arcade) of jejunal arteries

Straight arteries

Serosa (visceral peritoneum)

Longitudinal muscle layer

Circular muscle layer

Submucosa

Mucosa

Circular folds (valves of Kerckring)

Solitary lymphoid nodule

Ileum

Mesentery

Anastomotic loops (arcades) of ileal arteries

Straight arteries

Serosa (visceral peritoneum)

Longitudinal muscle layer

Circular muscle layer

Submucosa

Mucosa

Circular folds (valves of Kerckring)

Solitary lymphoid nodules

Aggregate lymphoid nodules (Peyer's patches)

Figure 6.7 JEJUNUM AND ILEUM

6.8 COLON

Once absorption occurs in the small intestine, the remaining products of digestion move into the **large intestine (colon)**. Water absorption continues in the colon to produce solid waste (feces) that is eliminated through the anal canal. The colon begins at the **cecum**, which is associated with a wormlike appendage called the **appendix**. The position of the appendix is variable and, at times, is located posterior to the cecum (retrocecal appendix). The remaining parts of the colon are the **ascending, transverse, descending**, and **sigmoid colons**. The ascending and descending colons are relatively fixed in location as they are retroperitoneal. The transverse and sigmoid colons are more mobile because they are intraperitoneal and are suspended from the body wall by mesenteries (**transverse mesocolon** and **sigmoid mesocolon**, respectively). The transition between the ascending and transverse colons is characterized by an abrupt bend called the **right colic (hepatic) flexure**. The **left colic (splenic) flexure** marks the junction between the transverse and descending colons. Most regions of the GI tract have a continuous layer of longitudinally arranged smooth muscle in their wall; however, in the colon, the longitudinal muscle is concentrated in three distinct bands called **taeniae coli**. Other features of the colon include **haustra** (sacculations) and small fatty appendages called **omental appendices**. The interior of the colon features **semilunar folds** that do not form a complete circle around the lumen. The difference in the fold pattern of the small versus large bowel helps to distinguish these organs on x-ray images.

Clinical Focus

The appendix is prone to inflammation because it is blind-ended and has a narrow lumen. If the lumen becomes blocked (e.g., by a seed or hard piece of fecal matter), bacteria can quickly multiply and cause infection (**appendicitis**). Tenderness or pain from appendicitis is typically felt in the region of **McBurney point**—a site two-thirds of the way along a line from the umbilicus to the anterior superior iliac spine (ASIS) that indicates the typical position of the appendix with respect to the abdominal wall. However, pain can refer to other locations such as the back if the appendix is in an atypical location.

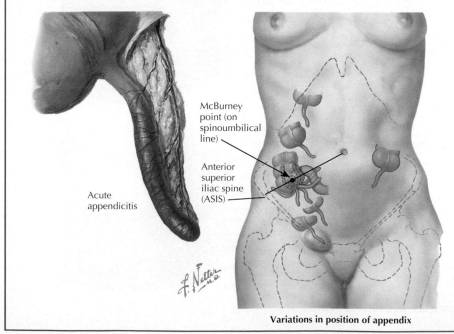

Acute appendicitis

McBurney point (on spinoumbilical line)

Anterior superior iliac spine (ASIS)

Variations in position of appendix

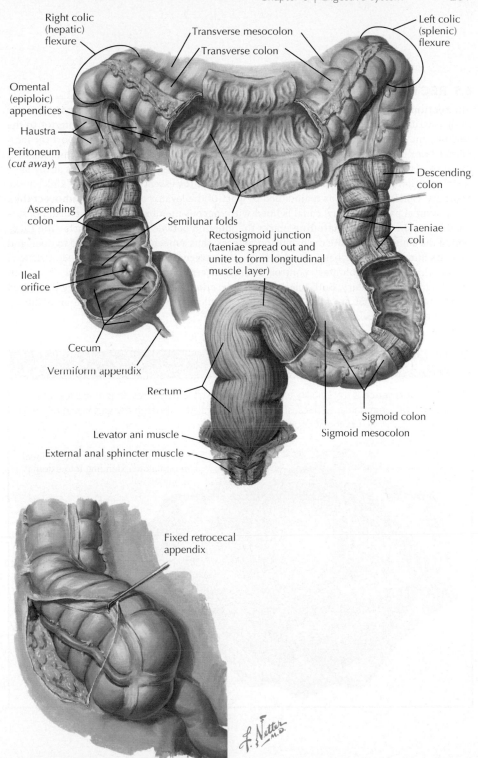

Right colic (hepatic) flexure

Transverse mesocolon

Transverse colon

Left colic (splenic) flexure

Omental (epiploic) appendices

Haustra

Peritoneum (*cut away*)

Descending colon

Ascending colon

Semilunar folds

Taeniae coli

Ileal orifice

Rectosigmoid junction (taeniae spread out and unite to form longitudinal muscle layer)

Cecum

Vermiform appendix

Rectum

Sigmoid colon

Levator ani muscle

Sigmoid mesocolon

External anal sphincter muscle

Fixed retrocecal appendix

Figure 6.8 COLON

6.9 RECTUM AND ANAL CANAL

The **rectum** begins at the rectosigmoid junction and descends into the pelvic cavity anterior to the sacrum. The rectum is described as subperitoneal because it is located inferior to the peritoneum. The rectal mucosa exhibits three **transverse folds** that help to support the fecal matter prior to elimination. At its distal end, the rectum narrows to become continuous with the anus at the **anorectal junction**. An angle of approximately 90 degrees exists at the anorectal junction to aid in the maintenance of continence (by essentially putting a "kink" in the anorectal canal). The angle is maintained by part of the levator ani muscle (**puborectalis**). The proximal part of the anal canal is lined with mucous membrane, while the distal part is lined with skin. The **pectinate line** marks the junction between these two parts. The function of the anus is to regulate the expulsion of feces; thus a mechanism is needed to open and close its lumen. The anus has two sphincters—an **external sphincter** composed of skeletal muscle that is under voluntary control, and **an internal sphincter** composed of smooth muscle that is involuntary. Both relax during defecation. The anus is bordered by the paired **ischioanal fossae** that are filled with fat, which allows for expansion of the anus during evacuation of the fecal mass.

Clinical Focus

Fecal incontinence is the inability to control bowel movements, resulting in leakage of stool. Childbirth is a common cause because the passage of a fetus through the vagina can tear adjacent musculature such as the levator ani and anal sphincters.

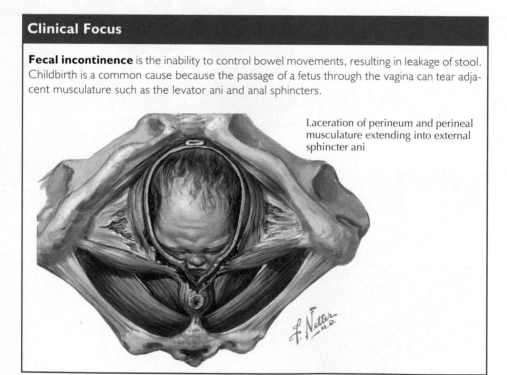

Laceration of perineum and perineal musculature extending into external sphincter ani

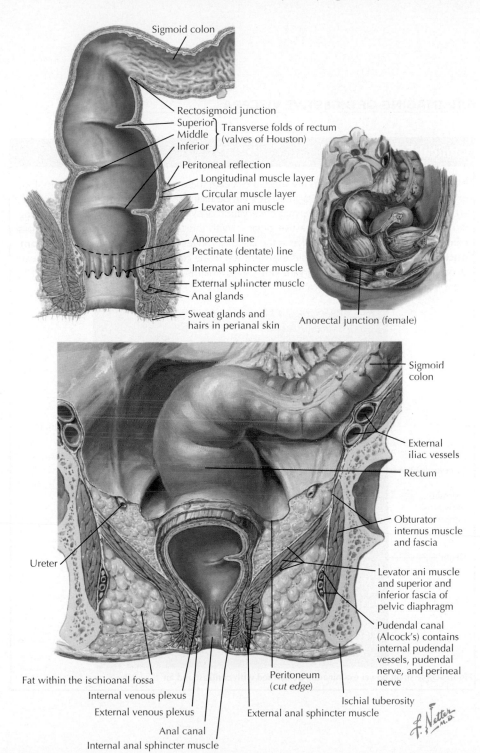

Sigmoid colon

Rectosigmoid junction
Superior
Middle   Transverse folds of rectum
Inferior   (valves of Houston)

Peritoneal reflection
Longitudinal muscle layer
Circular muscle layer
Levator ani muscle

Anorectal line
Pectinate (dentate) line
Internal sphincter muscle
External sphincter muscle
Anal glands
Sweat glands and
hairs in perianal skin

Anorectal junction (female)

Sigmoid
colon

External
iliac vessels

Rectum

Obturator
internus muscle
and fascia

Ureter

Levator ani muscle
and superior and
inferior fascia of
pelvic diaphragm

Pudendal canal
(Alcock's) contains
internal pudendal
vessels, pudendal
nerve, and perineal
nerve

Fat within the ischioanal fossa
Internal venous plexus
External venous plexus
Anal canal
Internal anal sphincter muscle

Peritoneum
(cut edge)

External anal sphincter muscle

Ischial tuberosity

f. Netter
M.D.

Figure 6.9 RECTUM AND ANAL CANAL

6.10 IMAGING OF DIGESTIVE VISCERA

Clinical Focus

Many different imaging modalities are used to evaluate the organs of the digestive system. Hollow organs such as the stomach or intestines can be examined with **radiography** when they are filled with air. **Fluoroscopy** permits observation of dynamic processes such as swallowing, peristalsis, and motility of the digestive organs. With this technique, the patient ingests oral contrast and images are captured live as the contrast moves through the digestive tract. **Computed tomography (CT)** provides excellent soft tissue contrast and can be used to evaluate structural changes in individual organs (e.g., inflammation, enlargement) that are caused by pathology such as infections or cancer.

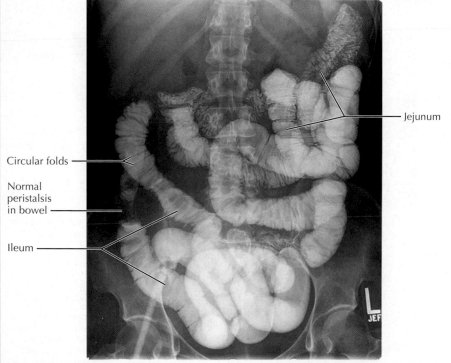

Circular folds

Normal peristalsis in bowel

Ileum

Jejunum

Fluoroscopic small bowel examination performed with contrast and air (*Courtesy Nancy McNulty, M.D.*).

Clinical Focus (Continued)

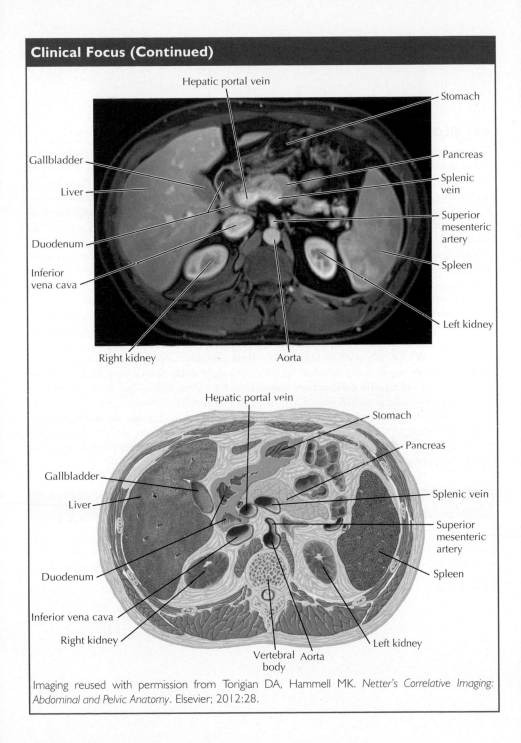

Imaging reused with permission from Torigian DA, Hammell MK. *Netter's Correlative Imaging: Abdominal and Pelvic Anatomy.* Elsevier; 2012:28.

6.11 BLOOD SUPPLY OF DIGESTIVE VISCERA

The thoracic portion of the esophagus mainly receives arterial blood from multiple branches of the **descending thoracic aorta**. The blood supply of the abdominal viscera is provided by three branches of the abdominal aorta that arise from its anterior surface. Each branch is associated with one of the embryonic divisions of the gut tube: the **celiac trunk** supplies organs derived from the foregut, the **superior mesenteric artery (SMA)** supplies midgut organs, and the **inferior mesenteric artery (IMA)** supplies organs of the hindgut. After arising from the aorta, the celiac trunk immediately divides into three terminal branches. The **left gastric artery** follows the lesser curvature of the stomach and supplies the stomach and abdominal part of the esophagus. The **splenic artery** travels along the superior border of the pancreas and gives branches to the stomach, pancreas, and spleen (an organ of the immune system). The **common hepatic artery** has multiple branches that supply the stomach, duodenum, pancreas, liver, and gallbladder; two primary branches are the **gastroduodenal** and **proper hepatic arteries**. The SMA supplies all three parts of the small intestine, the cecum, appendix, ascending colon, and the proximal two-thirds of the transverse colon. Its branches are logically named: **jejunal** and **ileal arteries** supply the small intestine; the **ileocolic artery** supplies the ileocecal junction; the **right colic artery** supplies the ascending colon; and the **middle colic artery** supplies the transverse colon. The IMA supplies the remaining parts of the bowel, specifically the distal one-third of the transverse colon and descending colon via the **left colic artery**, the sigmoid colon through **sigmoid arteries,** and the superior part of the rectum by the **superior rectal artery**. The rectum also receives blood supply from **middle** and **inferior rectal branches** of the internal iliac artery that arise within the pelvis.

Clinical Focus

Anastomoses exist in areas of transition; for example, the **marginal artery** of the colon links the middle colic branch of the SMA and the left colic branch of the IMA in the region of the splenic flexure. However, collateral flow is often limited in these "watershed" areas, and thus they are at risk for **ischemia** in situations of hypoperfusion or arterial blockage.

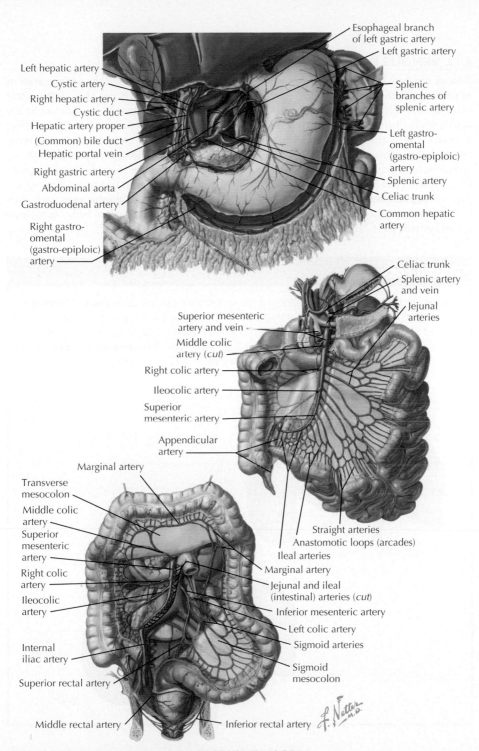

Figure 6.11 BLOOD SUPPLY OF DIGESTIVE VISCERA

6.12 VENOUS DRAINAGE OF DIGESTIVE VISCERA

Venous drainage of the thoracic esophagus occurs through tributaries of the **azygos system of veins**, while the abdominal portion drains into the esophageal branches of the **left gastric vein**. Venous blood from the abdominal organs contains nutrients that were absorbed by the capillaries in the intestinal tract. This blood needs to enter the liver for metabolic processing; thus blood is directed to the **hepatic portal vein**. The **superior mesenteric** and **splenic veins** merge to form the portal vein. The **inferior mesenteric vein** typically drains into the splenic vein. Once the blood enters the liver, it passes through the sinusoidal capillaries so that nutrients can be absorbed by hepatic cells. Venous blood is then transported out of the liver via **hepatic veins**, which are systemic veins that drain into the inferior vena cava. This unique arrangement—where a system of veins exists between two capillary beds—is called a portal system (see 4.1).

Clinical Focus

Pathology that slows the flow of blood through the liver can produce **portal hypertension**—high blood pressure in the portal vein or its tributaries. Causes can be intrahepatic (e.g., cirrhosis of the liver) or extrahepatic (e.g., clot in the portal vein). As blood backs up in tributaries of the portal vein, resulting complications include **esophageal varices** (dilated esophageal veins that may bleed) and **splenomegaly** (enlarged spleen).

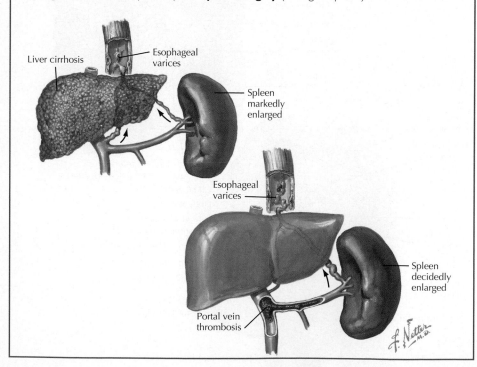

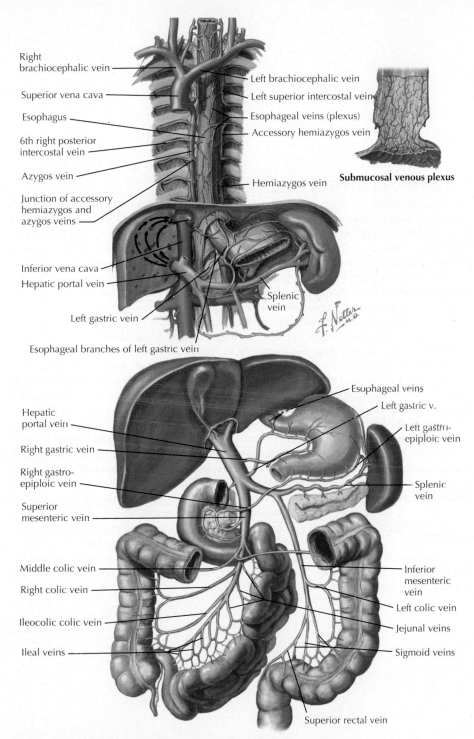

Submucosal venous plexus

Figure 6.12 VENOUS DRAINAGE OF DIGESTIVE VISCERA

6.13 INNERVATION OF DIGESTIVE VISCERA

The musculature of the esophagus is innervated by branches of the **vagus nerves**. Somatic efferent neurons innervate the superior part composed of skeletal muscle, while parasympathetic neurons supply the remaining portion consisting of smooth muscle. The innervation of the abdominal viscera is provided by autonomic nerves that intermingle within the **aortic plexus** on the anterior surface of the abdominal aorta. **Sympathetic neurons** originate in the thoracolumbar spinal cord and travel to the aortic plexus via the **thoracic** and **lumbar splanchnic nerves**; the three thoracic splanchnic nerves are named greater, lesser, and least splanchnics. These preganglionic neurons synapse in sympathetic ganglia that are located near the major branches of the aorta (e.g., celiac ganglion). The postganglionic neurons follow branches of the major vessels to reach their target organs. Sympathetic activity stimulates the body's "fight or flight" response, preparing the body for intense situations; thus it inhibits the digestive process. Its effects on the gastrointestinal system include shunting blood away from the intestines (vasoconstriction), inhibiting gastrointestinal motility by relaxing smooth muscle, contracting sphincters, and inhibiting glandular secretion. **Parasympathetic neurons** that innervate the gastrointestinal organs are from two sources. The vagus nerves enter the abdomen through the esophageal hiatus with the esophagus and become the **vagal trunks**. These nerves convey parasympathetic neurons to the viscera supplied by the celiac trunk and SMA (vagal innervation ends approximately at the splenic flexure). The parasympathetic neurons that innervate the remainder of the gastrointestinal tract arise in the sacral region of the spinal cord and travel superiorly to the viscera within the **pelvic splanchnic nerves**. Preganglionic parasympathetic neurons typically synapse in ganglia that are in the wall of the target organ between the layers of smooth muscle. Parasympathetic neurons promote "resting and digesting"—processes that conserve and restore the body's energy. Thus parasympathetic stimulation increases peristalsis in the gastrointestinal tract, stimulates glandular secretion, and relaxes smooth muscle sphincters to promote digestion and defecation. The external anal sphincter (skeletal muscle) is innervated by **inferior rectal nerves**, which are branches of the pudendal nerves.

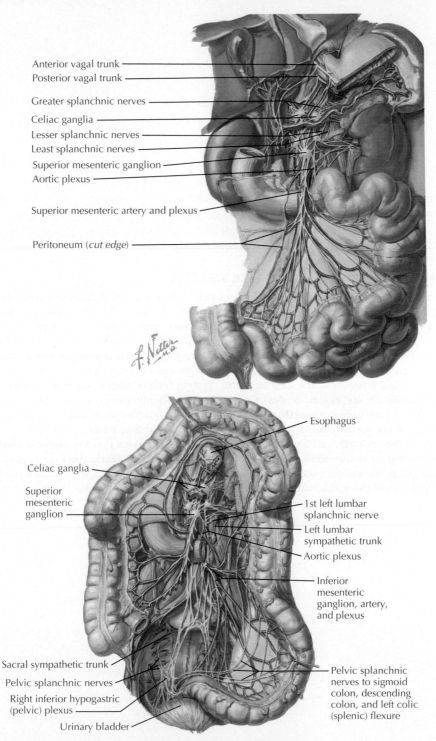

Anterior vagal trunk

Posterior vagal trunk

Greater splanchnic nerves

Celiac ganglia

Lesser splanchnic nerves

Least splanchnic nerves

Superior mesenteric ganglion

Aortic plexus

Superior mesenteric artery and plexus

Peritoneum (*cut edge*)

Esophagus

Celiac ganglia

Superior mesenteric ganglion

1st left lumbar splanchnic nerve

Left lumbar sympathetic trunk

Aortic plexus

Inferior mesenteric ganglion, artery, and plexus

Sacral sympathetic trunk

Pelvic splanchnic nerves

Right inferior hypogastric (pelvic) plexus

Urinary bladder

Pelvic splanchnic nerves to sigmoid colon, descending colon, and left colic (splenic) flexure

Figure 6.13 INNERVATION OF DIGESTIVE VISCERA

6.14 LYMPHATICS OF DIGESTIVE VISCERA

Because the esophagus extends from the neck to the abdomen, lymph from this organ drains into a variety of lymph nodes including **deep cervical nodes** in the neck, **posterior mediastinal nodes** in the thorax, and **left gastric nodes** in the abdomen. Lymphatic drainage from the abdominal organs resembles the pattern of the vasculature. Lymph initially drains to lymph nodes that are adjacent to particular organs (e.g., **gastric nodes, paracolic nodes**). Lymphatic vessels from these nodes converge on groups of lymph nodes that are adjacent to the primary vessels of the gastrointestinal system (**celiac nodes, superior mesenteric nodes, inferior mesenteric nodes**). Collectively these lymph nodes on the anterior surface of the aorta are called **preaortic nodes**, in contrast to lymph nodes located on the lateral aspects of the aorta, which are called **lateral aortic** or **lumbar nodes**. Lymph that passes through the preaortic and lateral aortic nodes ultimately drains into the **cisterna chyli**, a saclike dilation at the inferior end of the thoracic duct. The **thoracic duct** conveys all the lymph from the abdominal organs to the circulation by merging with the venous system at the junction of the subclavian and internal jugular veins.

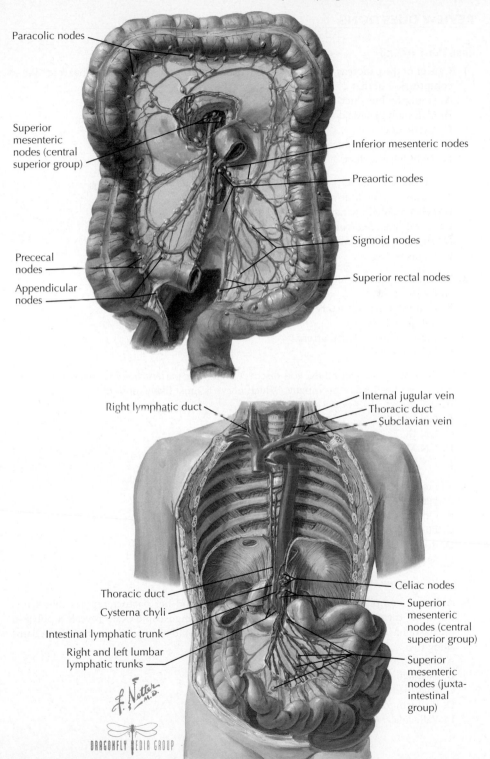

Figure 6.14 LYMPHATICS OF DIGESTIVE VISCERA

REVIEW QUESTIONS

Test Your Recall

1. Cancer of the pancreas could prevent bile from entering the gastrointestinal tract due to compression of the:
   A. Common bile duct
   B. Common hepatic duct
   C. Cystic duct
   D. Main pancreatic duct
   E. Right hepatic duct

2. Peristalsis (contraction) of the descending colon would be facilitated by:
   A. Lumbar splanchnic nerves
   B. Pelvic splanchnic nerves
   C. Sacral splanchnic nerves
   D. Thoracic splanchnic nerves
   E. Vagus nerves

3. Which artery travels along the lesser curvature of the stomach?
   A. Celiac trunk
   B. Common hepatic artery
   C. Left gastric artery
   D. Right gastro-omental artery
   E. Splenic artery

4. While testing the gag reflex, you discover that your patient has lost sensation on the posterior one-third of his tongue. Which nerve is most likely injured?
   A. CN V
   B. CN VII
   C. CN IX
   D. CN X
   E. CN XII

5. The internal lining of the jejunum exhibits:
   A. Haustra
   B. Omental appendices
   C. Plicae circulares
   D. Rugae
   E. Semilunar folds

Apply Your Knowledge

6. A patient complains of chronic nasal congestion, and her partner reports that she is breathing through her mouth while she sleeps. Laryngoscopic exam reveals a polyp in the nasopharynx. While removing this polyp, you would be most concerned about damaging the:
   A. Epiglottis
   B. Eustachian tube
   C. Palatine tonsil
   D. Piriform fossa
   E. Vallecula

7. A patient has cancer in the superior part of his rectum. If you wanted to assess metastatic spread via the lymphatic system, which group of lymph nodes should you examine first?
   A. External iliac nodes
   B. Inferior mesenteric nodes
   C. Internal iliac nodes
   D. Lateral aortic (lumbar) nodes
   E. Sacral nodes

8. A patient with a history of atherosclerosis tells her primary care physician that she often experiences pain after eating that eventually goes away within several hours. Angiography reveals that branches of the superior mesenteric artery are narrowed by plaque, and the pain is due to ischemia. Which of the following organs is most likely affected by the ischemia?
   A. Descending colon
   B. Duodenum
   C. Ileum
   D. Pancreas
   E. Rectum

9. A patient complains of difficulty swallowing and reports that she feels liquid entering her nose. A barium swallow study indicates that the soft palate is not elevating properly. This could be the result of damage to:
   A. CN V
   B. CN VII
   C. CN IX
   D. CN X
   E. CN XII

10. A man brings his partner to the emergency room because he has been vomiting blood. Endoscopic exam reveals that the patient has esophageal varices (dilated esophageal veins) in the distal part of his esophagus that ruptured causing internal bleeding. These varices are most likely the result of increased blood volume in the:
    A. Gastroduodenal vein
    B. Inferior vena cava
    C. Left gastric vein
    D. Right hepatic vein
    E. Splenic vein

See Appendix for answers.

ENDOCRINE SYSTEM

7.1 THE ENDOCRINE SYSTEM

The endocrine system consists of organs, glands, and tissues that produce and secrete hormones. Hormones influence the activity of numerous cells in the body and regulate processes such as growth, development, reproduction, and the response of the body to stress. Some organs, such as the heart, have an endocrine function because they secrete one or more hormones; however, this is not their primary function in the body. Other endocrine tissue is scattered throughout the body. For example, fat is endocrine tissue because its cells secrete a hormone that regulates food intake and fat storage. In this chapter we will focus on five major endocrine glands: the **pituitary gland**, **thyroid gland**, **parathyroid glands**, **adrenal glands**, and the **pancreas**. The **ovaries** and **testes** are important endocrine glands associated with reproduction; they are discussed in Chapter 9—The Reproductive System. Unlike exocrine glands that secrete their products into ducts, endocrine glands release hormones directly into the bloodstream or the lymphatic system. Thus endocrine glands typically have well-developed vasculature and lymphatic drainage.

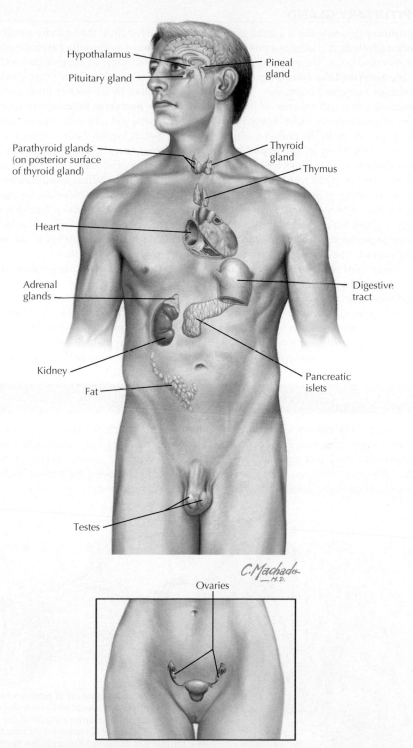

Figure 7.1 THE ENDOCRINE SYSTEM

7.2 PITUITARY GLAND

The **pituitary** (hypophysis) is a small gland that is suspended from the brain by a stalk called the **infundibulum**. It resides in a protective bony fossa known as the **sella turcica** that is part of the sphenoid bone. The pituitary gland has two lobes that differ in composition and function. The **anterior lobe** (adenohypophysis) is composed of glandular tissue that synthesizes and releases numerous hormones. This activity is regulated by hormones produced in the hypothalamus that can enhance or inhibit secretion. The **posterior lobe** (neurohypophysis) consists of neural tissue—specifically axons, axon terminals, and glial cells. The neuronal cell bodies of the axons in the posterior pituitary are located in hypothalamic nuclei; the axons are known collectively as the **hypothalamohypophyseal tract**. Hormones synthesized in the hypothalamus are transported along the axons of the hypothalamohypophyseal tract and stored in nerve terminals within the posterior lobe of the pituitary. When stimulated by neural impulses, secretory granules are released and the hormones enter the bloodstream via fenestrated capillaries of the posterior pituitary. Thus the posterior lobe of the pituitary is not an endocrine gland but rather a storage site for hormones. The pituitary receives arterial blood from the **superior** and **inferior hypophyseal arteries**, which are branches of the internal carotid arteries. The circulatory pattern in the posterior pituitary is typical—arteries branch to form arterioles and eventually capillaries, and then capillaries form **hypophyseal veins** that drain into the cavernous sinus. In contrast, the anterior pituitary is associated with the **hypophyseal portal system**, which consists of a system of veins between a primary capillary plexus in the hypothalamus and a secondary capillary bed in the anterior lobe. This system allows direct communication between the hypothalamus and anterior pituitary that is necessary for the regulatory function of the hypothalamus. Hormones that are secreted by the anterior lobe enter the bloodstream through hypophyseal veins that drain to the cavernous sinus.

Clinical Focus

Pituitary tumors (**pituitary adenomas**) are the most common cause of pituitary dysfunction. Because the pituitary gland is almost completely surrounded by bone, tumors often expand superiorly into the cranial cavity and may cause visual disturbances by compressing the optic chiasm. If surgical intervention is necessary, the relationship between the pituitary gland and sphenoidal sinus allows access through the nasal cavity (transsphenoidal approach).

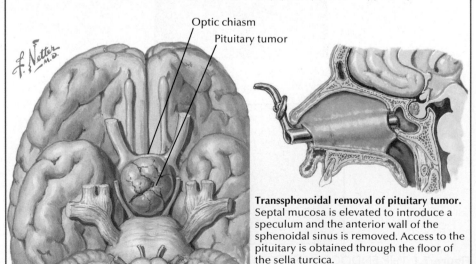

Optic chiasm

Pituitary tumor

Transsphenoidal removal of pituitary tumor. Septal mucosa is elevated to introduce a speculum and the anterior wall of the sphenoidal sinus is removed. Access to the pituitary is obtained through the floor of the sella turcica.

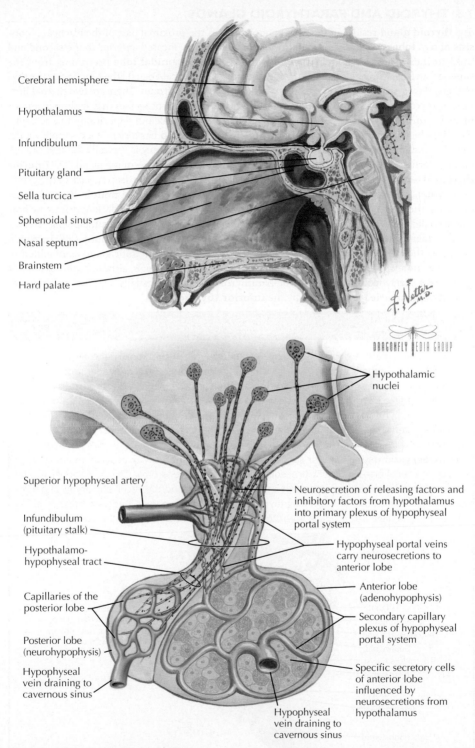

Cerebral hemisphere

Hypothalamus

Infundibulum

Pituitary gland

Sella turcica

Sphenoidal sinus

Nasal septum

Brainstem

Hard palate

Hypothalamic nuclei

Superior hypophyseal artery

Neurosecretion of releasing factors and inhibitory factors from hypothalamus into primary plexus of hypophyseal portal system

Infundibulum (pituitary stalk)

Hypothalamo-hypophyseal tract

Hypophyseal portal veins carry neurosecretions to anterior lobe

Anterior lobe (adenohypophysis)

Capillaries of the posterior lobe

Secondary capillary plexus of hypophyseal portal system

Posterior lobe (neurohypophysis)

Hypophyseal vein draining to cavernous sinus

Specific secretory cells of anterior lobe influenced by neurosecretions from hypothalamus

Hypophyseal vein draining to cavernous sinus

Figure 7.2 PITUITARY GLAND

7.3 THYROID AND PARATHYROID GLANDS

The **thyroid gland** resides in the neck anterolateral to the proximal part of the trachea. It consists of two **lobes** connected by an **isthmus** that is typically located anterior to the second and third tracheal rings. Some individuals also have a thin **pyramidal lobe** protruding from the superior surface, which is a developmental remnant (see Clinical Focus). The function of the thyroid gland is to produce and secrete thyroid hormones and calcitonin. There are two thyroid hormones, thyroxine (T_4) and triiodothyronine (T_3), which regulate processes that are important for metabolism, growth, and development. Calcitonin promotes calcium deposition in bones, thus reducing the amount of calcium in the blood. The thyroid gland has a rich blood supply via the superior and inferior thyroid arteries. The **superior thyroid artery** is typically the first branch of the external carotid artery, and it travels along the superior surface of the gland. The **inferior thyroid artery** arises from the thyrocervical trunk and ascends to the deep surface of the gland. Three pairs of thyroid veins drain the thyroid gland. The **superior** and **middle thyroid veins** drain into the internal jugular vein, while the **inferior thyroid veins** typically empty into the brachiocephalic veins. Notice that the middle thyroid vein does not have an accompanying artery.

The **parathyroid glands** manufacture and secrete parathyroid hormone (PTH), which increases the amount of calcium in the blood. There are typically four glands embedded in the posterior surface of the thyroid, a superior pair and inferior pair, although the number of glands and their location can vary. The parathyroid glands are usually supplied by the **inferior thyroid arteries** and drained by the **inferior thyroid veins**.

Clinical Focus

During development, thyroid tissue migrates inferiorly from the floor of the pharynx to the neck, tethered by the thyroglossal duct. The thyroglossal duct usually degenerates; however, portions may persist as a tract or **thyroglossal cyst**. In some individuals, thyroid tissue does not fully migrate. **Ectopic thyroid tissue** can be found anywhere along the path of migration, and the pyramidal lobe is one example of this. Occasionally the thyroid gland receives additional arterial supply from a small artery called the **thyroid ima artery**. If this artery is present, it typically branches from the aortic arch or brachiocephalic trunk and ascends to the thyroid gland on the anterior surface of the trachea. Thus it may provide an unexpected source of arterial bleeding during procedures such as a tracheostomy. Clinicians should also be aware of the close relationship between the thyroid gland and the recurrent laryngeal nerves to avoid damage to the nerves during thyroid surgery. These nerves innervate muscles of the larynx; thus damage can produce vocal cord paralysis and hoarseness of the voice.

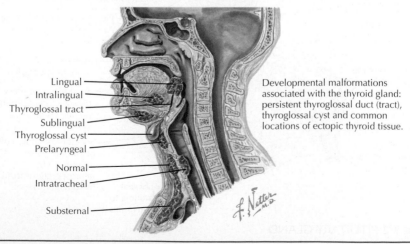

Lingual
Intralingual
Thyroglossal tract
Sublingual
Thyroglossal cyst
Prelaryngeal
Normal
Intratracheal
Substernal

Developmental malformations associated with the thyroid gland: persistent thyroglossal duct (tract), thyroglossal cyst and common locations of ectopic thyroid tissue.

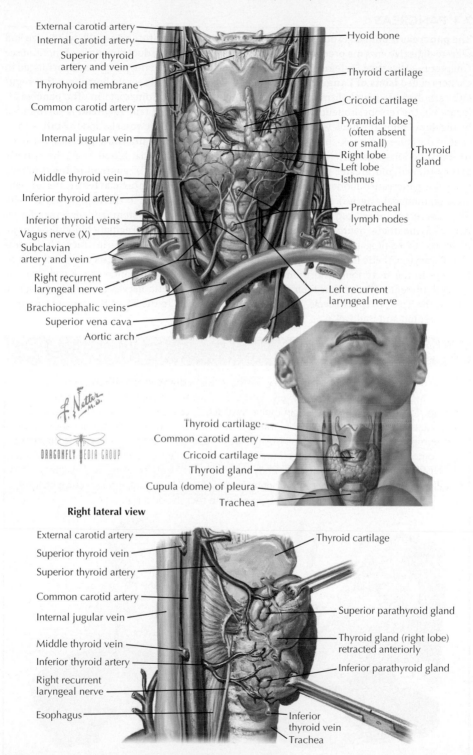

External carotid artery
Internal carotid artery
Superior thyroid artery and vein
Thyrohyoid membrane
Common carotid artery
Internal jugular vein
Middle thyroid vein
Inferior thyroid artery
Inferior thyroid veins
Vagus nerve (X)
Subclavian artery and vein
Right recurrent laryngeal nerve
Brachiocephalic veins
Superior vena cava
Aortic arch

Hyoid bone
Thyroid cartilage
Cricoid cartilage
Pyramidal lobe (often absent or small)
Right lobe
Left lobe
Isthmus
} Thyroid gland
Pretracheal lymph nodes
Left recurrent laryngeal nerve

Thyroid cartilage
Common carotid artery
Cricoid cartilage
Thyroid gland
Cupula (dome) of pleura
Trachea

Right lateral view

External carotid artery
Superior thyroid vein
Superior thyroid artery
Common carotid artery
Internal jugular vein
Middle thyroid vein
Inferior thyroid artery
Right recurrent laryngeal nerve
Esophagus

Thyroid cartilage
Superior parathyroid gland
Thyroid gland (right lobe) retracted anteriorly
Inferior parathyroid gland
Inferior thyroid vein
Trachea

Figure 7.3 THYROID AND PARATHYROID GLANDS

7.4 PANCREAS

The **pancreas** is both an exocrine and endocrine gland. Pancreatic acinar cells synthesize and secrete digestive enzyme precursors into a system of pancreatic ducts (exocrine function; see Chapter 6—Digestive System). Cells of the endocrine portion of the pancreas are arranged in clusters called **islets of Langerhans**. The islet cells produce and secrete hormones that regulate carbohydrate metabolism, namely insulin, glucagon, and somatostatin. The pancreas is located in the retroperitoneum and has a head, neck, body, and tail. The **head** is surrounded by the duodenum, the **neck** is anterior to the superior mesenteric vessels, and the **tail** is adjacent to the spleen. A hook-shaped protuberance of the head, the **uncinate process**, lies deep to the superior mesenteric vessels. The pancreas receives arterial blood from the **splenic artery** (dorsal and greater pancreatic arteries, artery to the tail), **gastroduodenal artery** (superior pancreaticoduodenal arteries), and the **superior mesenteric artery** (inferior pancreaticoduodenal arteries). Corresponding veins ultimately drain to the hepatic portal vein. The pancreas is innervated by efferent nerves of the autonomic system, and visceral afferent nerves. Sympathetic neurons within **thoracic splanchnic nerves** regulate blood flow to the pancreas; these preganglionic neurons synapse in the celiac and superior mesenteric ganglia. Parasympathetic innervation of the endocrine pancreas via the **vagus nerves** causes an increase in the secretion of hormones. Pain sensations from the pancreas are conveyed by visceral afferent neurons that typically travel with sympathetic nerves and enter the spinal cord at the T5–T10 spinal levels. Thus pain can be referred to the T5–T10 dermatomes (epigastric region and midback).

Clinical Focus

The most common disorder of the endocrine pancreas is **diabetes mellitus**, a condition that results in elevated blood glucose levels. There are two major types of diabetes that differ in etiology. In **type I diabetes**, autoimmune destruction of pancreatic islet cells causes insulin deficiency. Patients must obtain insulin through other means, such as injections or using an insulin pump that periodically releases insulin into the subcutaneous tissue. In **type II diabetes**, cells do not respond appropriately to insulin, a condition called insulin resistance. Many factors affect insulin resistance, such as excess body weight, lack of sleep, smoking, and inactivity. Thus type II diabetes can be managed by adopting healthy habits (e.g., diet and exercise); however, some patients also need medication to help regulate their blood sugar.

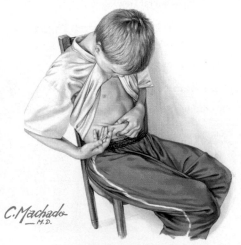
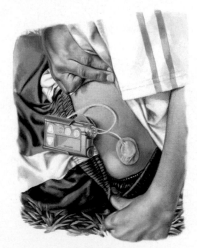

| Insulin pump | Multiple daily insulin injection |

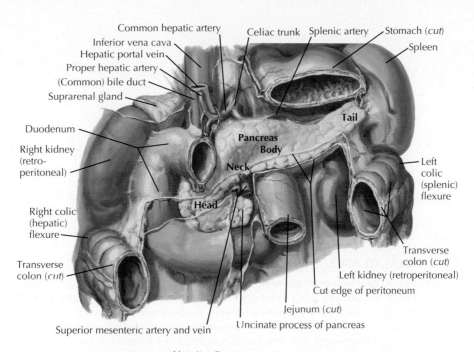

Common hepatic artery
Celiac trunk
Splenic artery
Stomach (*cut*)
Inferior vena cava
Hepatic portal vein
Proper hepatic artery
(Common) bile duct
Suprarenal gland
Spleen
Tail
Duodenum
Pancreas
Body
Right kidney
(retro-
peritoneal)
Neck
Left
colic
(splenic)
flexure
Head
Right colic
(hepatic)
flexure
Transverse
colon (*cut*)
Transverse
colon (*cut*)
Left kidney (retroperitoneal)
Cut edge of peritoneum
Jejunum (*cut*)
Uncinate process of pancreas
Superior mesenteric artery and vein

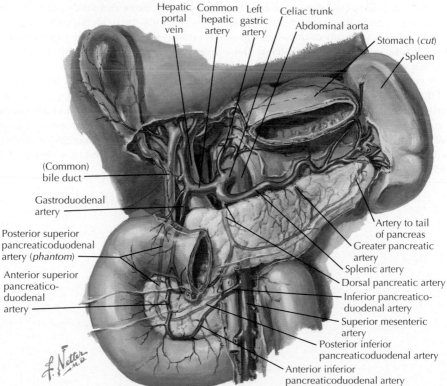

Hepatic
portal
vein
Common
hepatic
artery
Left
gastric
artery
Celiac trunk
Abdominal aorta
Stomach (*cut*)
Spleen
(Common)
bile duct
Gastroduodenal
artery
Posterior superior
pancreaticoduodenal
artery (*phantom*)
Anterior superior
pancreatico-
duodenal
artery
Artery to tail
of pancreas
Greater pancreatic
artery
Splenic artery
Dorsal pancreatic artery
Inferior pancreatico-
duodenal artery
Superior mesenteric
artery
Posterior inferior
pancreaticoduodenal artery
Anterior inferior
pancreaticoduodenal artery

Figure 7.4 PANCREAS

7.5 ADRENAL GLAND

The paired **suprarenal (adrenal) glands** are located in the retroperitoneum adjacent to the superior poles of the kidneys. Each gland consists of an **outer cortex** and **inner medulla**, and the cells of these parts have different functions. Cortical cells manufacture and secrete steroid hormones that aid in regulating numerous processes in the body such as metabolism, maintenance of blood pressure and electrolyte balance, bone formation, and the immune response. Medullary cells synthesize catecholamines (epinephrine and norepinephrine) that are secreted during the sympathetic "fight or flight" response to reinforce and prolong its effects. The arterial supply of the adrenal glands is extensive, provided by the **superior, middle**, and **inferior suprarenal arteries**. These arteries are branches of the inferior phrenic, abdominal aorta, and renal arteries, respectively. In contrast to the arterial pattern, there is a single **suprarenal vein** for each gland that drains to the renal vein on the left side of the body, and the inferior venae cava (IVC) on the right side of the body. The suprarenal glands are primarily innervated by sympathetic neurons within the **greater thoracic splanchnic nerves**. Some of the preganglionic sympathetic neurons synapse in the celiac ganglia and postganglionic neurons terminate on blood vessels to regulate blood flow. Others synapse directly on medullary cells that are equivalent to postganglionic sympathetic neurons. Stimulation of the medullary cells causes release of epinephrine and norepinephrine.

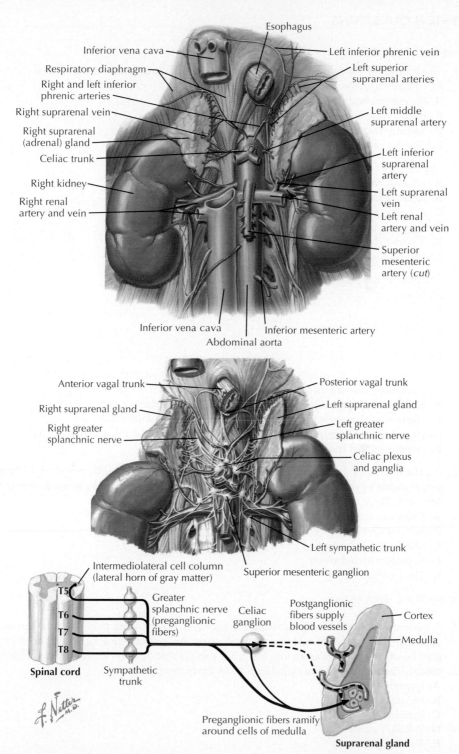

Figure 7.5 ADRENAL GLAND

REVIEW QUESTIONS

Test Your Recall

1. The isthmus of the thyroid gland is typically found on the anterior surface of the:
   A. Cricoid cartilage
   B. Fourth tracheal ring
   C. Hyoid bone
   D. Second tracheal ring
   E. Thyroid cartilage

2. The cells that synthesize and secrete epinephrine are part of the:
   A. Adrenal cortex
   B. Adrenal medulla
   C. Anterior pituitary
   D. Posterior pituitary
   E. Thyroid gland
   F. Parathyroid glands

3. The head of the pancreas is most closely associated with the:
   A. Duodenum
   B. Liver
   C. Right kidney
   D. Spleen
   E. Stomach

4. The secretory activity of cells of the anterior lobe of the pituitary is regulated by:
   A. Hormones that are manufactured in the infundibulum
   B. Hormones that are released into the superior hypophyseal artery
   C. Hormones that are synthesized in the posterior lobe of the pituitary
   D. Hormones that are transported in axons of the hypothalamohypophyseal tract
   E. Hormones that travel in the hypophyseal portal veins

5. A patient has an enlarged parathyroid gland that needs to be surgically removed. During removal, one or more clips are placed across the arteries supplying the gland to prevent bleeding. These arteries are most likely direct branches of the:
   A. External carotid artery
   B. Inferior thyroid artery
   C. Middle thyroid artery
   D. Superior thyroid artery
   E. Thyrocervical trunk

Apply Your Knowledge

6. A patient who was formerly addicted to opioids is experiencing pain due to a chronic condition. The patient would like to avoid using oral pain medication; thus her physician injects a neurolytic agent into the celiac ganglia that destroys axons (celiac ganglion block). The patient's chronic condition most likely involves the:
   A. Hypothalamus
   B. Pancreas
   C. Parathyroid glands
   D. Pituitary gland
   E. Thyroid gland

7. A resident is performing a midline tracheostomy on a trauma patient and encounters some bleeding during the procedure. The source of bleeding is most likely:

A. Arterial blood from the inferior thyroid artery

B. Arterial blood from the superior thyroid artery

C. Venous blood from the inferior thyroid vein

D. Venous blood from the middle thyroid vein

E. Venous blood from the superior thyroid vein

8. A patient has a tumor of the infundibulum of the pituitary gland that is compressing the hypothalamohypophyseal tract. This would most likely affect:

A. Secretion of hormones produced in the anterior lobe of the pituitary

B. Secretion of hormones produced in the hypothalamus

C. Secretion of hormones produced in the infundibulum

D. Secretion of hormones produced in the posterior lobe of the pituitary

9. A patient develops a retroperitoneal abscess. If left untreated, the pathogens in the abscess could spread to other areas in the retroperitoneum. Which of the following best describes organs that could become infected?

A. Pancreas

B. Pancreas and suprarenal glands

C. Suprarenal glands

D. Thyroid gland

E. Thyroid and parathyroid glands

10. A woman lacerated her spleen during an automobile accident. She is in surgery to have her spleen removed, and the surgeon temporarily clamps the splenic artery near its origin from the celiac trunk. During this procedure, the pancreas is not at risk for ischemia due to anastomotic connections between the three sources of arterial supply. If these connections did not exist, which parts of the pancreas would be experiencing a reduction in blood supply?

A. Head and uncinate process

B. Head, uncinate process, and neck

C. Neck and body

D. Neck, body, and tail

E. Body and tail

See Appendix for answers.

URINARY SYSTEM

8.1 THE URINARY SYSTEM

The **urinary system** is tasked with collecting and eliminating waste from the body. It also assists with maintaining homeostasis by regulating the amount of water, electrolytes, metabolites, and red blood cells in the blood. The urinary system is composed of the **kidneys**, **ureters**, **urinary bladder**, and **urethra**. The kidneys filter the blood to produce urine, while the other three organs transport and store urine until it can be eliminated. The kidneys are located in the retroperitoneum adjacent to muscles of the posterior abdominal wall and the twelfth rib. They are closely associated with the adrenal glands, although these organs do not share common functions. The kidneys are well protected by **pararenal and perirenal fat** and **renal fascia**. The ureters extend from the medial aspects of the kidneys to the bladder. The bladder and urethra are located inferior to the peritoneum in the pelvis.

Clinical Focus

The **costovertebral angle (CVA)** is the angle formed by the twelfth rib and vertebral column. The kidney is adjacent to the CVA, and pain or tenderness in this region is usually due to pathology of the kidney such as infection (pyelonephritis) or kidney stones.

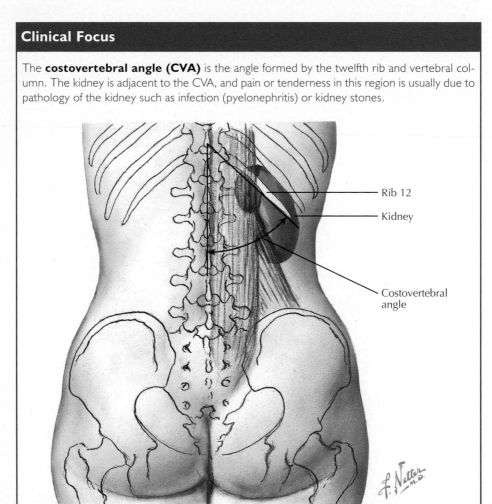

Rib 12

Kidney

Costovertebral angle

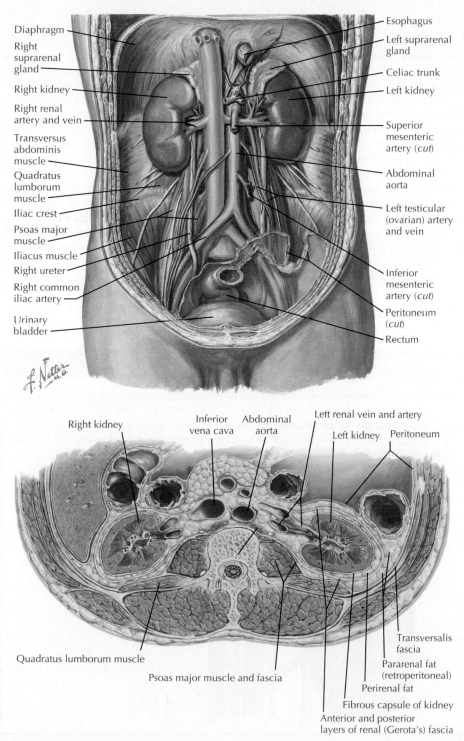

Diaphragm

Right suprarenal gland

Right kidney

Right renal artery and vein

Transversus abdominis muscle

Quadratus lumborum muscle

Iliac crest

Psoas major muscle

Iliacus muscle

Right ureter

Right common iliac artery

Urinary bladder

Esophagus

Left suprarenal gland

Celiac trunk

Left kidney

Superior mesenteric artery (*cut*)

Abdominal aorta

Left testicular (ovarian) artery and vein

Inferior mesenteric artery (*cut*)

Peritoneum (*cut*)

Rectum

Right kidney

Inferior vena cava

Abdominal aorta

Left renal vein and artery

Left kidney   Peritoneum

Quadratus lumborum muscle

Psoas major muscle and fascia

Transversalis fascia

Pararenal fat (retroperitoneal)

Perirenal fat

Fibrous capsule of kidney

Anterior and posterior layers of renal (Gerota's) fascia

Figure 8.1 THE URINARY SYSTEM

8.2 KIDNEY

Each **kidney** is surrounded by a capsule and has superior and inferior poles. Vessels and nerves enter and leave the medial aspect of the kidney, an area known as the **renal hilum**. The ureter also emerges from the kidney in this location. The space surrounding the structures of the hilum is filled with fat and is called the **renal sinus**. Internally the kidney consists of an outer cortex and inner medulla. Medullary tissue is organized into pyramidal-shaped clusters (**renal pyramids**) with the apex of each pyramid oriented towards the center of the kidney; each apex exhibits a **renal papilla**. Cortical tissue extends between the medullary pyramids as **renal columns**. Urine that is produced by the kidney is collected by a series of ducts that ultimately terminate in a dilated area called the **renal pelvis**. The smallest ducts are called **minor calyces**, and each minor calyx collects urine from one medullary pyramid. Minor calyces merge to form **major calyces**, and these subsequently join to form the renal pelvis. The renal pelvis narrows and continues as the **ureter** at the ureteropelvic junction (UPJ). The kidneys receive arterial blood from the paired **renal arteries** that branch from the lateral aspects of the abdominal aorta at approximately the L1 vertebral level. Each artery subsequently divides into approximately five segmental branches that supply different regions of the kidney. The **renal veins** that drain the kidneys are tributaries of the inferior vena cava (IVC). The right renal vein drains directly into the IVC; however, because the left renal vein begins on the left side of the body, it crosses the aorta deep to the superior mesenteric artery during its course from the kidney to the IVC.

Clinical Focus

During embryonic development, the kidneys ascend into the abdomen from the pelvis and numerous transient arteries supply the kidneys during their ascent. Typically these arteries degenerate, but **accessory renal arteries** are seen in approximately 25% of the population. Arteriosclerosis is common in the renal arteries, and a reduction in renal blood flow may lead to **chronic kidney disease (CKD)**.

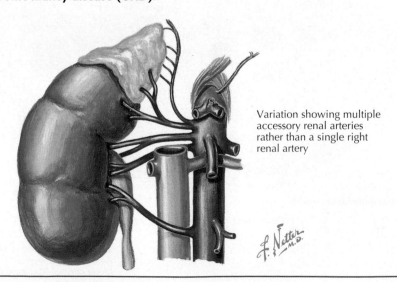

Variation showing multiple accessory renal arteries rather than a single right renal artery

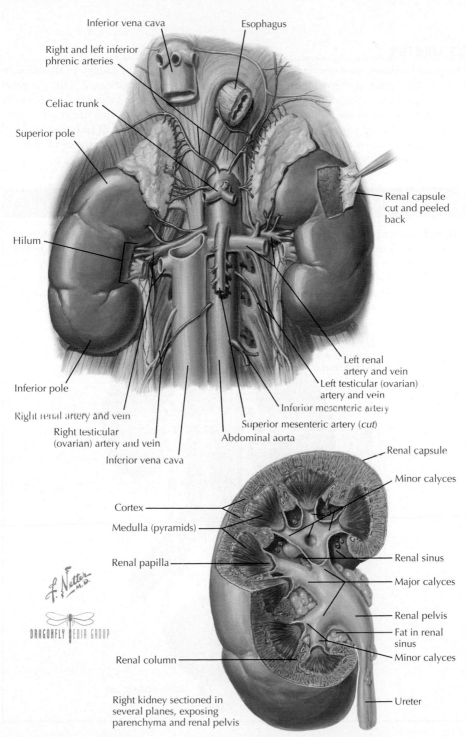

Inferior vena cava

Esophagus

Right and left inferior
phrenic arteries

Celiac trunk

Superior pole

Renal capsule
cut and peeled
back

Hilum

Inferior pole

Right renal artery and vein

Right testicular
(ovarian) artery and vein

Inferior vena cava

Left renal
artery and vein

Left testicular (ovarian)
artery and vein

Inferior mesenteric artery

Superior mesenteric artery (*cut*)

Abdominal aorta

Renal capsule

Minor calyces

Cortex

Medulla (pyramids)

Renal papilla

Renal sinus

Major calyces

Renal pelvis

Fat in renal
sinus

Minor calyces

Renal column

Ureter

Right kidney sectioned in
several planes, exposing
parenchyma and renal pelvis

Figure 8.2 THE KIDNEY

8.3 URETER

The paired **ureters** are muscular tubes that convey urine from the kidney to the bladder. Each ureter begins at the **ureteropelvic junction**, where it is continuous with the renal pelvis of the kidney. The ureters descend in the retroperitoneum and enter the pelvic cavity by passing anterior to the bifurcations of the common iliac arteries. Each ureter terminates by merging with the posterior wall of the bladder at the **ureterovesical junction**. Arterial blood to the ureters is provided by multiple small arteries that arise from the renal arteries, abdominal aorta, gonadal vessels, and the iliac arteries.

Clinical Focus

Kidney stones (renal calculi) can form in the kidney, for example in individuals with concentrated urine. Small stones often pass through the urinary system and are voided; however, large stones may lodge in the ureter and cause pain ("**renal colic**"). The UPJ is a common site of obstruction for kidney stones due to the transition in the size of the ductal lumen from the renal pelvis. Two additional sites where stones often lodge are where the ureters pass anterior to the common iliac artery and at the ureterovesical junction.

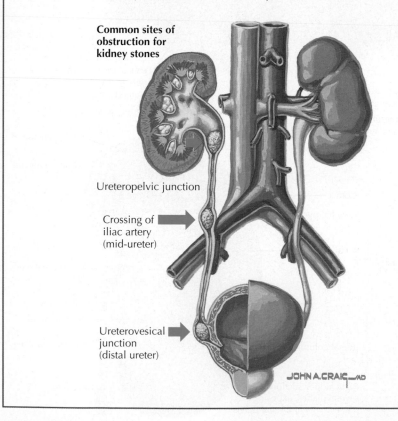

Common sites of obstruction for kidney stones

Ureteropelvic junction

Crossing of iliac artery (mid-ureter)

Ureterovesical junction (distal ureter)

JOHN A.CRAIG—AD

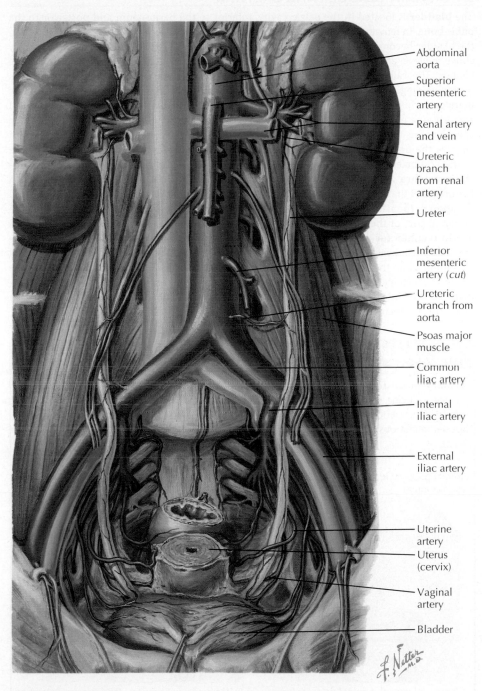

- Abdominal aorta
- Superior mesenteric artery
- Renal artery and vein
- Ureteric branch from renal artery
- Ureter
- Inferior mesenteric artery (*cut*)
- Ureteric branch from aorta
- Psoas major muscle
- Common iliac artery
- Internal iliac artery
- External iliac artery
- Uterine artery
- Uterus (cervix)
- Vaginal artery
- Bladder

Figure 8.3 URETER

8.4 URINARY BLADDER AND URETHRA

The **bladder** is located in the pelvic cavity, inferior to the peritoneum and posterior to the pubic bone. In females it is anterior to the vagina; in males it is anterior to the rectum. When the bladder becomes distended with urine, the superior surface (**dome**) extends superiorly above the level of the pubic symphysis. The narrow inferior portion is called the **neck** of the bladder. The wall of the bladder is composed primarily of the **detrusor muscle** that contracts during voiding. The posterior wall of the bladder exhibits openings for the ureters (**ureteric orifices**), while the neck surrounds the **internal urethral orifice**. The triangular-shaped smooth area outlined by these three openings is the **trigone**. The internal urethral orifice is continuous with the **urethra**, which conveys urine out of the bladder to the exterior. In females the urethra is short and straight and terminates at the **external urethral orifice** in the vestibule of the vulva. In males the urethra is long and has four parts: the **prepro-static urethra** within the neck of the bladder; the **prostatic urethra** that passes through the prostate; the **membranous urethra** between the prostate and perineal membrane; and the **spongy (penile) urethra** that is located within the corpus spongiosum of the penis. The proximal part of the urethra within the neck of the bladder is surrounded by an **internal urethral sphincter** composed of smooth muscle. An **external urethral sphincter** consisting of striated muscle is located distal to the internal sphincter and allows conscious control of voiding. A urethral suspensory mechanism composed of multiple ligaments supports the urethra to help maintain urinary continence. One primary ligament is the **pubovesical liga-ment** that anchors the neck of the bladder and urethra to the pubic bone (see Fig. 9.3); in males this ligament is also known as the puboprostatic ligament.

Clinical Focus

Urinary incontinence is involuntary leakage of urine. There are multiple causes of incon-tinence including loss of support to the bladder neck and urethra (urethral hypermobility), sphincter deficiency, detrusor overactivity ("overactive bladder"), detrusor underactivity, or bladder outlet obstruction (e.g., due to benign prostatic enlargement; see Clinical Focus on 9.12).

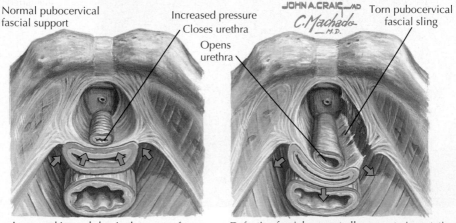

Normal pubocervical fascial support

Increased pressure Closes urethra

Opens urethra

Torn pubocervical fascial sling

Increased intra-abdominal pressure forces urethra against intact pubocervical fascia, closing urethra and maintaining continence

Defective fascial support allows posterior rotation of U-V junction with increased pressure, opening urethra and causing urine loss

Female: midsagittal section

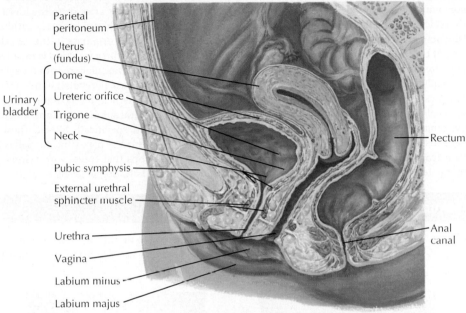

Parietal peritoneum

Uterus (fundus)

Urinary bladder
- Dome
- Ureteric orifice
- Trigone
- Neck

Pubic symphysis

External urethral sphincter muscle

Urethra

Vagina

Labium minus

Labium majus

Rectum

Anal canal

Male: midsagittal section

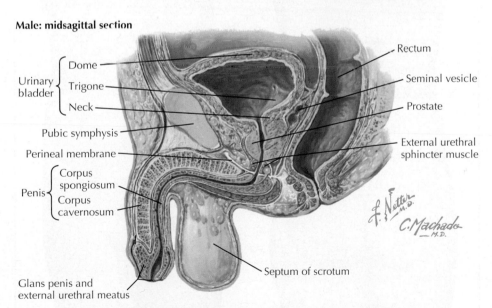

Urinary bladder
- Dome
- Trigone
- Neck

Pubic symphysis

Perineal membrane

Penis
- Corpus spongiosum
- Corpus cavernosum

Glans penis and external urethral meatus

Rectum

Seminal vesicle

Prostate

External urethral sphincter muscle

Septum of scrotum

Figure 8.4 URINARY BLADDER AND URETHRA (see Figs. 9.4 and 9.12)

8.5 INNERVATION OF THE URINARY SYSTEM

The organs of the urinary system are innervated by visceral neurons that travel within the **aortic plexus** on the anterior surface of the abdominal aorta and the **pelvic plexuses** associated with the lateral aspects of the pelvic viscera. Sympathetic neurons arise from the lower thoracic and upper lumbar segments of the spinal cord and travel to relevant plexuses within **thoracic and lumbar splanchnic nerves**. Parasympathetic neurons originate in the sacral part of the spinal cord and travel in the **pelvic splanchnic nerves**. Kidney function is mainly regulated by hormones; however, sympathetic neurons do innervate vascular smooth muscle to regulate blood flow to the kidney. Sympathetic neurons also increase peristalsis in the ureter. Parasympathetic neurons cause contraction of the detrusor muscle and relaxation of the internal urethral sphincter to facilitate voiding. The external urethral sphincter is innervated by somatic neurons that arise in the sacral levels of the spinal cord, specifically S2–S4. These neurons travel in the **pudendal nerve**, which is a branch of the sacral plexus in the pelvis. Pain from urinary organs is conveyed by visceral afferent neurons that travel with sympathetic neurons and join the spinal cord at approximately the T11–L2 spinal levels.

Clinical Focus

Pain in the kidney or ureter (e.g., from kidney stones) is referred to the T11–L2 dermatomes; thus it is felt over a wide area including the lower back, abdominal wall, groin, and medial thigh.

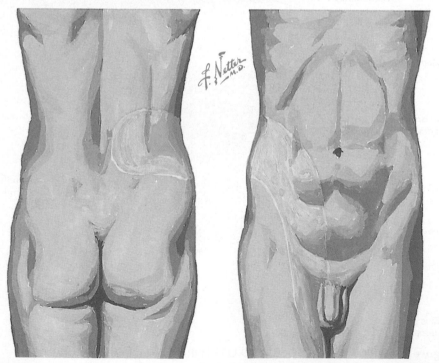

Distribution of pain in renal colic

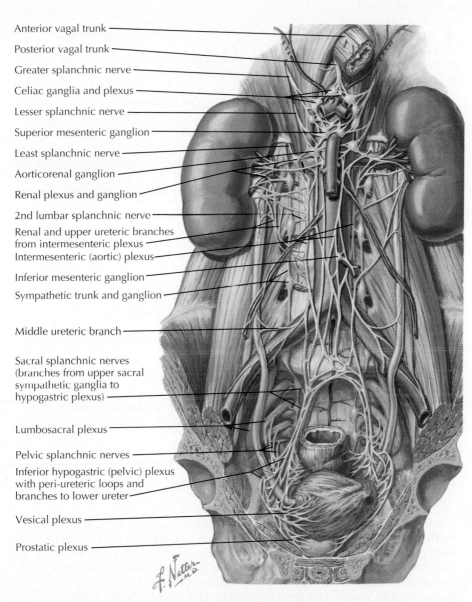

Anterior vagal trunk

Posterior vagal trunk

Greater splanchnic nerve

Celiac ganglia and plexus

Lesser splanchnic nerve

Superior mesenteric ganglion

Least splanchnic nerve

Aorticorenal ganglion

Renal plexus and ganglion

2nd lumbar splanchnic nerve

Renal and upper ureteric branches
from intermesenteric plexus

Intermesenteric (aortic) plexus

Inferior mesenteric ganglion

Sympathetic trunk and ganglion

Middle ureteric branch

Sacral splanchnic nerves
(branches from upper sacral
sympathetic ganglia to
hypogastric plexus)

Lumbosacral plexus

Pelvic splanchnic nerves

Inferior hypogastric (pelvic) plexus
with peri-ureteric loops and
branches to lower ureter

Vesical plexus

Prostatic plexus

Figure 8.5 INNERVATION OF THE URINARY SYSTEM

REVIEW QUESTIONS

Test Your Recall

1. The kidneys are well protected by multiple layers of fat. Which of the following contains some of this fat?
   A. Major calyx
   B. Renal column
   C. Renal pelvis
   D. Renal pyramid
   E. Renal sinus

2. Which of the following best describes the ureteropelvic junction?
   A. Junction between the bladder neck and urethra
   B. Junction between the kidney and ureter
   C. Junction between the ureter and bladder
   D. Location where the ureter enters the pelvic cavity anterior to the common iliac vessels
   E. Location where the ureter enters the pelvic cavity anterior to the external iliac vessels

3. Urine that is released from the renal papilla is first collected by:
   A. Major calyx
   B. Minor calyx
   C. Renal column
   D. Renal pelvis
   E. Renal sinus

4. Which of the following is innervated by parasympathetic neurons?
   A. Detrusor muscle
   B. External urethral sphincter
   C. Minor calyx
   D. Renal artery
   E. Smooth muscle of ureter

5. Which of the following best describes the position of the bladder in females?
   A. Posterior to the common iliac vessels
   B. Posterior to the peritoneum
   C. Posterior to the pubic bone
   D. Posterior to the rectum
   E. Posterior to the uterus

Apply Your Knowledge

6. A patient with a large kidney stone in the renal pelvis undergoes a percutaneous nephrolithotomy to remove the stone. During this procedure, a needle is introduced into the renal pelvis via the retroperitoneum using image guidance. Which of the following best describes the layers traversed by the needle after passing through the abdominal wall?
   A. Pararenal fat, renal fascia, perirenal fat, capsule of kidney
   B. Pararenal fat, perirenal fat, renal fascia, capsule of kidney
   C. Perirenal fat, renal fascia, pararenal fat, capsule of kidney
   D. Perirenal fat, pararenal fat, renal fascia, capsule of kidney
   E. Renal fascia, pararenal fat, perirenal fat, capsule of kidney
   F. Renal fascia, perirenal fat, pararenal fat, capsule of kidney

7. A physician orders an intravenous pyelogram (x-ray of the urinary system with contrast) to evaluate a patient with blood in their urine. Which structure is indicated by the number *3* on the x-ray?

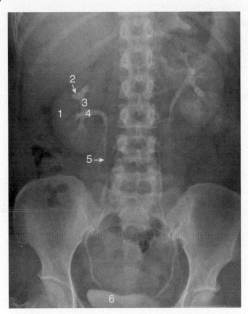

   A. Major calyx
   B. Minor calyx
   C. Renal column
   D. Renal pelvis
   E. Renal sinus

8. A patient was diagnosed with superior mesenteric artery (SMA) syndrome, which can lead to compression of structures passing between the SMA and abdominal aorta. Which of the following could be a consequence of this condition?
   A. Back up of blood in the left kidney
   B. Back up of blood in the right kidney
   C. Back up of urine in the left kidney
   D. Back up of urine in the right kidney
   E. Lack of blood supply to the left kidney
   F. Lack of blood supply to the right kidney

9. During childbirth, the nerves in the pelvis and perineum (genital region) can be stretched, leading to temporary or permanent loss of function. A patient who recently gave birth is experiencing urinary incontinence (loss of bladder control) due to impaired innervation of the external urethral sphincter. Which of the following nerves was most likely stretched during childbirth?
   A. Lumbar splanchnic nerves
   B. Pelvic splanchnic nerves
   C. Pudendal nerve
   D. Thoracic splanchnic nerves
   E. Visceral afferent nerves

10. A patient who is experiencing pain visits an outpatient clinic. The nurse practitioner performs a physical exam and detects tenderness in the region of the costovertebral angle (CVA). Which of the following is the most likely source of the patient's pain?

A. Bladder infection (cystitis)

B. Detrusor overactivity ("overactive bladder")

C. Kidney infection (pyelonephritis)

D. Kidney stone lodged in the ureterovesical junction

E. Prostatic hypertrophy that is compressing the urethra

See Appendix for answers.

CHAPTER 9

REPRODUCTIVE SYSTEM

9.1 THE REPRODUCTIVE SYSTEM

The organs and glands of the reproductive system function to create and nourish new life. In the female these include the **ovaries, uterus, uterine tubes, vagina**, and **mammary glands**. In the male the primary structures are the **testes, epididymis, vas deferens, seminal vesicles, prostate glands**, and **penis**. Apart from the mammary glands, the reproductive structures are located in the **pelvis** or **perineum**. The pelvic region is composed of a cavity surrounded by the bony pelvis. The pelvic cavity is continuous superiorly with the abdominal cavity and bordered inferiorly by the muscular pelvic diaphragm. The superior limit of the pelvic cavity is indicated by a bony margin called the **pelvic inlet**. This separates the true pelvic cavity from a region called the "false pelvis," which is the inferior part of the abdominal cavity bordered by the iliac crests. The perineum is the region inferior to the pelvic diaphragm that contains the external genitalia and the anus.

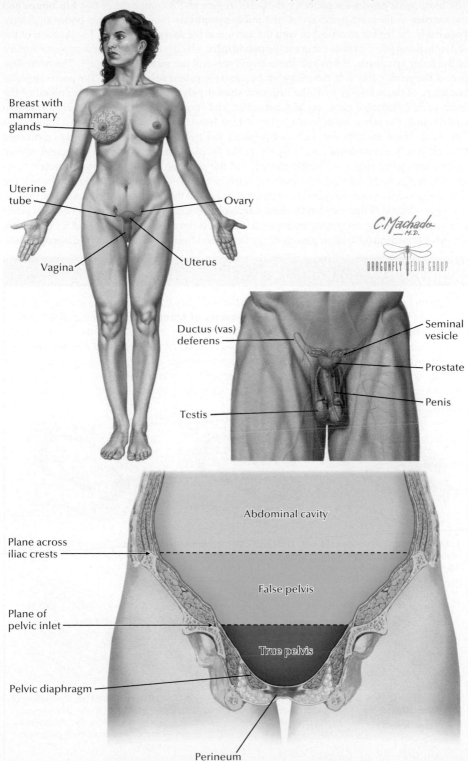

Breast with mammary glands

Uterine tube

Ovary

Vagina

Uterus

C. Machado M.D.

DRAGONFLY MEDIA GROUP

Ductus (vas) deferens

Seminal vesicle

Prostate

Penis

Testis

Abdominal cavity

Plane across iliac crests

False pelvis

Plane of pelvic inlet

True pelvis

Pelvic diaphragm

Perineum

Figure 9.1 THE REPRODUCTIVE SYSTEM

The bony pelvis provides support for the pelvic region and is composed of two **hip bones** and the **sacrum**. A fibrocartilaginous disc, the **pubic symphysis**, joins the two hip bones anteriorly. Posteriorly the hip bones articulate with the sacrum at the **sacroiliac joints**. The junction of the abdominal and pelvic cavities occurs at the **pelvic inlet**, which is composed of the superior surface of the pubic symphysis, the paired lineae terminales and the sacral promontory. The narrowest part of the pelvic cavity is in the midpelvis between the paired ischial spines. The posteroinferior boundary of the pelvic cavity is the diamond-shaped **pelvic outlet**, which is composed of the pubic arch, ischiopubic rami, ischial tuberosities, and coccyx. The sacrotuberous ligaments also contribute to the pelvic outlet because they extend between the sacrum and ischial tuberosities (see 3.38). There are different shapes of pelvises, and two of the most common are **gynecoid** ("female type") and **android** ("male type"). In the female type, the pelvic inlet is round or oval shaped, the ischial spines are widely spaced, and the pubic arch is 80 degrees or greater; these features facilitate childbirth. In the male type, the pelvic inlet is triangular or heart shaped, the distance between the ischial spines is relatively narrow, and the pubic arch is typically less than 70 degrees—all features that may hinder childbirth. Not all women have a gynecoid pelvis; thus pelvic measurements during pregnancy are important to assess the adequacy of the pelvis for childbirth. If a pelvis is inadequate to allow passage of the fetus, this is termed **cephalopelvic disproportion**.

Clinical Focus

Childbirth involves passage of the fetus through the bony pelvis, which requires positional changes of the fetal head called the **cardinal movements of labor**. Engagement is defined as descent of the fetal head into the pelvic inlet. Typically this occurs with the fetus either facing the left or right side of the mother because the transverse diameter of the pelvic inlet is wider than the anteroposterior diameter. In the midpelvis, the anteroposterior diameter is larger than the interspinous distance; thus the head turns (internal rotation) to facilitate passage. As the fetus leaves the pelvis through the pelvic outlet, the head typically extends to pass under the pubic arch.

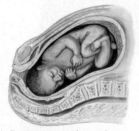 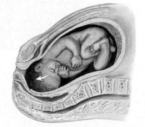 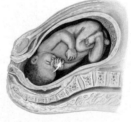

1. Engagement: The widest part of the fetal head enters the pelvic inlet (generally in the transverse position).

2. Descent: Often occurs with flexion.

3. Flexion: Descent causes the fetus to move to a chin-on-chest position.

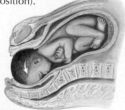 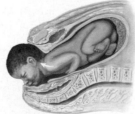 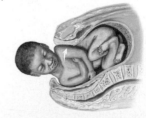

4. Internal rotation: Rotation to the occiput-anterior position (generally).

5. Extension: The head extends as it emerges below the maternal symphysis.

6. External rotation: Restitution of the fetal head to the transverse position to allow the shoulders to emerge in the anterior-posterior plane.

7. Expulsion: The delivery of the infant.

f. Netter M.D.   K. marzejn

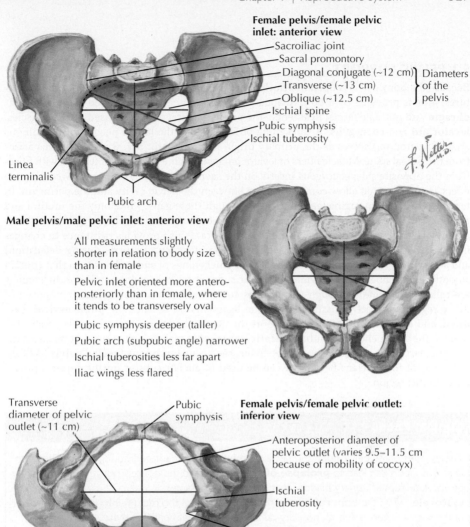

Female pelvis/female pelvic inlet: anterior view
- Sacroiliac joint
- Sacral promontory
- Diagonal conjugate (~12 cm)
- Transverse (~13 cm) } Diameters of the pelvis
- Oblique (~12.5 cm)
- Ischial spine
- Pubic symphysis
- Ischial tuberosity

F. Netter M.D.

Linea terminalis

Pubic arch

Male pelvis/male pelvic inlet: anterior view

All measurements slightly shorter in relation to body size than in female

Pelvic inlet oriented more anteroposteriorly than in female, where it tends to be transversely oval

Pubic symphysis deeper (taller)

Pubic arch (subpubic angle) narrower

Ischial tuberosities less far apart

Iliac wings less flared

Transverse diameter of pelvic outlet (~11 cm)

Pubic symphysis

Female pelvis/female pelvic outlet: inferior view

- Anteroposterior diameter of pelvic outlet (varies 9.5–11.5 cm because of mobility of coccyx)
- Ischial tuberosity
- Ischial spine

Tip of coccyx

Sacral promontory

True conjugate is ~1.5 cm shorter than diagonal conjugate

Diagonal conjugate is only diameter of pelvic inlet that can be measured clinically

Female: sagittal section

Plane of pelvic inlet

True conjugate diameter of pelvic inlet (~11 cm)

Diagonal conjugate

Plane of pelvic outlet

Anteroposterior diameter of pelvic outlet (9.5–11.5 cm)

Transverse diameter is the widest distance of pelvic inlet

Figure 9.2 BONY PELVIS

9.3 PELVIC SUPPORT

Because the bony pelvis is open inferiorly, the pelvic organs need support from other structures. This is provided by a bowl-shaped group of striated muscles called the **pelvic diaphragm** and multiple fascial ligaments. The pelvic diaphragm is composed of two muscles, **levator ani** and **coccygeus**. A thickening of fascia along the lateral pelvic wall (tendinous arch of levator ani) serves as the primary origin for the levator ani, while coccygeus arises from the ischial spine. Muscle fibers of levator ani insert in the midline by blending with fibers from the opposite side; coccygeus inserts on the sacrum and coccyx. Gaps between muscle fibers are present that allow communication between the pelvic cavity and the perineum. In females, the urethra, vagina, and anus pass through these gaps, while only the urethra and anus pass through the openings in males. Contraction of the pelvic diaphragm causes it to elevate, which provides support for the pelvic viscera. It also provides resistance to changes in intrapelvic pressure during contraction of abdominal muscles (e.g., during defecation) and aids with voluntary control of micturition. Thickenings of endopelvic fascia that contain smooth muscle fibers also provide important support for pelvic viscera. These thickenings are called "ligaments", although this term is confusing because they are not composed of dense regular connective tissue like skeletal ligaments. In females the **pubocervical**, **cardinal**, and **uterosacral ligaments** support the uterine body, cervix, and vagina, anchoring them to the bony pelvis. The **puboprostatic ligament** in males helps to support the prostate. A particularly dense band of connective tissue, the **arcus tendineus fasciae pelvis (ATFP)**, is significant to clinicians because it can be used to anchor sutures during surgical procedures in this region.

Clinical Focus

The muscles of the pelvic floor and fascial ligaments can be damaged during natural childbirth. Loss of support can lead to **prolapse of the uterus** and the nonreproductive organs in the pelvis. A prolapsed urinary bladder that bulges into the anterior wall of the vagina is called a **cystocele**, while the term **rectocele** refers to bulging of the rectum into the posterior wall of the vagina. There are both nonsurgical and surgical treatments for these conditions.

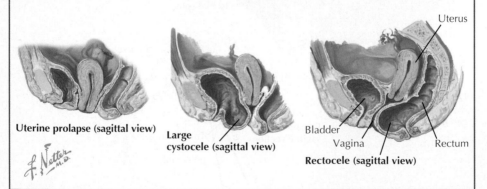

Uterine prolapse (sagittal view)

Large cystocele (sagittal view)

Bladder   Vagina   Rectum

Rectocele (sagittal view)

Uterus

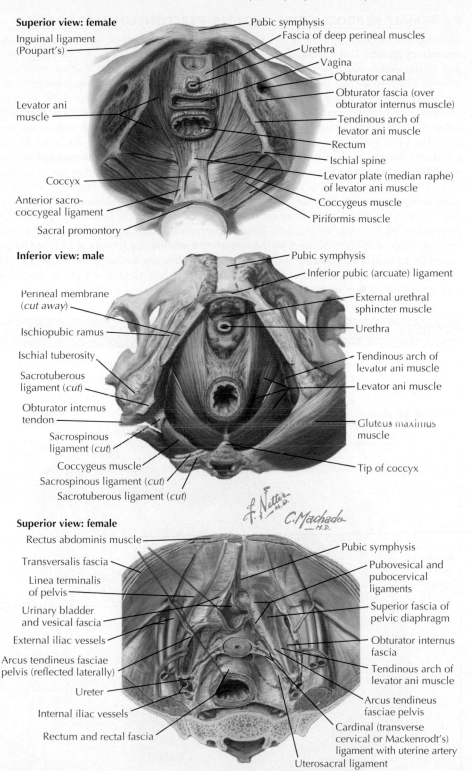

Superior view: female

- Pubic symphysis
- Fascia of deep perineal muscles
- Inguinal ligament (Poupart's)
- Urethra
- Vagina
- Obturator canal
- Obturator fascia (over obturator internus muscle)
- Levator ani muscle
- Tendinous arch of levator ani muscle
- Rectum
- Ischial spine
- Coccyx
- Levator plate (median raphe) of levator ani muscle
- Anterior sacro-coccygeal ligament
- Coccygeus muscle
- Sacral promontory
- Piriformis muscle

Inferior view: male

- Pubic symphysis
- Inferior pubic (arcuate) ligament
- Perineal membrane (cut away)
- External urethral sphincter muscle
- Ischiopubic ramus
- Urethra
- Ischial tuberosity
- Tendinous arch of levator ani muscle
- Sacrotuberous ligament (cut)
- Levator ani muscle
- Obturator internus tendon
- Sacrospinous ligament (cut)
- Gluteus maximus muscle
- Coccygeus muscle
- Tip of coccyx
- Sacrospinous ligament (cut)
- Sacrotuberous ligament (cut)

Superior view: female

- Rectus abdominis muscle
- Pubic symphysis
- Transversalis fascia
- Pubovesical and pubocervical ligaments
- Linea terminalis of pelvis
- Superior fascia of pelvic diaphragm
- Urinary bladder and vesical fascia
- External iliac vessels
- Obturator internus fascia
- Arcus tendineus fasciae pelvis (reflected laterally)
- Tendinous arch of levator ani muscle
- Ureter
- Arcus tendineus fasciae pelvis
- Internal iliac vessels
- Rectum and rectal fascia
- Cardinal (transverse cervical or Mackenrodt's) ligament with uterine artery
- Uterosacral ligament

Figure 9.3 PELVIC SUPPORT

9.4 FEMALE REPRODUCTIVE ORGANS: PERITONEUM AND ADNEXA

The reproductive organs in the female are the **uterus**, **uterine tubes**, **ovaries**, **vagina**, and **mammary glands**. These are all located in the pelvic cavity, with the exception of the lower part of the vagina which is in the perineum, and the mammary glands that are within the breasts. The bladder and rectum are also in the pelvic cavity, anterior and posterior to the uterus, respectively. The **peritoneum** of the abdominal cavity reflects over the superior surfaces of the pelvic organs creating "pouches" between them—the **vesicouterine pouch** between the bladder and uterus, and the **rectouterine pouch** between the uterus and rectum. The peritoneum over the uterus, uterine tubes, and ovaries forms a double-layered mesentery known as the **broad ligament**. The terms **mesometrium**, **mesosalpinx**, and **mesovarium** are used to describe specific parts of the broad ligament that are associated with the uterine body, uterine tube, and ovary, respectively. The broad ligament, as well as other structures such as the ovary and uterine tube, are part of the **adnexa**—a clinical term that refers to the region adjacent to the uterus. The **ovaries** are the sites of egg production (oogenesis). Mature eggs are ovulated into the peritoneal cavity and directed into the adjacent openings of the uterine tubes by the fingerlike **fimbriae**. Each ovary is attached to the uterus by an **ovarian ligament**. The paired **uterine tubes** are anchored to the body of the uterus. Each tube has a dilated region (**ampulla**) that is typically the site of fertilization if both an egg and sperm are present.

Clinical Focus

The rectouterine pouch is the most inferior part of the peritoneal cavity. Fluid collections or abscesses in the pouch can be drained by inserting a needle through the posterior vaginal fornix, which is a part of the vagina that is adjacent to the pouch.

Cul-de-sac abscess

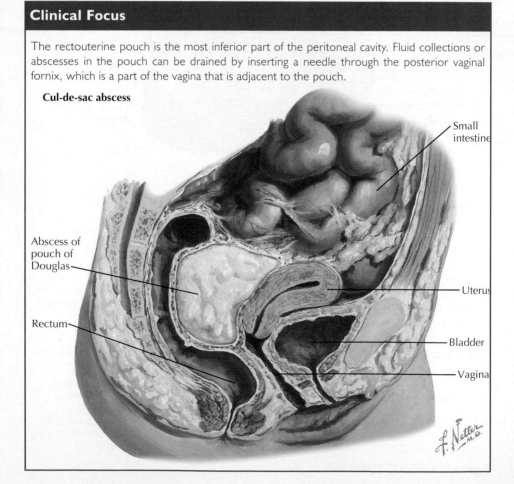

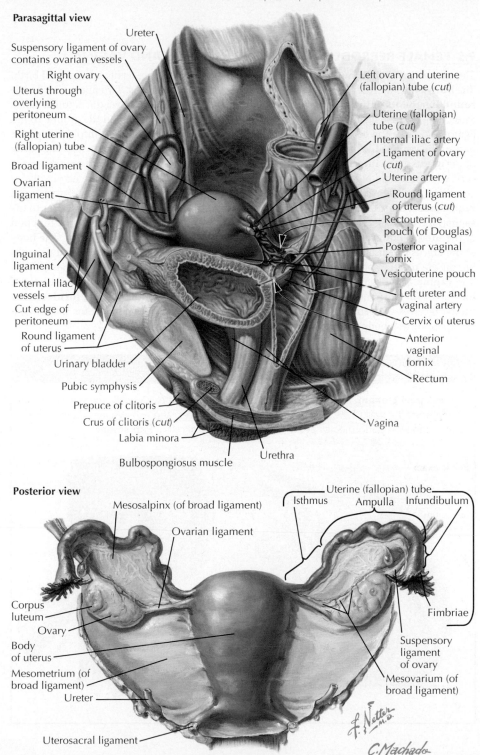

Parasagittal view

Ureter

Suspensory ligament of ovary contains ovarian vessels

Right ovary

Uterus through overlying peritoneum

Right uterine (fallopian) tube

Broad ligament

Ovarian ligament

Inguinal ligament

External iliac vessels

Cut edge of peritoneum

Round ligament of uterus

Urinary bladder

Pubic symphysis

Prepuce of clitoris

Crus of clitoris (*cut*)

Labia minora

Bulbospongiosus muscle

Left ovary and uterine (fallopian) tube (*cut*)

Uterine (fallopian) tube (*cut*)

Internal iliac artery

Ligament of ovary (*cut*)

Uterine artery

Round ligament of uterus (*cut*)

Rectouterine pouch (of Douglas)

Posterior vaginal fornix

Vesicouterine pouch

Left ureter and vaginal artery

Cervix of uterus

Anterior vaginal fornix

Rectum

Vagina

Urethra

Posterior view

Mesosalpinx (of broad ligament)

Ovarian ligament

Uterine (fallopian) tube

Isthmus   Ampulla   Infundibulum

Corpus luteum

Ovary

Body of uterus

Mesometrium (of broad ligament)

Ureter

Uterosacral ligament

Fimbriae

Suspensory ligament of ovary

Mesovarium (of broad ligament)

Figure 9.4 FEMALE REPRODUCTIVE ORGANS: PERITONEUM AND ADNEXA

9.5 FEMALE REPRODUCTIVE ORGANS: UTERUS AND VAGINA

The **uterus** is a hollow muscular organ that functions to nourish a fertilized egg until birth. The **body** of the uterus has a rounded superior part called the **fundus**. Two fibrous cords, the **round ligaments of the uterus**, anchor the uterus to the groin region via the inguinal canal. Stretching of these ligaments during pregnancy can be a source of pain in the groin ("round ligament pain"). The **cervix** is the inferior part of the uterus that projects into the superior part of the vagina. The lumen of the cervix, the **cervical canal**, is continuous with the cavity of the uterus at the **internal os** and with the vagina at the **external os**. During pregnancy the cervix forms a rigid barrier that helps to keep the fetus in utero. At birth the cervix dilates and thins to allow passage of the baby. The cervix is typically bent anteriorly relative to the vagina (**anteverted**), although its position can vary. If the axis of the cervix is posterior to the vagina, the uterus is described as **retroverted**. This does not generally impact the function of the uterus; however, it may be more difficult to palpate during physical exam. The body of the uterus can also be bent with respect to the cervix (**anteflexed** or **retroflexed** depending on the position of the fundus). In the typical position, the uterus is slightly anteflexed. The **vagina** is a distensible muscular tube that extends from the cervix to the vestibule of the vulva. The portions of the vagina that surround the cervix are the **vaginal fornices**. The vagina receives the penis during sexual intercourse and serves as a conduit for the fetus to exit the mother's body during parturition.

Clinical Focus

During a **pelvic exam**, many structures can be visualized and palpated via the vagina, including the posterior wall of the bladder, cervix, vaginal fornices, and ischial spines. Screening for cervical cancer is performed by taking a sample of cervical cells ("**Pap smear**").

Pelvic exam

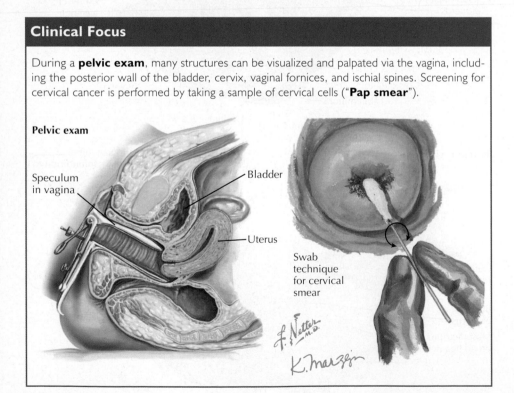

Speculum in vagina

Bladder

Uterus

Swab technique for cervical smear

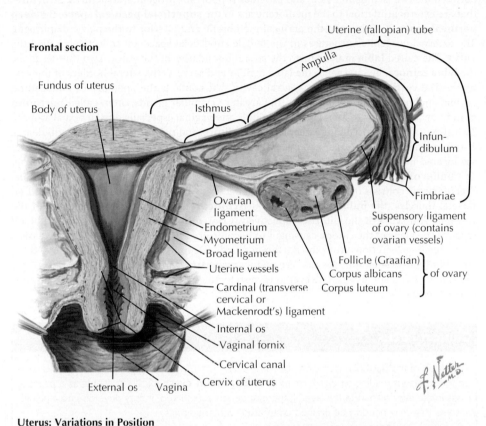

Frontal section

Fundus of uterus

Body of uterus

Isthmus

Ampulla

Uterine (fallopian) tube

Infundibulum

Fimbriae

Suspensory ligament of ovary (contains ovarian vessels)

Ovarian ligament
Endometrium
Myometrium
Broad ligament
Uterine vessels

Follicle (Graafian)
Corpus albicans } of ovary
Corpus luteum

Cardinal (transverse cervical or Mackenrodt's) ligament

Internal os

Vaginal fornix

Cervical canal

Cervix of uterus

External os   Vagina

Uterus: Variations in Position

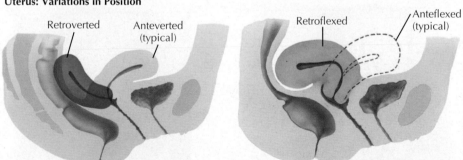

Retroverted   Anteverted (typical)

Retroflexed   Anteflexed (typical)

Figure 9.5 FEMALE REPRODUCTIVE ORGANS: UTERUS AND VAGINA

9.6 FEMALE PERINEUM

The urogenital region in both males and females is divided into superficial and deep spaces by a sheet of connective tissue called the **perineal membrane**. This membrane extends between the two ischiopubic rami and provides support for urogenital structures. Structures that are external (inferior) to the membrane are in the **superficial perineal space**; the **deep perineal space** is superior to the perineal membrane and inferior to the pelvic diaphragm. The external urogenital structures in the female superficial space are collectively called the **vulva**. The paired **labia majora** form the lateral boundaries of the vulva. Two thinner folds, the **labia minora**, lie internal to the labia majora and serve as the lateral borders of the vestibule. The **vestibule** is a shallow central cavity that contains the openings of the urethra, vagina, and greater vestibular glands. The greater vestibular glands, often called **Bartholin glands**, secrete mucus to lubricate the vestibule and vagina, especially during sexual arousal. Two structures composed of erectile tissue, the clitoris and paired bulbs of the vestibule, are also important for the sexual response. The **clitoris** is composed of a glans and body that are located in the midline, and two crura that anchor the clitoris to the ischiopubic rami. The **bulbs of the vestibule** lie deep to the skin of the labia on either side of the vestibule. Erectile tissue consists of vascular cavities that become filled with blood during arousal. Two skeletal muscles, the **bulbospongiosus** and **ischiocavernosus**, surround the bulbs of the vestibule and crura of the clitoris, respectively. Contraction of these muscles directs blood towards the glans of the clitoris causing it to become erect. The bulbospongiosus also assists with expelling secretions from the Bartholin glands. Deep to the perineal membrane, there are additional striated muscles that are mainly associated with the urinary system (e.g., the external urethral sphincter); however, one muscle, the sphincter urethrovaginalis, also constricts the vagina.

Clinical Focus

The ducts of the Bartholin glands can become obstructed, which can cause secretions to back up in the glands leading to cyst formation. A **Bartholin cyst** typically presents as a painless mass in the inferior part of the labia. If the cyst becomes infected, it may develop into a painful abscess that may need to be drained or treated with antibiotics.

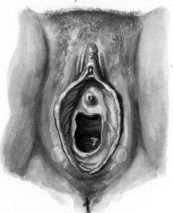

Bartholin's glands located at 5:00 and 7:00 o'clock positions

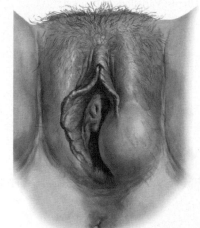

Bartholin's cyst at 5:00 position

Female Perineum

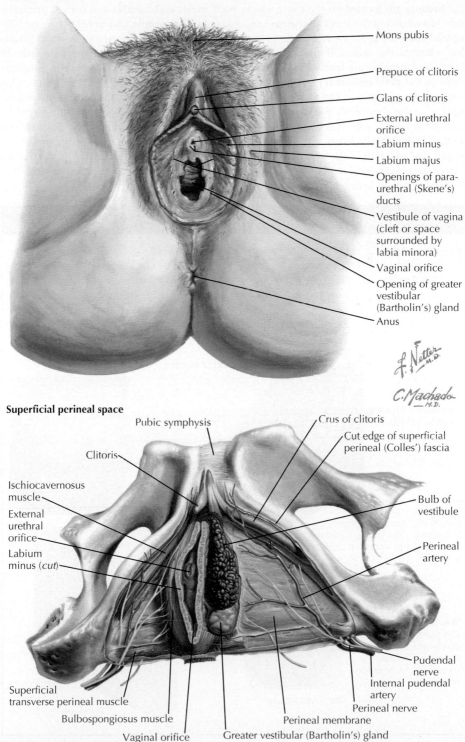

Mons pubis

Prepuce of clitoris

Glans of clitoris

External urethral orifice

Labium minus

Labium majus

Openings of para-urethral (Skene's) ducts

Vestibule of vagina (cleft or space surrounded by labia minora)

Vaginal orifice

Opening of greater vestibular (Bartholin's) gland

Anus

Superficial perineal space

Pubic symphysis

Crus of clitoris

Cut edge of superficial perineal (Colles') fascia

Clitoris

Ischiocavernosus muscle

External urethral orifice

Labium minus (*cut*)

Bulb of vestibule

Perineal artery

Pudendal nerve

Internal pudendal artery

Perineal nerve

Superficial transverse perineal muscle

Bulbospongiosus muscle

Vaginal orifice

Greater vestibular (Bartholin's) gland

Perineal membrane

Figure 9.6 FEMALE PERINEUM

9.7 BREASTS

The **breasts** are located on the chest wall in both males and females and consist primarily of fat surrounding the lobes of the mammary glands. The **nipple** and **areola** (circular pigmented area) are prominent features in the center of the breast. The areola contains glands that lubricate the skin of the nipple. Each **mammary gland** consists of approximately 20 glandular lobes that are located in the superficial fascia of the breast. Deep to the glandular tissue is the **retromammary space** that contains a layer of loose connective tissue. This connective tissue allows the mammary gland to move independently from the underlying muscles of the chest wall. The lobes of the mammary gland are separated and supported by connective tissue septa called **suspensory retinacula**. Each individual lobe is drained by a single **lactiferous duct** that expands to form a **lactiferous sinus** near its termination at the nipple. The function of the mammary glands is to produce milk to nourish infants. Glands only become functional in females due to hormonal influences; as the glandular tissue develops, additional fat is deposited around the glands.

Clinical Focus

Breast cancer is a common cancer in females. For the purpose of breast examinations, the breast is divided into four quadrants defined by horizontal and vertical lines through the nipple. The glandular tissue in the upper outer quadrant extends into the axilla (the "axillary tail"); thus it is important to remember to palpate the axilla as well as the breast during exams. Depending on where a cancer forms, it may put tension on lactiferous ducts or suspensory retinacula, causing retraction of the nipple or dimpling of the skin.

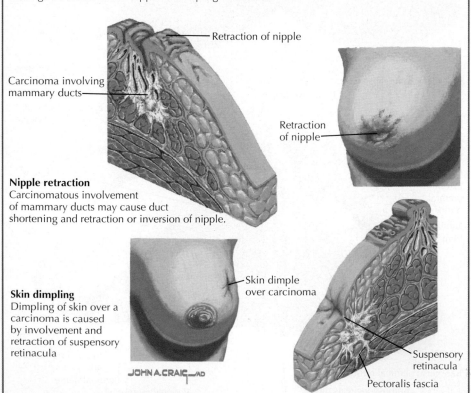

Retraction of nipple

Carcinoma involving mammary ducts

Retraction of nipple

Nipple retraction
Carcinomatous involvement of mammary ducts may cause duct shortening and retraction or inversion of nipple.

Skin dimpling
Dimpling of skin over a carcinoma is caused by involvement and retraction of suspensory retinacula

Skin dimple over carcinoma

Suspensory retinacula

Pectoralis fascia

JOHN A.CRAIG—AD

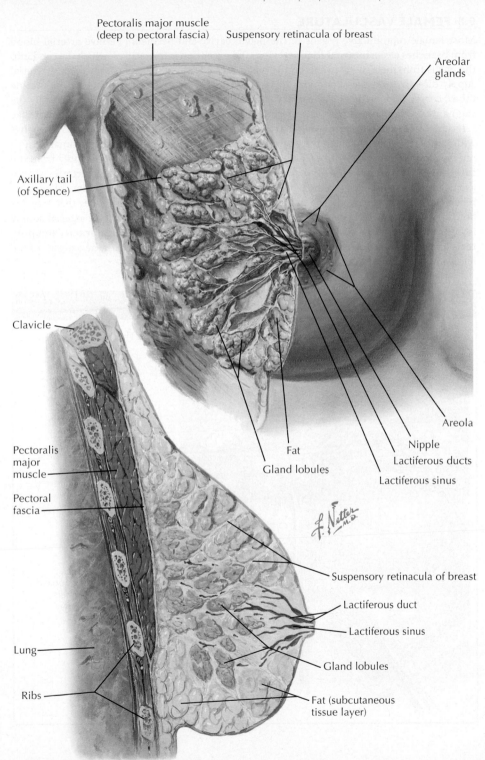

Pectoralis major muscle
(deep to pectoral fascia)

Suspensory retinacula of breast

Areolar glands

Axillary tail
(of Spence)

Clavicle

Pectoralis
major
muscle

Pectoral
fascia

Lung

Ribs

Areola

Nipple

Lactiferous ducts

Lactiferous sinus

Fat

Gland lobules

Suspensory retinacula of breast

Lactiferous duct

Lactiferous sinus

Gland lobules

Fat (subcutaneous
tissue layer)

Figure 9.7 BREASTS

9.8 FEMALE VASCULATURE

Most female reproductive organs in the pelvic cavity and perineum receive arterial blood from branches of the **internal iliac arteries**. The exception is the ovaries, which descend into the pelvis from their site of origin on the posterior abdominal wall; thus they receive arterial supply directly from the abdominal aorta. The **uterine arteries** supply the uterus, uterine tubes, cervix, and portions of the ovary and vagina. The **vaginal arteries** supply mainly the vagina; they may branch from the uterine arteries or independently from the internal iliac arteries. The **ovarian arteries** branch from the abdominal aorta and descend into the pelvis within a peritoneal fold called the **suspensory ligament of the ovary**; they primarily supply the ovaries and uterine tubes. Structures in the perineum receive blood supply from the **internal pudendal arteries**. These arteries branch from the internal iliac arteries within the pelvic cavity, pass deep to the pelvic diaphragm, and travel within the pudendal canal to reach the urogenital region. The internal pudendal arteries give off branches that traverse both the superficial and deep perineal spaces. The mammary glands receive arterial supply from the arteries of the chest, specifically the **internal thoracic**, **lateral thoracic**, and **posterior intercostal arteries** (see 3.34). Veins of the same name travel with the arteries of the female reproductive tract and ultimately drain into the vena cavae.

Clinical Focus

In females the ureter passes between the uterine and vaginal arteries. Thus care must be taken during a hysterectomy to avoid cutting the ureter.

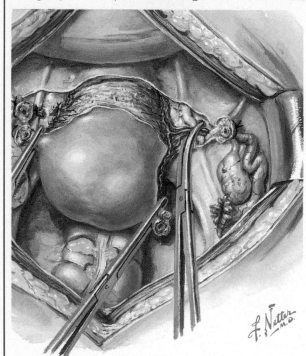

Ureter caught in clamp applied to overlying uterine vessels in course of hysterectomy

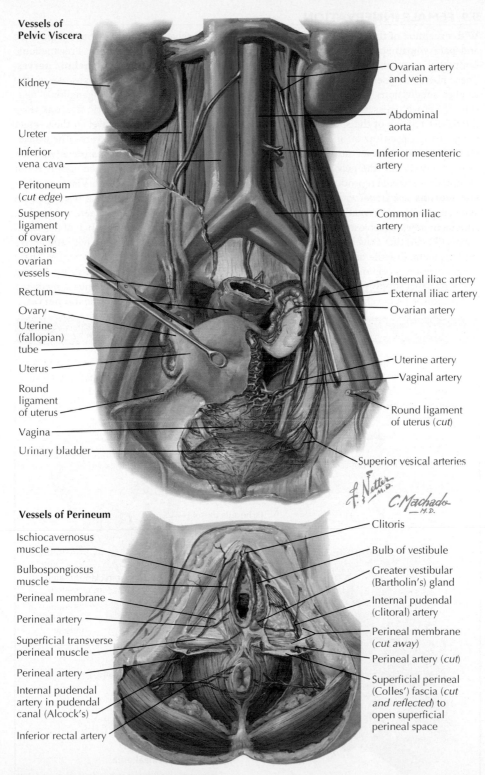

Vessels of Pelvic Viscera

Kidney

Ureter

Inferior vena cava

Peritoneum (*cut edge*)

Suspensory ligament of ovary contains ovarian vessels

Rectum

Ovary

Uterine (fallopian) tube

Uterus

Round ligament of uterus

Vagina

Urinary bladder

Ovarian artery and vein

Abdominal aorta

Inferior mesenteric artery

Common iliac artery

Internal iliac artery

External iliac artery

Ovarian artery

Uterine artery

Vaginal artery

Round ligament of uterus (*cut*)

Superior vesical arteries

Vessels of Perineum

Ischiocavernosus muscle

Bulbospongiosus muscle

Perineal membrane

Perineal artery

Superficial transverse perineal muscle

Perineal artery

Internal pudendal artery in pudendal canal (Alcock's)

Inferior rectal artery

Clitoris

Bulb of vestibule

Greater vestibular (Bartholin's) gland

Internal pudendal (clitoral) artery

Perineal membrane (*cut away*)

Perineal artery (*cut*)

Superficial perineal (Colles') fascia (*cut and reflected*) to open superficial perineal space

Figure 9.8 FEMALE VASCULATURE

9.9 FEMALE INNERVATION

With exception of the ovaries, the female pelvic organs receive innervation from sympathetic and parasympathetic nerves of the **pelvic (inferior hypogastric) plexuses**. Preganglionic sympathetic neurons leave the sympathetic chains as **lumbar** and **sacral splanchnic nerves**. These fibers synapse in sympathetic ganglia that are located within the pelvic plexuses or the smaller subdivisions of the pelvic plexuses (e.g., uterovaginal plexus); postganglionic neurons travel with vessels to their target organ. Preganglionic parasympathetic neurons leave the S2–S4 regions of the spinal cord as **pelvic splanchnic nerves** and travel to their target organs to synapse near or on the target organ wall with postganglionic neurons. The ovaries receive autonomic innervation mainly from the **aortic plexus**, and neurons travel with the ovarian vessels into the pelvis. The effect of efferent innervation on the pelvic organs is not clear because female reproductive function is mainly under hormonal control. **Visceral afferent neurons** also travel within the pelvic plexus and convey sensations of pain (e.g., the pain associated with menstruation and childbirth). Somatic structures in the perineum (e.g., skin, skeletal muscles) receive innervation from the **pudendal nerve**, which is a branch of the sacral plexus (S2–S4) that travels adjacent to the ischial spine as it leaves the pelvic cavity and enters the perineum. Erectile tissue in the perineum is innervated by pelvic splanchnic nerves. These nerves cause erection of the clitoris and engorgement of the bulbs of the vestibule by dilating the vessels that supply these tissues. The secretory activity of the mammary glands is regulated by hormones; however, the skin of the breast receives innervation from **intercostal nerves**.

Clinical Focus

The skin of the perineum can be anesthetized for surgical procedures or to alleviate pain during childbirth with a **pudendal nerve block**. This involves injecting local anesthetic around the pudendal nerve where it travels adjacent to the ischial spine. The ischial spine can be located by palpation via the vagina or using ultrasound.

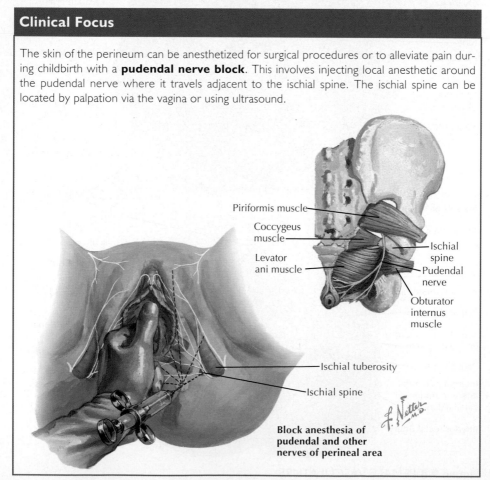

Piriformis muscle
Coccygeus muscle
Levator ani muscle
Ischial spine
Pudendal nerve
Obturator internus muscle
Ischial tuberosity
Ischial spine

Block anesthesia of pudendal and other nerves of perineal area

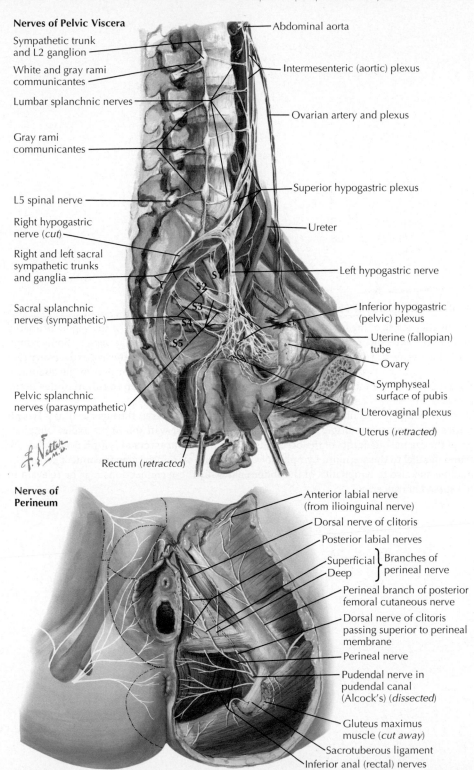

Nerves of Pelvic Viscera

Sympathetic trunk and L2 ganglion

White and gray rami communicantes

Lumbar splanchnic nerves

Gray rami communicantes

L5 spinal nerve

Right hypogastric nerve (cut)

Right and left sacral sympathetic trunks and ganglia

Sacral splanchnic nerves (sympathetic)

Pelvic splanchnic nerves (parasympathetic)

Abdominal aorta

Intermesenteric (aortic) plexus

Ovarian artery and plexus

Superior hypogastric plexus

Ureter

Left hypogastric nerve

Inferior hypogastric (pelvic) plexus

Uterine (fallopian) tube

Ovary

Symphyseal surface of pubis

Uterovaginal plexus

Uterus (retracted)

Rectum (retracted)

S1
S2
S3
S4
S5

Nerves of Perineum

Anterior labial nerve (from ilioinguinal nerve)

Dorsal nerve of clitoris

Posterior labial nerves

Superficial
Deep
} Branches of perineal nerve

Perineal branch of posterior femoral cutaneous nerve

Dorsal nerve of clitoris passing superior to perineal membrane

Perineal nerve

Pudendal nerve in pudendal canal (Alcock's) (dissected)

Gluteus maximus muscle (cut away)

Sacrotuberous ligament

Inferior anal (rectal) nerves

Figure 9.9 FEMALE INNERVATION

9.10 FEMALE LYMPHATICS

Lymphatic vessels of the uterus, uterine tubes, cervix, and upper part of the vagina primarily drain to the **external** and **internal iliac nodes** that travel with the iliac vessels. Some lymph from the uterine tubes and fundus of the uterus may join drainage pathways of the ovary that follow the ovarian vessels to the **lateral aortic nodes** in the posterior part of the abdomen. Structures in the perineum mainly drain to the **superficial** and **deep inguinal nodes** in the groin.

Most lymphatic drainage from the mammary glands passes through **axillary lymph nodes** that comprise multiple groups of nodes on the chest wall and in the axilla. Lymphatics of the medial quadrants of the breast also drain to the **parasternal lymph nodes** that are found parallel to the sternum. Lymphatic vessels of the mammary glands connect across the midline and also to lymphatics of the abdominal wall. These connections may be relevant in the spread of cancer.

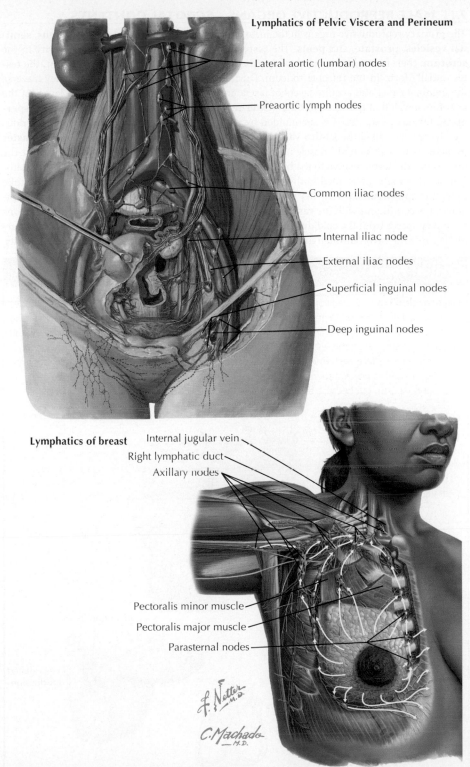

Lymphatics of Pelvic Viscera and Perineum

Lateral aortic (lumbar) nodes

Preaortic lymph nodes

Common iliac nodes

Internal iliac node

External iliac nodes

Superficial inguinal nodes

Deep inguinal nodes

Lymphatics of breast

Internal jugular vein

Right lymphatic duct

Axillary nodes

Pectoralis minor muscle

Pectoralis major muscle

Parasternal nodes

Figure 9.10 FEMALE LYMPHATICS

9.11 MALE REPRODUCTIVE ORGANS—SCROTAL CONTENTS

The primary reproductive organs in the male are the **testes, epididymis, vas deferens, seminal vesicles, prostate**, and **penis**. The **testes** are located outside of the pelvic cavity in the **scrotum**; their function is to produce spermatozoa. During embryonic development, the testes initially form in the retroperitoneum. During their descent to the scrotum, they traverse the inguinal canal and acquire layers of fascia and muscle that are derived from layers of the abdominal wall that they pass through (**external spermatic, cremasteric**, and **internal spermatic fascias**). Each testis is surrounded by a capsule (**tunica albuginea**) as well as a double-layered sac called the **tunica vaginalis** that is derived from peritoneum. The **cremaster muscle**, as well as smooth muscle in the wall of the scrotum (dartos muscle), can adjust the position of the testis relative to the body to maintain the optimum temperature for spermatogenesis. Spermatozoa formed in the testis pass through **efferent ductules** into a coiled tube called the **epididymis**, where they undergo a maturation process. The terminal part of the epididymis is continuous with the **vas (ductus) deferens**, which is a muscular tube that functions to convey sperm from the epididymis to the pelvic cavity. The vas deferens ascends in the spermatic cord and travels through the inguinal canal to obtain access to the abdominopelvic cavity.

Clinical Focus

Cryptorchidism is a condition in which one or both testes do not descend properly. An undescended testis can be found anywhere along the path of migration, although the most common location is within the inguinal canal. This condition is usually identified at birth with palpation and can be corrected surgically if the testis does not complete the descent on its own. **Vasectomy** is a minor surgical procedure performed in males to prevent pregnancy. Both vas deferens are identified and then divided to prevent sperm from entering the semen. After a vasectomy the testes continue to produce sperm, but because they cannot be transported they are absorbed by the body.

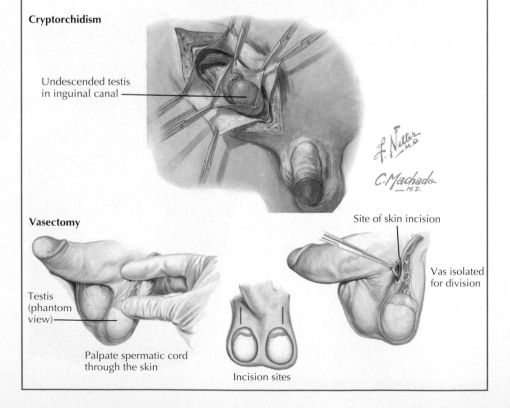

Cryptorchidism

Undescended testis in inguinal canal

Vasectomy

Site of skin incision

Vas isolated for division

Testis (phantom view)

Palpate spermatic cord through the skin

Incision sites

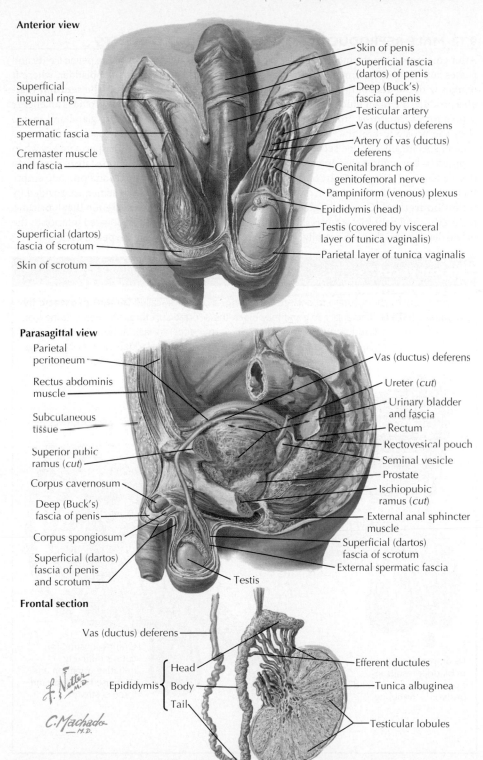

Anterior view

Skin of penis

Superficial fascia (dartos) of penis

Deep (Buck's) fascia of penis

Testicular artery

Vas (ductus) deferens

Artery of vas (ductus) deferens

Genital branch of genitofemoral nerve

Pampiniform (venous) plexus

Epididymis (head)

Testis (covered by visceral layer of tunica vaginalis)

Parietal layer of tunica vaginalis

Superficial inguinal ring

External spermatic fascia

Cremaster muscle and fascia

Superficial (dartos) fascia of scrotum

Skin of scrotum

Parasagittal view

Parietal peritoneum

Rectus abdominis muscle

Subcutaneous tissue

Superior pubic ramus (*cut*)

Corpus cavernosum

Deep (Buck's) fascia of penis

Corpus spongiosum

Superficial (dartos) fascia of penis and scrotum

Testis

Vas (ductus) deferens

Ureter (*cut*)

Urinary bladder and fascia

Rectum

Rectovesical pouch

Seminal vesicle

Prostate

Ischiopubic ramus (*cut*)

External anal sphincter muscle

Superficial (dartos) fascia of scrotum

External spermatic fascia

Frontal section

Vas (ductus) deferens

Epididymis { Head, Body, Tail }

Efferent ductules

Tunica albuginea

Testicular lobules

f. Netter M.D.

C. Machado M.D.

Figure 9.11 MALE REPRODUCTIVE ORGANS: SCROTAL CONTENTS

9.12 MALE REPRODUCTIVE ORGANS—PELVIC CONTENTS

After emerging from the inguinal canal, each **vas deferens** descends into the pelvic cavity and passes superior to the ureter. The vas deferens terminates posterior to the bladder, where it merges with the duct of the seminal vesicle to form the **ejaculatory duct**. The **seminal vesicles** produce the main fluid components of semen, including fructose that provides an energy source for spermatozoa. The ejaculatory ducts travel through the prostate gland and merge with the prostatic urethra. The **prostate gland** also synthesizes fluid that contributes to semen, specifically alkaline secretions that provide a protective effect for spermatozoa when exposed to the acidic environment of the female reproductive tract. The prostate is inferior to the bladder and surrounds part of the urethra. Both the ejaculatory ducts and prostate empty their secretions into this portion of the urethra. The final component of semen is provided by the **bulbourethral (Cowper's) glands**, which produce a mucus-rich secretion that lubricates the urethra and neutralizes any residual urine. Because these glands are located inferior to the pelvic diaphragm, they are actually within the perineum rather than the pelvic cavity.

Clinical Focus

It is common for the prostate to enlarge with aging, a condition called **benign prostatic hyperplasia (BPH)**. The enlarged gland may block the prostatic urethra, preventing urine from flowing out of the bladder. As a result, men may experience a weak urine stream, dribbling at the end of urination, or frequent urges to urinate because the bladder never fully empties.

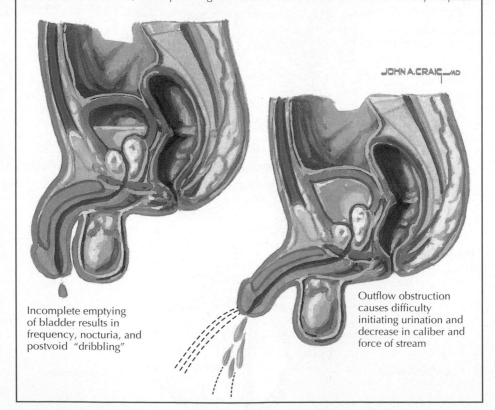

JOHN A. CRAIG⎯AD

Incomplete emptying of bladder results in frequency, nocturia, and postvoid "dribbling"

Outflow obstruction causes difficulty initiating urination and decrease in caliber and force of stream

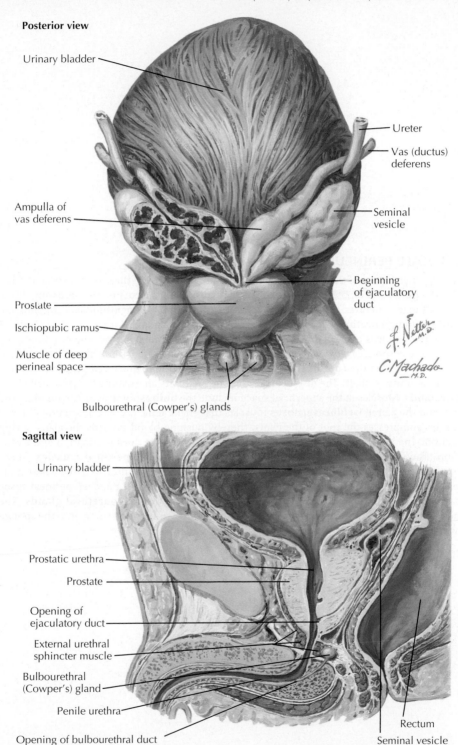

Posterior view

Urinary bladder

Ureter

Vas (ductus) deferens

Ampulla of vas deferens

Seminal vesicle

Beginning of ejaculatory duct

Prostate

Ischiopubic ramus

Muscle of deep perineal space

Bulbourethral (Cowper's) glands

Sagittal view

Urinary bladder

Prostatic urethra

Prostate

Opening of ejaculatory duct

External urethral sphincter muscle

Bulbourethral (Cowper's) gland

Penile urethra

Opening of bulbourethral duct

Rectum

Seminal vesicle

Figure 9.12 MALE REPRODUCTIVE ORGANS: PELVIC CONTENTS

9.13 MALE PERINEUM

The superficial space of the male perineum contains the penis and three paired striated muscles. The **penis** is composed of two **corpora cavernosa** and the **corpus spongiosum**. These three tubular structures consist of erectile tissue; the corpus spongiosum also contains the **penile (spongy) urethra**. The proximal part of the corpus spongiosum is called the **bulb of the penis**, and it is anchored to the perineal membrane. The **crura** are the proximal portions of the corpora cavernosa that are attached to the ischiopubic rami. The bulb and crura together are called the **root of the penis**, in contrast to the unanchored portion, which is called the **body** or shaft. The distal part of the body exhibits an expanded portion called the **glans penis**. Muscles in the superficial space include the **bulbospongiosus** surrounding the bulb, and the paired **ischiocavernosus** muscles that encircle the crura. Contraction of these muscles compresses the root of the penis, thereby pushing blood towards the glans during erection. The bulbospongiosus also helps to empty the urethra during urination and ejaculation. The final pair of muscles are the **superficial transverse perineal muscles**. These muscles help to stabilize the **perineal body**, which is a mass of connective tissue where multiple muscles of the perineum intersect. The primary structures in the deep perineal space of males are the **external urethral sphincter** muscle and the **bulbourethral glands**. The ducts of the bulbourethral glands penetrate the perineal membrane to empty into the spongy part of the urethra.

Male Perineum

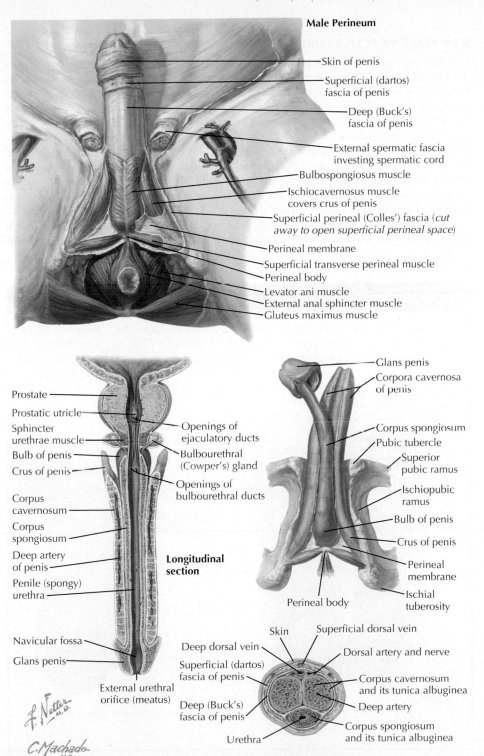

Skin of penis

Superficial (dartos) fascia of penis

Deep (Buck's) fascia of penis

External spermatic fascia investing spermatic cord

Bulbospongiosus muscle

Ischiocavernosus muscle covers crus of penis

Superficial perineal (Colles') fascia (*cut away to open superficial perineal space*)

Perineal membrane

Superficial transverse perineal muscle

Perineal body

Levator ani muscle

External anal sphincter muscle

Gluteus maximus muscle

Prostate

Prostatic utricle

Sphincter urethrae muscle

Bulb of penis

Crus of penis

Corpus cavernosum

Corpus spongiosum

Deep artery of penis

Penile (spongy) urethra

Navicular fossa

Glans penis

Longitudinal section

Openings of ejaculatory ducts

Bulbourethral (Cowper's) gland

Openings of bulbourethral ducts

External urethral orifice (meatus)

Glans penis

Corpora cavernosa of penis

Corpus spongiosum

Pubic tubercle

Superior pubic ramus

Ischiopubic ramus

Bulb of penis

Crus of penis

Perineal membrane

Ischial tuberosity

Perineal body

Skin

Superficial dorsal vein

Deep dorsal vein

Dorsal artery and nerve

Superficial (dartos) fascia of penis

Corpus cavernosum and its tunica albuginea

Deep (Buck's) fascia of penis

Deep artery

Urethra

Corpus spongiosum and its tunica albuginea

Cross section through body of penis

Figure 9.13 MALE PERINEUM

9.14 MALE VASCULATURE

The male reproductive organs in the pelvic cavity receive arterial blood from branches of the **internal iliac arteries**. The **inferior vesical arteries** supply the prostate and seminal vesicles. The vas deferens has its own artery, the **artery to vas deferens**, that typically arises from either the umbilical or superior vesical branches of the internal iliac artery. Because the testes develop adjacent to the posterior abdominal wall, the **testicular arteries** branch from the abdominal aorta. These arteries pass through the inguinal canal and descend into the scrotum within the **spermatic cord**. The structures in the superficial and deep perineal spaces receive blood supply from the **internal pudendal arteries**. Veins of the same name travel with the arteries and in most cases have a similar pattern. The testicular veins are unique because they form a plexus around each testicular artery (**pampiniform plexus**) that functions not only to drain blood from the testis but also to absorb heat from the testicular artery to maintain an optimal temperature for spermatogenesis. The left testicular vein drains into the left renal vein, while the right testicular vein drains directly into the inferior vena cava.

Clinical Focus

If the veins in the pampiniform plexus become abnormally dilated, the condition is called a **varicocele**. Causes include backup of blood in the testicular veins or incompetent valves. Varicoceles are more common on the left side of the body because the left testicular vein drains into the left renal vein, rather than directly into the inferior vena cava. The superior mesenteric artery passes anterior to the left renal vein and may be a source of compression.

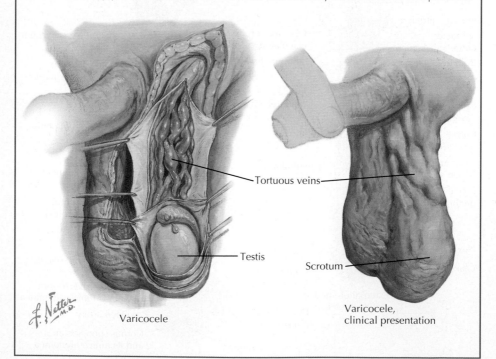

Tortuous veins

Testis

Scrotum

Varicocele

Varicocele,
clinical presentation

Vessels of Pelvic Viscera

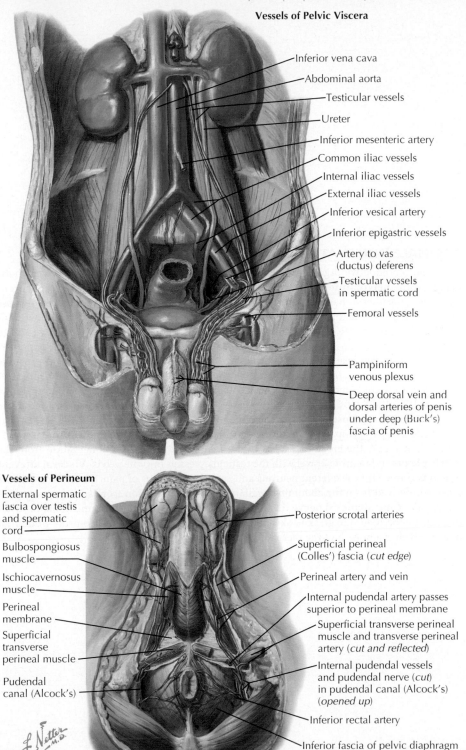

Inferior vena cava

Abdominal aorta

Testicular vessels

Ureter

Inferior mesenteric artery

Common iliac vessels

Internal iliac vessels

External iliac vessels

Inferior vesical artery

Inferior epigastric vessels

Artery to vas (ductus) deferens

Testicular vessels in spermatic cord

Femoral vessels

Pampiniform venous plexus

Deep dorsal vein and dorsal arteries of penis under deep (Buck's) fascia of penis

Vessels of Perineum

External spermatic fascia over testis and spermatic cord

Bulbospongiosus muscle

Ischiocavernosus muscle

Perineal membrane

Superficial transverse perineal muscle

Pudendal canal (Alcock's)

Posterior scrotal arteries

Superficial perineal (Colles') fascia (*cut edge*)

Perineal artery and vein

Internal pudendal artery passes superior to perineal membrane

Superficial transverse perineal muscle and transverse perineal artery (*cut and reflected*)

Internal pudendal vessels and pudendal nerve (*cut*) in pudendal canal (Alcock's) (*opened up*)

Inferior rectal artery

Inferior fascia of pelvic diaphragm (roof of ischioanal fossa)

Figure 9.14 MALE VASCULATURE

9.15 MALE INNERVATION

The male reproductive organs receive innervation from sympathetic and parasympathetic nerves of the **pelvic (inferior hypogastric) plexuses**. Preganglionic sympathetic neurons leave the sympathetic chains as **lumbar** and **sacral splanchnic nerves**. These fibers synapse in sympathetic ganglia that are located within the pelvic plexuses or the smaller subdivisions of the pelvic plexuses (e.g., prostatic plexus); postganglionic neurons travel with vessels to their target organ. Sympathetic neurons cause contraction of smooth muscle in the vas deferens, seminal vesicles, ejaculatory ducts, and prostate for emission of semen into the prostatic urethra. During ejaculation, sympathetic neurons constrict the internal urethral sphincter to prevent retrograde movement of sperm into the bladder. Preganglionic parasympathetic neurons leave the S2–S4 regions of the spinal cord as **pelvic splanchnic nerves** and travel to their targets to synapse near or on the target organ wall with postganglionic neurons. The major effect of parasympathetic innervation in males is erection of the penis by dilating the vessels that supply the erectile tissues. The testes receive autonomic innervation from the **aortic plexus** and neurons travel with the testicular vessels into the pelvis. **Visceral afferent neurons** travel with the efferent neurons and convey sensations of pain. Since the cremaster muscle is derived from the abdominal wall, it receives innervation from spinal nerves, specifically the **genitofemoral nerve** that is formed by the L1–L2 anterior rami. Somatic structures in the perineum (e.g., skin, skeletal muscles) receive innervation from the **pudendal nerve**, which is a branch of the sacral plexus (S2–S4).

Nerves of Pelvic Viscera

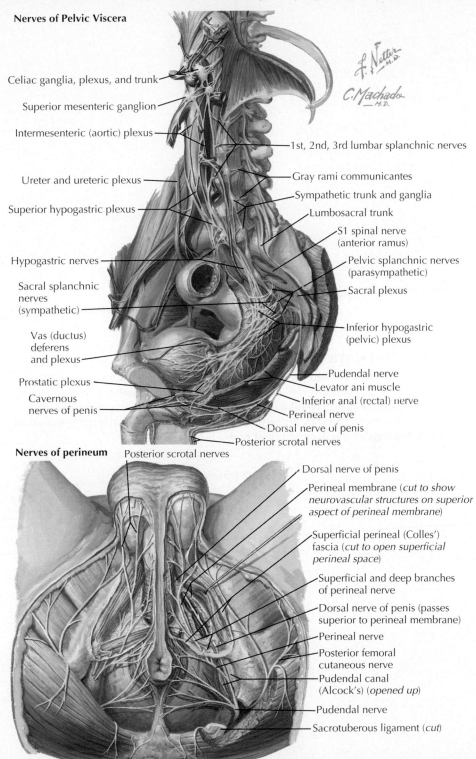

Celiac ganglia, plexus, and trunk

Superior mesenteric ganglion

Intermesenteric (aortic) plexus

1st, 2nd, 3rd lumbar splanchnic nerves

Ureter and ureteric plexus

Gray rami communicantes

Superior hypogastric plexus

Sympathetic trunk and ganglia

Lumbosacral trunk

S1 spinal nerve (anterior ramus)

Hypogastric nerves

Pelvic splanchnic nerves (parasympathetic)

Sacral splanchnic nerves (sympathetic)

Sacral plexus

Inferior hypogastric (pelvic) plexus

Vas (ductus) deferens and plexus

Prostatic plexus

Pudendal nerve

Levator ani muscle

Cavernous nerves of penis

Inferior anal (rectal) nerve

Perineal nerve

Dorsal nerve of penis

Posterior scrotal nerves

Nerves of perineum

Posterior scrotal nerves

Dorsal nerve of penis

Perineal membrane (*cut to show neurovascular structures on superior aspect of perineal membrane*)

Superficial perineal (Colles') fascia (*cut to open superficial perineal space*)

Superficial and deep branches of perineal nerve

Dorsal nerve of penis (*passes superior to perineal membrane*)

Perineal nerve

Posterior femoral cutaneous nerve

Pudendal canal (Alcock's) (*opened up*)

Pudendal nerve

Sacrotuberous ligament (*cut*)

Fig. 9.15 MALE INNERVATION

9.16 MALE LYMPHATICS

Lymphatic vessels of the seminal vesicles and prostate take multiple routes; however, the primary path is along the inferior vesical vessels to the **internal iliac nodes**. In contrast, lymph from the testes drains to the **lateral aortic nodes** in the posterior part of the abdomen via lymphatic vessels that travel with the testicular vessels. Structures in the perineum mainly drain to the **superficial** and **deep inguinal nodes** in the groin.

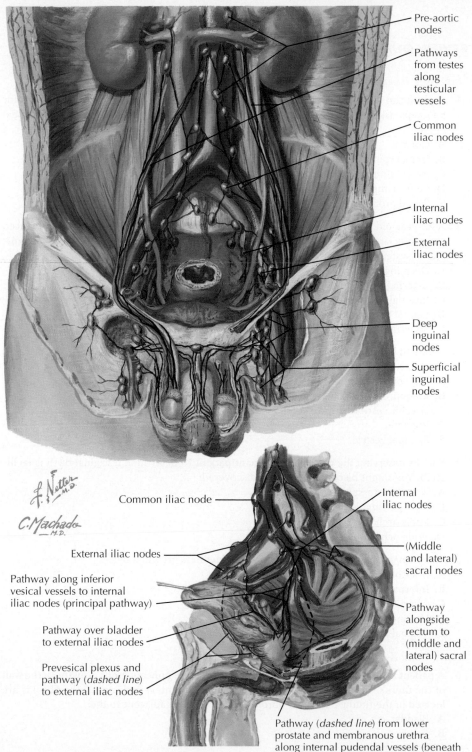

Figure 9.16 MALE LYMPHATICS

Pre-aortic nodes

Pathways from testes along testicular vessels

Common iliac nodes

Internal iliac nodes

External iliac nodes

Deep inguinal nodes

Superficial inguinal nodes

Common iliac node

External iliac nodes

Pathway along inferior vesical vessels to internal iliac nodes (principal pathway)

Pathway over bladder to external iliac nodes

Prevesical plexus and pathway (*dashed line*) to external iliac nodes

Internal iliac nodes

(Middle and lateral) sacral nodes

Pathway alongside rectum to (middle and lateral) sacral nodes

Pathway (*dashed line*) from lower prostate and membranous urethra along internal pudendal vessels (beneath pelvic diaphragm) to internal iliac nodes

REVIEW QUESTIONS

Test Your Recall

1. A physician administers a pudendal block on a patient to anesthetize the perineum for a forceps-assisted birth. What palpable landmark could be used to locate the pudendal nerve?
   A. Coccyx
   B. Ischial spine
   C. Ischial tuberosity
   D. Pubic symphysis
   E. Sacral promontory

2. A 22-year-old male notices a lump in his testicle and is diagnosed with testicular cancer. His physician orders some imaging to determine if the cancer has spread via the lymphatic system. Which group of lymph nodes should be examined first?
   A. Deep inguinal nodes
   B. External iliac nodes
   C. Internal iliac nodes
   D. Lateral aortic nodes
   E. Superficial inguinal nodes

3. A patient has a bacterial infection in their deep perineal space. Which of the following is most likely infected?
   A. Bulb of the vestibule
   B. Bulbourethral (Cowper's) gland
   C. Greater vestibular (Bartholin) gland
   D. Prostate
   E. Seminal vesicle

4. You are assessing the pelvis of a pregnant patient to determine if vaginal birth is facilitated. You might be concerned if you discovered:
   A. Narrow interspinous distance
   B. Oval pelvic inlet
   C. Pubic arch of 80 degrees
   D. Wide pelvic outlet

5. The primary blood supply to the female perineum is provided by:
   A. Inferior vesical artery
   B. Internal pudendal artery
   C. Ovarian artery
   D. Uterine artery
   E. Vaginal artery

Apply Your Knowledge

6. A patient is diagnosed with uterine fibroids, which are noncancerous growths in the wall of the uterus. In this particular patient, who has an anteverted uterus, the fibroids are located in the fundus. Thus the fibroids are most likely adjacent to the:
   A. Bladder
   B. Cervix
   C. Posterior fornix
   D. Rectum
   E. Vagina

7. A male patient presents with a swollen left testicle. The physician assistant diagnoses the condition as a varicocele—dilated veins of the left pampiniform plexus—that is due to an obstruction in the vasculature. Which of the following is most likely obstructed in this patient?

   A. Left common iliac vein
   B. Left external iliac vein
   C. Left inferior vesical vein
   D. Left internal iliac vein
   E. Left renal vein

8. A patient presents to her family physician complaining of loss of urine when coughing and sneezing. Her medical history states that, during the delivery of her third child, she sustained damage to her pelvic floor. Which of the following was most likely damaged during childbirth?

   A. Broad ligament
   B. Coccygeus
   C. Levator ani
   D. Perineal membrane
   E. Pubocervical ligament

9. A technician inserts a cystoscope in a male patient's urethra to remove a small tumor in the bladder. Unfortunately, the urethra is accidentally punctured within the deep perineal space. The portion of the urethra that was damaged is the:

   A. Membranous urethra
   B. Preprostatic urethra
   C. Prostatic urethra
   D. Spongy urethra

10. A patient with a fractured pelvis has torn their perineal membrane. This would allow communication between:

   A. Deep perineal space and false pelvis
   B. Deep perineal space and pelvic cavity
   C. Superficial perineal space and deep perineal space
   D. Superficial perineal space and pelvic cavity
   E. Superficial perineal space and false pelvis

See Appendix for answers.

APPENDIX

ANSWERS TO REVIEW QUESTIONS

CHAPTER 2, NERVOUS SYSTEM

Test Your Recall

1. C, Subarachnoid space
2. E, CN IX, CN X, and CN XI
3. A, CN I
4. E, Transverse sinus
5. A, Facial nerve

Apply Your Knowledge

6. **B, Loss of sensation just inferior to the eye.** The maxillary nerve (CN V_2) passes through the foramen rotundum before entering the pterygopalatine fossa; thus it is the nerve that is compressed. CN V_2 provides sensory innervation to the middle one-third of the face, including the region inferior to the eye, which is innervated by its infraorbital branch.
7. **A, Anterior wall.** Excess fluid in the tympanic cavity normally drains through the eustachian tube, which is located on the anterior wall of the tympanic cavity.
8. **B, Inability to abduct the eye.** The internal carotid artery and abducens nerve travel through the cavernous sinus. CN VI innervates the lateral rectus muscle, thus compression of this nerve would lead to the loss of abduction of the eye on the affected side.
9. **A, Lens becomes round due to contraction of the ciliary muscle by parasympathetics.** Focusing on close objects (accommodation) requires the lens to become rounder. This occurs when the ciliary muscle contracts and releases tension on the zonular fibers. The ciliary muscle is innervated by the parasympathetic neurons in CN III.
10. **E, Superior cervical ganglion.** Ptosis is drooping of the eyelid, indicating that one of the two muscles that elevates the eyelid is not working properly (levator palpebrae superioris or superior tarsal muscle). If the pupil is constricted, this indicates that the dilator pupillae is not functioning. Sympathetic neurons innervate the dilator pupillae and superior tarsal muscle; thus damage to the superior cervical ganglion (containing cell bodies for sympathetic neurons in the head) provides a valid explanation for the observed signs.

CHAPTER 3, MUSCULOSKELETAL SYSTEM

Test Your Recall

1. D, Proximal radioulnar joint
2. A, Coronal suture
3. D, Semitendinosus
4. C, Inversion
5. C, Lateral pterygoid

Apply Your Knowledge

6. **B, Head of the femur.** The branches of the deep femoral artery include the medial and lateral circumflex arteries, and the perforating branches of the thigh. The medial circumflex artery is the primary blood supply to the head of the femur. The gluteal region is supplied by branches of the internal iliac artery, while the popliteal fossa and leg receive blood from the popliteal artery. The deep femoral artery does contribute to the blood supply of the quadriceps muscle; however, this muscle also receives blood from the femoral artery directly.

7. **D, Weakness in lateral (external) rotation of the arm.** The suprascapular nerve travels through the suprascapular notch; thus the two muscles it innervates (supraspinatus and infraspinatus) are likely impaired. The infraspinatus is the primary muscle that laterally rotates the humerus. The suprascapular artery is not affected by the spur because it travels superficial to the transverse scapular ligament and does not pass through the notch.

8. **B, Aponeuroses of external oblique and half of internal oblique.** Because the wound is superior to the umbilicus, it is also superior to the arcuate line. Thus the anterior layer of the rectus sheath is comprised of the external oblique aponeurosis and half of the internal oblique aponeurosis. The posterior layer of the sheath, composed of the aponeuroses of half of the internal oblique and transversus abdominis, is deep to the rectus muscle and thus not affected by the piece of metal.

9. **A, Loss of abduction of the middle finger.** Distal to the wrist, the ulnar nerve innervates numerous intrinsic muscles of the hand that could be affected by this injury, including the hypothenar muscles, interossei, and the adductor pollicis. The dorsal interossei are responsible for abduction of digits 2 to 4; thus abduction of the middle finger is impaired. The long abductor of the thumb and extensor of the little finger are innervated by the radial nerve; the median nerve innervates the abductor pollicis brevis. The flexor digiti minimi brevis is impaired with this injury; however, there are other muscles in the forearm that flex the little finger that are functioning.

10. **A, Difficulty with swallowing and/or eating.** The ansa cervicalis innervates most of the infrahyoid muscles; thus the patient would have difficulty with actions that require depression of the hyoid such as swallowing and speaking. The muscles that move the vocal cords are innervated by the vagus nerves, and the accessory nerve innervates muscles that turn the chin and elevate the shoulder. The skin of the neck is innervated by cutaneous branches of the cervical plexus.

CHAPTER 4, CARDIOVASCULAR SYSTEM

Test Your Recall

1. **D, Parietal serous pericardium and visceral serous pericardium**
2. **E, Right coronary artery**
3. **D, Purkinje fibers**
4. **C, Pulmonary semilunar valve**
5. **B, Left anterior descending artery**

Apply Your Knowledge

6. **C, 2.** The clot would travel towards the heart in the venous system and eventually reach the inferior vena cava. After traveling in the inferior vena cava, it enters the right atrium of the heart, passes through the tricuspid valve, and enters the right ventricle. It leaves the right ventricle through the pulmonary semilunar valve and travels to the lungs via

branches of the pulmonary arteries. The clot would encounter its first capillary bed in the lungs, where it would become lodged.

7. **C, Pulmonary semilunar valve.** Hypertrophy refers to an increase in size of muscle cells that occurs in response to increased demand. This explains why lifting weights in a gym is an effective way to increase muscle size. In this case the cardiac muscle of the right ventricle demonstrated hypertrophy, which indicates that the right ventricle experienced increased demand. Because the right ventricle pushes blood out the pulmonary semilunar valve, this valve must be the one that is stenotic because a narrower opening makes it harder for blood to pass through.

8. **C, Inflammation of the parietal pericardium (pericarditis).** The patient's pain is sharp in nature rather than dull or vague, indicating that the source is a somatic structure rather than a visceral structure. In addition, the pain is referred to the shoulder (C3–C5 dermatomes); thus the neurons conveying the pain sensations must be traveling in branches of the C3–C5 spinal nerves. The heart is a visceral structure, and its pain neurons travel with sympathetic neurons that arise in the T1–T5 spinal levels. In contrast, the parietal pericardium is somatic and its pain neurons travel in the phrenic nerves, which arise from the C3–C5 spinal nerves.

9. **A, Closure of the ductus arteriosus.** The coarctation is located distal to the blood supply of the upper extremities and proximal to the blood supply of the lower extremities, thus explaining the differences in the pulses. A higher volume of blood is reaching the head and upper extremities than is typical, causing high blood pressure. Leg pain and weakness are due to lack of blood supply (claudication). In the fetus, the ductus arteriosus connects to the aorta in the vicinity of where the coarctation developed. The ductus normally closes after birth by contraction of the muscle in its wall. One theory of the cause of coarctation is that during this remodeling, cells migrate into the wall of the aorta, causing the lumen to narrow.

10. **D, Right atrium.** The two major structures that contribute to the right heart border on a posteroanterior (PA) chest x-ray are the superior vena cava (superiorly) and the right atrium (inferiorly). The left ventricle contributes to the left heart border. The other two chambers of the heart do not contribute significantly to the cardiac silhouette on a PA view; however, they do form borders on a lateral view.

CHAPTER 5, RESPIRATORY SYSTEM

Test Your Recall

1. **E, Trachea**
2. **B, Middle nasal meatus**
3. **D, Between the parietal pleura and visceral pleura**
4. **E, Vocal folds**
5. **D, Ophthalmic nerve**

Apply Your Knowledge

6. **C, 7th intercostal space at midclavicular line.** At the midclavicular line the inferior border of the lung is found at the sixth rib, while the pleura extends as far as the eighth rib. Thus, to puncture the pleural cavity and not the lung, the penetrating object would need to enter either the sixth or seventh intercostal space.

7. **A, Left hemidiaphragm would be abnormally high.** Each hemidiaphragm is innervated independently; thus they also contract separately. In this patient, the left hemidiaphragm would not be functioning due to loss of innervation from the left phrenic nerve.

Thus, during inspiration, the right hemidiaphragm would descend normally but the left hemidiaphragm would remain in an elevated location, thus appearing abnormally high in comparison with the right side.

8. **B, Middle meatus.** Pain in the sinuses is often due to the accumulation of fluid that creates pressure. The location of the pain indicates that the frontal and maxillary sinuses are infected, because they are located in the forehead and cheek, respectively. These both drain into the middle meatus; thus this is the space likely obstructed by the polyp.

9. **E, Costal cartilage of rib 2.** The sternal angle is the junction between the manubrium and body of the sternum. The second rib articulates with the lateral aspect of the sternum in this location via its costal cartilage.

10. **A, Aortic arch aneurysm.** Almost all intrinsic laryngeal muscles are innervated by the recurrent laryngeal nerve; thus compression or injury to this nerve is a frequent cause of vocal cord paralysis. The left nerve travels around the inferior surface of the arch of the aorta, then ascends in the neck lateral to the trachea. Thus the aortic arch aneurysm is the most likely source of damage to this nerve.

CHAPTER 6, DIGESTIVE SYSTEM

Test Your Recall

1. **A, Common bile duct**
2. **B, Pelvic splanchnic nerves**
3. **C, Left gastric artery**
4. **C, CN IX**
5. **C, Plicae circulares**

Apply Your Knowledge

6. **B, Eustachian tube.** The eustachian tube is the only structure listed in the nasopharynx. The palatine tonsil and vallecula are in the oropharynx. The epiglottis marks the border between the oropharynx and laryngopharynx, and the piriform fossa is in the laryngopharynx.

7. **B, Inferior mesenteric nodes.** The blood supply to the superior part of the rectum is provided by the inferior mesenteric artery and venous drainage is via the inferior mesenteric vein. Lymphatic drainage follows these vessels; thus lymph first passes through the inferior mesenteric nodes. In contrast, the middle and inferior parts of the rectum are supplied by branches of the internal iliac artery in the pelvis; thus lymph from these regions typically drains first to internal iliac nodes.

8. **C, Ileum.** The superior mesenteric artery supplies the duodenum, ileum, and pancreas (as well as other organs not listed). However, the duodenum and pancreas also receive blood supply from branches of the celiac trunk; thus the ileum is most likely impacted by ischemia. The descending colon and rectum receive blood supply from the inferior mesenteric and internal iliac arteries.

9. **D, CN X.** The soft palate normally elevates during swallowing to seal off the opening between the oral cavity and nasopharynx. The muscle that performs this action is innervated by the vagus nerve. Because elevation of the palate is easily observed in a patient, evaluation of this function is one way clinicians test the integrity of the vagus nerve.

10. **C, Left gastric vein.** Blood in the esophageal veins normally flows into the left gastric vein and then the hepatic portal vein. If something prevents normal flow through the hepatic portal vein (e.g., liver disease), blood backs up in its tributaries and can cause dilated veins.

CHAPTER 7, ENDOCRINE SYSTEM

Test Your Recall

1. D, Second tracheal ring
2. B, Adrenal medulla
3. A, Duodenum
4. E, Hormones that travel in the hypophyseal portal veins
5. B, Inferior thyroid artery

Apply Your Knowledge

6. **B, Pancreas.** The celiac ganglia are located in the abdomen adjacent to the celiac trunk. Neurons conveying pain sensations that pass through the ganglia mainly arise in organs of the upper abdomen including the liver, gallbladder, pancreas, spleen, and adrenal glands.
7. **C, Venous blood from the inferior thyroid vein.** Most vessels that supply and drain the thyroid gland have origins and terminations lateral to the gland (i.e., not in the midline). Unless an aberrant thyroid ima artery is present, the inferior thyroid veins are the only vessels close to the midline.
8. **B, Secretion of hormones produced in the hypothalamus.** The neurons of the hypothalamohypophyseal tract contain hormones that are produced in the hypothalamus. They are transported to the posterior lobe of the pituitary via axonal transport.
9. **B, Pancreas and suprarenal glands.** The retroperitoneum is located in the abdomen, posterior to the peritoneum, and anterior to the muscles of the posterior abdominal wall. Organs in this region include the pancreas, kidneys, and suprarenal glands.
10. **D, Neck, body, and tail.** The splenic artery gives rise to the dorsal pancreatic artery, greater pancreatic artery, and artery to the tail of the pancreas. These arteries supply the neck, body, and tail. The head and uncinate process of the pancreas receive arterial supply mainly from the gastroduodenal and superior mesenteric arteries.

CHAPTER 8, URINARY SYSTEM

Test Your Recall

1. E, Renal sinus
2. B, Junction between the kidney and ureter
3. B, Minor calyx
4. A, Detrusor muscle
5. C, Posterior to the pubic bone

Apply Your Knowledge

6. **A, Pararenal fat, renal fascia, perirenal fat, capsule of kidney.** The prefix "para" means "alongside," and the prefix "peri" means "around"; thus perirenal fat is closest to the kidney because it is around it rather than next to it. The renal fascia separates the two different collections of fat.
7. **A, Major calyx.** The structure labeled with a 3 is part of the collecting system of the kidney. The renal pelvis is the final collecting area prior to the ureter (5); thus it must be the structure labeled with a 4. Major calyces (3) merge to form the renal pelvis, and

minor calyces (2) merge to form major calyces. The kidney itself is labeled with a 1, and the bladder with a 6.

8. **A, Back up of blood in the left kidney.** During its course to the kidney, the left renal vein passes between the superior mesenteric artery and abdominal aorta. If this vein was compressed, normal venous drainage would be impeded and blood would start to back up in the kidney. The renal artery and the ureter do not pass through this gap between the vessels; thus they would not be affected.

9. **C, Pudendal nerve.** The external urethral sphincter is composed of striated muscle and thus is under voluntary control. Therefore it is innervated by somatic neurons rather than visceral. Splanchnic nerves convey only visceral neurons, while branches of spinal nerves carry both somatic and visceral neurons. The pudendal nerve is a branch of the sacral plexus that is formed by anterior rami of spinal nerves.

10. **C, Kidney infection (pyelonephritis).** The costovertebral angle is located between the vertebral column and the twelfth rib and is an area that correlates with the position of the kidney. Although it is true that multiple pathologic conditions, including kidney stones and urethral obstruction, can cause tenderness in the costovertebral angle, the most common sources involve the kidney itself, such as pyelonephritis or a kidney stone that is within the kidney.

CHAPTER 9, REPRODUCTIVE SYSTEM

Test Your Recall
1. **B, Ischial spine**
2. **D, Lateral aortic nodes**
3. **B, Bulbourethral (Cowper's) gland**
4. **A, Narrow interspinous distance**
5. **B, Internal pudendal artery**

Apply Your Knowledge

6. **A, Bladder.** The fundus of the uterus is the dome-shaped portion near the origins of the uterine tubes. In a patient with an anteverted uterus, the fundus is adjacent to the bladder. If the uterus is retroverted, the fundus would be closer to the rectum. The cervix is located at the opposite end of the uterus, adjacent to the vagina and posterior fornix.

7. **E, Left renal vein.** Dilated veins (varices) are often the result of increased blood volume in veins due to back up of blood or incompetent valves. If blood does not drain out of the testicular vein, the result is a varicocele. On the right side of the body the testicular vein drains directly into the inferior vena cava, but on the left side it drains into the left renal vein. Thus conditions that cause stasis or obstruction in the left renal vein could impact drainage from the testis.

8. **C, Levator ani.** The pelvic floor (diaphragm) is composed of two muscles, levator ani and coccygeus. Levator ani is the more anterior muscle that surrounds the urethra and vagina, while coccygeus is posterior. The broad ligament, perineal membrane, and pubocervical ligament all provide support to pelvic viscera; however, they are not part of the pelvic floor. Because this patient is experiencing loss of urine, it indicates loss of support to the urethra/bladder, indicating that levator ani must be the muscle that was damaged.

9. **A, Membranous urethra.** The preprostatic urethra is inferior to the neck of the bladder, while the prostatic urethra is within the prostate gland. The membranous urethra

is within the deep perineal space, and the spongy urethra is in the superficial perineal space within the corpus spongiosum.

10. **C, Superficial perineal space and deep perineal space.** The perineal membrane separates the superficial perineal space from the deep perineal space. The pelvic diaphragm separates the deep perineal space from the pelvic cavity. There is no true separation between the false pelvis and pelvic cavity, although the pelvic inlet marks the transition between these two regions.

INDEX

Page number followed by *f* indicate figures; *t*, tables; *b*, boxes.